REVIEW

We woul

review.

VIRUSES AND

Basic Resear

(Hematology

Neal S. You

March 1993

416 pages,

ISBN# 0-8

$159.00

(price su

27

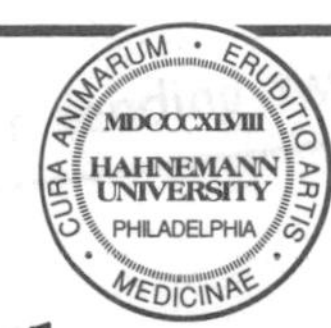




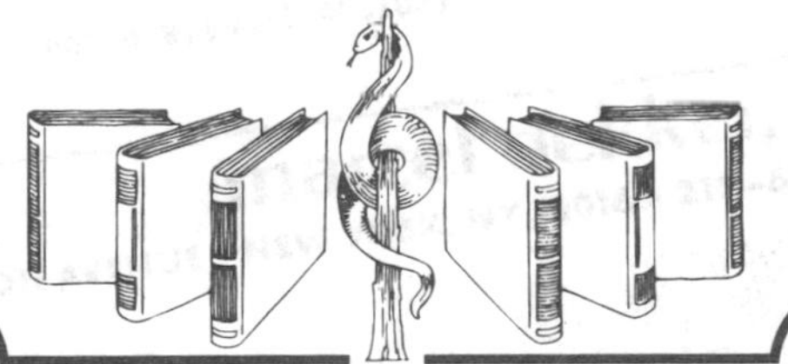

# Viruses and Bone Marrow

# HEMATOLOGY

*Series Editors*

**Kenneth M. Brinkhous, M.D.**
*Department of Pathology*
*University of North Carolina*
*School of Medicine*
*Chapel Hill, North Carolina*

**Sanford A. Stass, M.D.**
*Hematopathology Program*
*The University of Texas System Cancer Center*
*M. D. Anderson Hospital and Tumor Institute*
*Houston, Texas*

1. Prostaglandins and Leukotrienes: Blood and Vascular Cell Function, *Jonathan M. Gerrard*
2. Hematopoietic Stem Cells, *edited by David W. Golde and Fumimaro Takaku*
3. Bone Marrow Transplantation: Biological Mechanisms and Clinical Practice, *edited by Dirk W. van Bekkum and Bob Löwenberg*
4. Myelofibrosis: Pathophysiology and Clinical Management, *edited by S. M. Lewis*
5. Plasma Fibronectin: Structure and Function, *edited by Jan McDonagh*
6. The Acute Leukemias: Biologic, Diagnostic, and Therapeutic Determinants, *edited by Sanford A. Stass*
7. Hemostasis and Animal Venoms, *edited by Hubert Pirkle and Francis S. Markland, Jr.*
8. Hematopoiesis: Long-Term Effects of Chemotherapy and Radiation, *edited by Nydia G. Testa and Robert Peter Gale*
9. Coagulation and Bleeding Disorders, *edited by Theodore S. Zimmerman and Zaverio M. Ruggeri*
10. Disorders of the Spleen, *edited by Carl Pochedly, Richard H. Sills, and Allen D. Schwartz*
11. Red Blood Cell Membranes: Structure, Function, Clinical Implications, *edited by Peter Agre and John C. Parker*
12. Graft-vs.-Host Disease: Immunology, Pathophysiology, and Treatment, *edited by Steven J. Burakoff, H. Joachim Deeg, James Ferrara, and Kerry Atkinson*

13. Chronic Myelogenous Leukemia: Molecular Approaches to Research and Therapy, *edited by Albert B. Deisseroth and Ralph B. Arlinghaus*
14. Therapy of Hematopoietic Neoplasia, *edited by Emil J. Freireich and Hagop Kantarjian*
15. Biological Response Modifiers in the Treatment of Hematopoietic Neoplasia, *edited by Moshe Talpaz, Razelle Kurzrock, and Jordan U. Gutterman*
16. Viruses and Bone Marrow: Basic Research and Clinical Practice, *edited by Neal S. Young*

*Additional Volumes in Preparation*

# Viruses and Bone Marrow

## Basic Research and Clinical Practice

edited by

**Neal S. Young**

*National Heart, Lung and Blood Institute*
*National Institutes of Health*
*Bethesda, Maryland*

Marcel Dekker, Inc. New York • Basel • Hong Kong

**Library of Congress Cataloging-in-Publication Data**

Viruses and bone marrow : basic research and clinical practice /
edited by Neal S. Young.
p. cm. -- (Hematology ; 16)
Includes bibliographical references and index.
ISBN 0-8247-8833-8 (alk. paper)
1. Bone marrow--Infections. 2. Virus diseases. 3. Myelocytic leukemia. 4. Hematopoietic stem cell disorders. 5. Bone marrow cells. 6. Leukemia, Myeloid--etiology. 7. Virus Diseases--complications. I. Young, Neal S. II. Series. III. Series: Hematology (New York, N.Y.) ; v. 16.
[DNLM: 1. Bone Marrow--pathology. W1 HE873 v.16 1993 / WC 500 V8232 1993]
RC645.7.V56 1993
616.4'01094--dc20
DNLM/DLC
for Library of Congress 92-48418
CIP



Marcel Dekker, Inc.
270 Madison Avenue, New York, New York 10016

Current printing (last digit):
10 9 8 7 6 5 4 3 2 1

PRINTED IN THE UNITED STATES OF AMERICA

# Series Introduction

For most of this century, hematology has followed a pattern of major scientific discoveries, improved understanding of disease, and rapid application of new knowledge in the clinic. The rate of advance continues at an accelerating pace, so that all but the most zealous have difficulty in keeping up with the literature in even a limited area of specialized interest. As the explosive development of knowledge continues apace, it is a continuing challenge to keep abreast of significant new developments as they impact on clinical and laboratory hematology. The Hematology series is designed to help in this respect, by providing up-to-date and expert presentations on important subject areas in our field. It is hoped that these works, both individually and collectively, will become important volumes for updating information and for reference for the clinician, investigator, teacher, and student, and in this manner contribute to the advancement of hematology.

This volume provides a superb exposition of the state of the art of viruses and viral infections affecting the bone marrow. The coverage is broad, ranging from the discovery of the specific viruses and first recognition of their clinical manifestations to the characteristics of the viruses and cloning of their genes, with emphasis on pathogenetic mechanisms and therapeutic approaches. Major advances have been made in the field, through the applications of the new methodologies in molecular biology and immunology.

The result is a volume that is up to date and exciting to read, with the multiple recent advances melded into a well-organized presentation of the present state of the art.

Part I provides a general introduction to the field of pathogenic viruses that infect hematopoietic cells, covering mechanisms of viral action, the immune response, vaccination strategies, and malignant cell transformation. Parts II–V deal with the four major groups of viruses with hematopoietic effects, the parvoviruses, the herpesviruses, the flaviviruses, and the retroviruses, and the diverse disease states resulting from infection. There is skillful weaving of the old information with the new. For example, in 1948 Paul Owren, the pioneer in establishing the Roman numeral system for clotting factors, introduced the term "acute aplastic crises" to focus on the erythroid aplasia as the cause of the anemic crises in hereditary spherocytosis, rather than hemolysis. In retrospect, with the discovery of B19 parvovirus in 1975 as a human pathogen and the later discovery of the specificity of the virus for infecting marrow erythroid cells, it was likely Owren was dealing with an intercurrent B19 parvovirus infection as the basis for the cessation of red cell production in his patients. Human disease is emphasized throughout, with presentation of certain viral diseases of animals as models for study of pathophysiologic mechanisms and effectiveness of therapy. Part VI covers the role of these viruses in the rapidly developing field of gene therapy. Much of the power of molecular genetics and genetic engineering is due to the effectiveness of viral elements, lacking the ability to replicate, to transfer and express selected exogenous genes in target cells. This section provides a superb and comprehensive presentation of viral vector constructs and gene expression both in vitro in cell culture and in vivo.

This volume should appeal to a multidisciplinary audience including hematologists, clinical microbiologists, immunologists, pathologists, and clinicians in a range of specialties with interests in infectious disease, hematology, disease mechanisms, and/or gene therapy. It should be valuable to teacher and student alike for reading and reference. The editor, along with the authors, have indeed contributed a significant addition to the field.

*Kenneth M. Brinkhous*
*Series Coeditor*

# Preface

This volume was inspired by an increasing interest in the interaction of viruses and hematopoietic cells. Although it has long been known that viral infections in patients affect blood counts, the extremely specific interactions of some viruses with progenitors of blood cells are a more recent discovery. B19 parvovirus toxicity for erythroid precursors and HIV infection of lymphocytes are two clear and notable examples of interactions between viruses and target cells that are now relatively well understood at the intracellular and molecular level. The body of this volume contains chapters that review these and other individual viruses, their biology in tissue culture, and their medical role in patients or in animal models.

Studies of virus infections in humans have shown that viral effects on hematopoietic target cells are often regulated by the immune response. Humoral and cellular activity against viruses normally limit infection, but cytotoxic lymphocytes and cross-reactive antibodies can also damage the host. The absence of an adequate immune response in patients with the acquired immunodeficiency syndrome has dramatically illustrated the central role of immunity in controlling otherwise benign viral infections. New immunological concepts of molecular mimicry, superantigens, tolerance, apoptosis, and distant lymphokine effects on cell proliferation have suggested particularly exciting mechanisms by which viruses may induce immune-mediated disease. Therefore, several authoritative chapters are devoted to the role of the immune system in viral infection from the perspectives of infection control and immune-mediated pathology. Finally, the ability to manipulate the limited genomes of viruses has been profitably employed in the molecular biology of vector construction for gene therapy, the subject of a final chapter.

No previous monograph has dealt with the subject of virus infection of hematopoietic cells. This volume should appeal to both infectious disease specialists who care for patients with viral infections and hematologists who treat blood diseases of viral origin. Other basic scientists, especially virologists and immunologists, should be interested in the product harvest of fundamental research in the clinic and the utility of human disease as biological models.

*Neal S. Young*

# Contents

# Contributors

**Janis L. Abkowitz, M.D.** Associate Professor, Division of Hematology, Department of Medicine, University of Washington, Seattle, Washington

**Bruce G. Baranski, M.D.** Assistant Professor, Division of Hematology, Department of Medicine, University of Wisconsin—Madison, Madison, Wisconsin

**Pascal Bouffard, Ph.D.** Postdoctoral Fellow, Division of Gastroenterology. Department of Internal Medicine, University of California, Davis, Medical Center, Sacromento, California

**Robert S. Fujinami, Ph.D.** Professor, Department of Neurology, University of Utah School of Medicine, Salt Lake City, Utah

**Jonathan R. Hibbs, M.D.** National Research Service Award Fellow, Cell Biology Section, Clinical Hematology Branch, National Heart, Lung and Blood Institute, National Institutes of Health, Bethesda, Maryland

**Caroline I. B. Kurtz, B.S., Ph.D.** Postdoctoral Fellow, Department of Neurology, University of Utah School of Medicine, Salt Lake City, Utah

**Gary J. Kurtzman, M.D.** Group Leader, Virology, Gilead Sciences, Inc., Foster City, California

**Michael L. Linenberger, M.D.** Acting Instructor, Division of Hematology, Department of Medicine, University of Washington, Seattle, Washington

**Johnson Liu, M.D.** Medical Staff Fellow, Clinical Hematology Branch, National Heart, Lung and Blood Institute, National Institutes of Health, Bethesda, Maryland

**Jaroslaw P. Maciejewski, M.D., Ph.D.** Postdoctoral Fellow, Cell Biology Section, Clinical Hematology Branch, National Heart, Lung and Blood Institute, National Institutes of Health, Bethesda, Maryland

**Ian T. Magrath, M.D., FRCP, FRCPath** Head, Lymphoma Biology Section, Pediatric Branch, National Cancer Institute, National Institutes of Health, Bethesda, Maryland

**Hugh I. McFarland, Ph.D.** Postdoctoral Fellow, Department of Pathology, University of Massachusetts Medical Center, Worcester, Massachusetts

**Arthur W. Nienhuis, M.D.** Chief, Clinical Hematology Branch, National Heart, Lung and Blood Institute, National Institutes of Health, Bethesda, Maryland

**Barbara Potts, Ph.D.** Research Scientist, Department of Virology, Repligen Corporation, Cambridge, Massachusetts

**Stephen J. Rosenfeld, M.D.** Clinical Associate, Clinical Hematology Branch, National Heart, Lung and Blood Institute, National Institutes of Health, Bethesda, Maryland

**Sandra K. Ruscetti, Ph.D.** Senior Investigator, Laboratory of Molecular Oncology, National Cancer Institute, National Institutes of Health, Frederick, Maryland

**Stephen St. Jeor, Ph.D.** Professor and Director, Cell and Molecular Biology Program, Department of Microbiology, University of Nevada, Reno, Reno, Nevada

**Jerry L. Spivak, M.D.** Professor, Departments of Medicine and Oncology, and Director, Division of Hematology, Department of Medicine, Johns Hopkins University School of Medicine, Baltimore, Maryland

**Christopher Edward Walsh, M.D., Ph.D.** Medical Staff Fellow, Clinical Hematology Branch, National Heart, Lung and Blood Institute, National Institutes of Health, Bethesda, Maryland

**Raymond M. Welsh, Ph.D.** Professor, Department of Pathology, University of Massachusetts Medical Center, Worcester, Massachusetts

**Neal S. Young, M.D.** Chief, Cell Biology Section, Clinical Hematology Branch, National Heart, Lung and Blood Institute, National Institutes of Health, Bethesda, Maryland

**Jerome B. Zeldis, M.D., Ph.D.** Associate Professor, Division of Gastroenterology, Department of Internal Medicine, University of California, Davis, Medical Center, Sacramento, California

# Part I

## GENERAL ASPECTS OF VIRUS INFECTION OF HEMATOPOIETIC CELLS

# 1

# Mechanisms of Viral Pathogenesis

**Raymond M. Welsh and Hugh I. McFarland**

*University of Massachusetts Medical Center*
*Worcester, Massachusetts*

## INTRODUCTION

The term "pathogenesis" refers to the mechanisms associated with the origin and development of disease. In the context of viral infections this entails the entry of the virus into the host, the spread of the virus throughout the host, the host reponse to the infection, the damage to tissue by the virus or by the host reponse, the egress of the virus from the host, and the sequelae of the infection. The pathogenicity of a virus is defined by the host it infects; a virus is *pathogenic* to a host if it infects that host and causes symptoms of disease, and the features of a disease that are distinctive for a particular viral infection are its *pathognomonic* features. *Virulence* refers to the relative capacities of closely related viruses to cause disease; it is proper in this case to state that one such virus is more virulent, not more pathogenic, than the other. The damage to a cell that is a direct consequence of virus infection is the virus-induced cytopathic effect (CPE). Virus-induced CPE can take on many forms, ranging from minor changes in cell structure to cell dysfunction, lysis, or transformation.

Many factors are involved in the ability of a virus to infect a cell productively and to establish disease in a host. A case in point simply for the initiation of infection is the nature and stability of the virion. The protein coat or capsid must be sufficiently stable to protect the viral nucleic acid from degradation by extracellular nucleases in the environment, but the capsid structure should be sufficiently labile to release the nucleic acid after the virion enters the cell. Depending on its tropism, the virion may have to contend with an acid or protease-rich environment before infecting its cell target, and it would need to express appropriate attachment proteins for receptors present on the target cell.

When considering the topic of viral pathogenesis one must view the infection in the context of the whole body or organism level, but to fully understand the mechanisms at work one must also examine the molecular interactions between the virus and the infected cell. This chapter presents an overview of the subject of viral pathogenesis, taking into account both of these factors.

## ENTRY OF THE VIRUS INTO THE HOST

Viruses may enter the body through the skin, through the mucosal surfaces of the eye or respiratory, alimentary, and genitourinary tracts, or through the placenta (Fig. 1; for reviews, see Refs. 1–3). There usually is replication of the virus near the site of entry, and a number of viral and host factors determine whether the infection remains confined to the point of entry, spreads throughout an organ system, or disseminates throughout the body.

### Skin

The outer layer of the skin, or stratum corneum, consists of keratinized dead cells that do not support viral replication, but minor abrasions can expose living skin tissue to viruses, which initiate infection and replicate in the skin. These viruses include the papillomaviruses (wart) and the poxviruses cowpox, orf, and molluscum contagiosum. Many other viruses, such as measles, rubella, variola (smallpox), and varicella zoster (VZV, chickenpox), can replicate in the skin but usually initiate infection via the respiratory tract and disseminate to the skin later in infection. The most common natural route of infection through the skin is by means of an arthropod vector, such as a mosquito, tick, mite, or gnat. This allows access of the virus to the dermis and local blood vessels. Arthropod vectors may mechanically transfer virus from one host to another, but vector-borne viruses often replicate in the arthropods, allowing transmission of a much greater inoculum. Arthropod-borne human viruses include members of the flavivirus (yellow fever and dengue), togavirus (eastern equine encephalitis), and bunyavirus (Rift Valley fever) groups. A less common natural route of inoculation through the skin is by animal bite. Rabies virus is shed at high titers into dog saliva and is transmitted to a human by deep inoculation caused by the bite of a rabid dog. Of

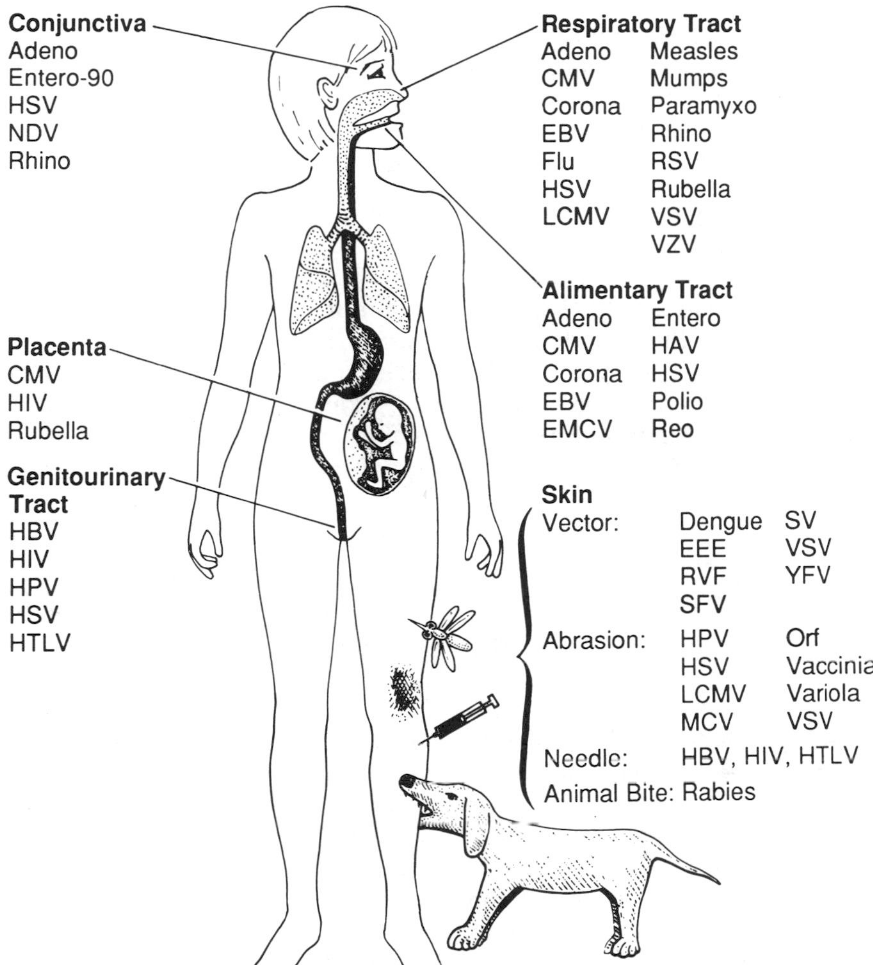


**Figure 1** Entry of virus into the host: the usual points of entry into the host of the viruses discussed in this chapter and of some other important human viruses. Note that this is an incomplete listing of human viral pathogens and that only the most common points of entry are listed for each virus. CMV, cytomegalovirus; EBV, Epstein-Barr virus; EEE, eastern equine encephalitis virus; EMCV, encephalomyocarditis virus; FLU, influenza virus; HAV, hepatitis A virus; HBV, hepatitis B virus; HIV, human immunodeficiency virus; HPV, human papillomavirus; HSV, herpes simplex virus; HTLV, human T cell leukemia virus; LCMV, lymphocytic choriomeningitis virus; MCV, molluscum contagiosum virus; NDV, Newcastle disease virus; RVF, Rift Valley fever virus; RSV, respiratory syncytial virus; SFV, Semliki Forest virus; SV, Sindbis virus; VSV, vesicular stomatitis virus; VZV, varicella zoster virus; YFV, yellow fever virus.

great current epidemiologic significance is the deep inoculation of viruses by hypodermic needles and by unsanitary acupuncture, ear piercing, or tattooing. These procedures, in particular hypodermic needle use by drug abusers, have contributed greatly to the spread of hepatitis B (HBV) and human immunodeficiency (HIV) viruses in the developed countries.

### Conjunctiva

The cleansing action of tears protects the eye from viral infections, but the conjunctiva may nevertheless serve as a port of entry for a variety of respiratory tract infections, including rhinoviruses, a cause of the common cold. Herpes simplex virus type 1 (HSV-1) can enter by this route, cause conjunctivitis, and be reactivated periodically, resulting in repetitive bouts of conjunctivitis and eventual scarring of the cornea. Conjunctivitis by way of initial infection can also be caused by some adenoviruses and enterovirus-70.

### Respiratory Tract

The respiratory tract is the most common port of entry for human viruses. These viruses, which are spread from one individual to another by droplets in respiratory secretions, include many members of the adeno-, corona-, herpes-, orthomyxo-, paramyxo, and picornavirus groups. To achieve infection the virus must penetrate a mucosal membrane, which is bathed in mucus and swept by cilia. Drugs that inhibit the mucociliary transport system increase susceptibility to respiratory infections (4). The virus must also escape inactivation by the high levels of secretory IgA and degradation after phagocytosis by alveolar macrophages. Of importance to viruses that grow in the upper respiratory tract is the ability to replicate at a relatively cool temperature. Rhinoviruses, for example, replicate well at 33 °C, which is the approximate temperature of the upper respiratory tract, whereas other members of the picornavirus group replicate better at 37 °C.

### Alimentary Tract

Transmission of enteric viruses is primarily via the oral-fecal route. These viruses, which include members of the adeno-, corona-, picorna-, and reovirus groups, must contend with acid pH, bile salts, and the proteolytic enzymes involved in the digestive process. Most enveloped viruses are inactivated by acid pH and by bile salts, and with the exception of the coronaviruses, the enteric viruses lack envelopes. The enteric picornaviruses differ from the rhinoviruses not only in temperature optima (already discussed) but also in pH optima. Rhinoviruses readily degrade at acid pH, whereas enteroviruses are stable. Some viruses have evolved to take advantage of the seemingly hostile environment of the alimentary tract. For example, proteolytic digestion of outer capsid proteins of reoviruses activates virion transcriptases that may enhance the productive infection of cells lining the gastrointestinal tract; reovirus mutants resistant to this cleavage lose their ability to infect by the gastrointestinal route (5).

### Genitourinary Tract

Some viruses may be transmitted sexually, and abrasions in the vaginal epithelium or urethra can allow infections with HBV, HIV, HSV-1 and 2, and the genital papillomaviruses.

### Placenta

The placenta must present an effective barrier against infection of the fetus, which is spared in most nonfatal viral infections of pregnant women. However, rubella virus, human cytomegalovirus (CMV), and HIV are important exceptions, and rubella and CMV are causes of congenital abnormalities and stillbirths. Studies with rubella virus have shown necrotic foci in the endothelium of placental blood vessels, indicating a breakdown in the integrity of the placenta that could allow viral passage from maternal blood (6).

## SPREAD OF INFECTION

For a virus to spread from its point of entry it must survive in the environment of the target cell, overcome natural defense mechanisms of the host, and replicate productively in a variety of cells (1–3). In addition to physical and chemical barriers, the virus must also contend with antiviral serum components. In secondary infections these include specific antiviral antibodies but, in primary infections, may include natural antibodies that interact directly with viral proteins or with lipids or carbohydrates on the viral envelope derived from the plasma membrane of the previous host (7). Many enveloped viruses are lysed by complement because they directly activate either the alternative (paramyxoviruses) or the classical (retroviruses) complement pathway without antibody involvement, and serum lipoproteins have been shown to inactivate viruses directly or to stimulate complement-dependent antiviral activity (7).

If a virus escapes this extracellular inactivation, it must be able to infect cells and replicate, and restrictions can occur at a variety of steps in the replicative cycle. Viruses must express attachment proteins interactive with cell receptors (1). These attachment proteins may be species specific, as in the poliovirus, which infects primate but not rodent cells, or they may be cell specific, as in HIV, which binds to the CD4 antigen expressed predominantly on helper T cells. Viruses must then interact with appropriate additional structures to facilitate entry into the cell and uncoating. The permissivity of a cell to virus infection may then relate to the availability of transcription factors, RNA splicing mechanisms, the stage of the cell cycle (which is stimulated by a variety of DNA viruses), RNA translational control mechanisms, and, notably, the availability of appropriate proteases to cleave virion proteins. Some paramyxoviruses and other enveloped viruses require host proteases to cleave viral glycoproteins to render the virion infectious (8). The permissivity of a cell to infection may also be influenced by low levels of interferons (IFN) produced in otherwise healthy individuals. Macrophages or hepatocytes isolated from healthy, uninfected mice may resist infection with influenza virus; cultivation of the cells removes them from the influence of interferon and renders them sensitive to productive infection (9).

Viruses usually replicate locally at the site of initial infection. Some viruses, such as the papillomaviruses and certain poxviruses, restrict their replication to discrete localized lesions, whereas others, such as many of the respiratory or alimentary tract viruses, spread more extensively along epithelial surfaces. Such infections can result in systemic symptomatology and severe illness yet remain localized to a given organ system. Other viruses spread to the lymphatics and/or to the bloodstream and thereby initiate *disseminated* infections. The ability of a viral infection to spread locally or to develop systemically may depend partially on the ability of viruses to grow in and resist degradation by the macrophages of the reticuloendothelial system. Studies have shown that poxviruses injected intravenously into mice are cleared rapidly from the blood by macrophages (10). Numerous other properties determine whether a viral infection will become systemic, including the ability of the virus to grow in several cell types and the pattern of its release from cells. Some enveloped viruses are released exclusively at the luminal surface of epithelial cells, thereby restricting spread laterally to other epithelial cells. Others bud into the subepithelial tissue and more easily disseminate (1). Viruses can be found free in the plasma or in association with erythrocytes, lymphocytes, monocytes, or platelets. The ability to productively replicate in leukocytes can serve to enhance viral spread.

Classic studies done with mouse poxvirus (ectromelia) have served as a model for viral dissemination (11). After local replication in the skin, the virus invades and replicates in the regional lymph node. From there it spreads into the bloodstream and causes a low-level "primary viremia." Blood virus seeds the major visceral organs, such as the liver and spleen, and grows to high titers. It is released into the bloodstream in a high-titer "secondary viremia," and then spreads from the blood to the pathognomonic target organ, the skin, which develops smallpoxlike lesions. Although it is usually not easy to distinguish a primary from a secondary viremia in human infections, it is likely that a similar sequence occurs in a variety of disseminated infections, such as measles, smallpox, rubella, and varicella.

Viral infections sometimes disseminate to the central nervous system (CNS). Frequently, as in poliovirus, CNS infection follows high-level viremia. Viruses usually invade the CNS across cerebral capillary endothelial cells. Some viruses replicate in these endothelial cells, others are transported across in infected leukocytes, and others may be passively transferred across the vascular endothelium by unknown mechanisms. Viruses may also enter the CNS by axonal transport through the peripheral nerve, as in rabies virus, HSV, and VZV. The rate of axonal transport differs with the virus, and the length of time before transport into the brain is a function of the rate of axonal transport and the length of the peripheral nerve (1). The strategy for immunizing against rabies virus after an animal bite is predicated on an immune response to the vaccine developing before the virus reaches and establishes significant levels of replication in the brain.

## HOST RESPONSE TO INFECTION

Viruses are potent biologic response modifiers that, particularly in systemic infections, stimulate a profound variety of nonspecific and virus-specific responses, as shown in Figure 2, which depicts the host response to acute lymphocytic choriomeningitis virus (LCMV) infection in the mouse. A brief summary of the host response, which is reviewed in greater detail in Chapter 2, is presented here. Soon after virus infection there is an induction of an IFN-$\alpha/\beta$ response (12,13). Most virus-infected cells produce IFN-$\alpha$ or $\beta$, although some studies indicate that dendritic cells and macrophages may be particularly adept in this capacity. IFN serves to limit viral replication; depletion of IFN-$\alpha/\beta$ in mice greatly enhances viral titers, and genetic resistance of mice to influenza virus and HSV is dependent on the IFN-$\alpha/\beta$ response (9). Concomitant with the synthesis of IFN-$\alpha/\beta$ in the LCMV infection is the synthesis of tumor necrosis factor (TNF)$\alpha$ (Ruddle and Welsh, unpublished), whose promoter region shares homology with the IFN promotor and whose synthesis is induced by IFN-inducing agents (20). TNF-$\alpha$ mediates antiviral activity in vitro, but its antiviral effects in vivo have not yet been established (21). Closely paralleling the IFN-$\alpha/\beta$ levels is augmentation of the natural killer (NK) cell response. IFN activates the cytotoxic capacities and induces the proliferation of NK cells, which accumulate at sites of virus replication early in infection. NK cells play a role in limiting the spread of many viruses, and it is thought that the combination of IFN-mediated inhibition in virus synthesis and NK cell-mediated lysis of virus-infected targets slows the spread of infection, giving time for specific immune responses to

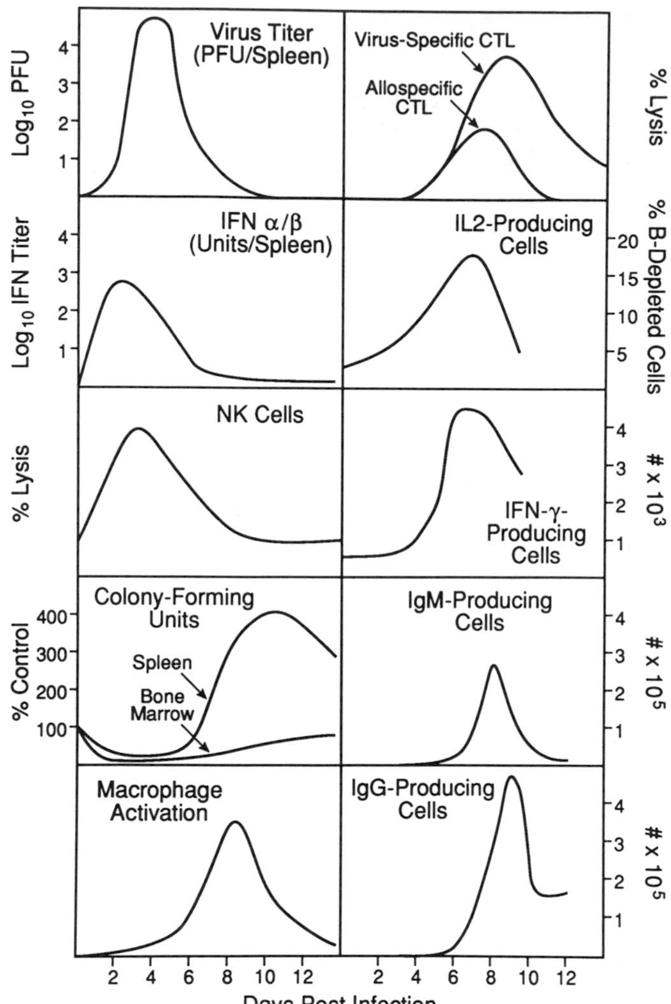


**Figure 2** Host response to LCMV infection: compilation of data from several laboratories regarding various aspects of the host response in the spleen to LCMV infection in the mouse. Although different strains of mice and LCMV were used, the kinetics of the responses in the different studies were sufficiently similar to compile this information, which is more extensive than that for any other infection. Data are presented as the log viral plaque-forming units (PFU) per spleen, the log IFN-$\alpha/\beta$ units per spleen homogenate (12,13), the relative levels of NK cell-mediated lysis (14), the hematopoietic function as determined by colony-forming units (CFU) derived from the spleen and bone marrow (15), the kinetics of the number of peritoneal macrophages and the activation state of spleen macrophages, which are virtually identical (12,16), the virus-specific and virus-induced allospecific spleen CTL responses (14), the percentage of non-B spleen cells expressing messenger RNA for IL-2 (17), the number of splenocytes secreting IFN-$\gamma$ (18), the number of LCMV-specific IgM-producing spleen B cells (19), and the number of LCMV-specific IgG-producing spleen B cells (19).

develop (22). Although neutrophils are found in very early lesions within hours after infection, they are rapidly replaced by mononuclear cells. A common consequence of severe systemic viral infections is a neutropenia associated with impaired bone marrow function (15). This is thought to be due to inhibition of bone marrow cell proliferation and differentiation mediated by a direct cytokine (such as IFN) or to lysis of hematopoietic precursor cells by NK cells activated during infection (15,22,23).

In the early stages of infection, dendritic cells, macrophages, and possibly B cells serve as antigen-presenting cells to stimulate the antigen-specific immune response (24). Viral infections characteristically elicit potent proliferative responses in the $CD4^+$ and $CD8^+$ T lymphocyte populations. High levels of virus-specific class I major histocompatibility complex (MHC)-restricted cytotoxic T cells (CTL) are generated, and as the CTL clonally expand the levels of virus usually decline (Fig. 2). Animal models attest to the importance of $CD8^+$ T cells in regulating viral infections, as adoptive transfers of $CD8^+$ CTL clear infections and selective depletions of $CD8^+$ cells from infected mice lead to persistence (22). $CD4^+$ CTL have also been documented, particularly after secondary stimulation in vitro, but their significance in controlling infections is not yet clearly established. Virus infections are also polyclonal CTL inducers, spontaneously stimulating the generation of allospecific CTL and even CTL reactive to viruses from previous infections (22).

The generation of the T cell response parallels the synthesis of interleukin-2 (IL-2) and IFN-$\gamma$, which are produced by T cells, and the IFN-$\gamma$ response as well as other macrophage-activating cytokines contribute to a high level of macrophage activation late in infection (Fig. 1). These activated macrophages may mediate tissue injury by secreting proteases and toxic cytokines, but there is little evidence that they play roles in controlling the infection (16). The functioning of the $CD8^+$ CTL response as well as the NK cell response may rely heavily on the IFN-$\alpha/\beta$ response induced early in infection. IFN upregulates class I MHC expression on target cells, rendering them more susceptible to lysis by $CD8^+$ CTL. Since, with the exception of the mature cells of the immune system, most cells in the body express very low levels of class I MHC antigens, this upregulation may be critical for the $CD8^+$ CTL to function efficiently to clear the infection. A strong correlation has been made between the susceptibility of a target cell to NK cells and the target cell's *lack* of exprcssion of class I MHC antigens, and IFN *protects* target cells from lysis by IFN-activated NK cells (25,26). Thus, the IFN response conditions cells in a virus-infected host to become resistant to the nonspecific activated NK cells as they become more sensitive to T cells. This mechanism would prevent unnecessary toxicity due to the activated NK cell response while improving the efficiency of T cell-mediated clearance of virus-infected cells. Some viruses downregulate class I MHC expression by inhibiting transcription or translation or, as in adenovirus infection, complexing with MHC in the cytoplasm and preventing its expression on the cell surface (27). Viruses, by virtue of their interference with cellular metabolism, may also impair the ability of IFN to induce the upregulation of class I antigens. These features provide mechanisms for NK cells to selectively lyse virus-infected targets (22).

As clones of virus-specific T cells respond to viral infection, so do clones of B cells, whose response is mostly dependent on $CD4^+$ T cells. The antibody response to infection occurs in the sequence IgM, IgG, IgA, and the peaks in serum levels of IgG and IgA are usually long after the infection has resolved. The peaks in antibody-producing B cells during the acute infection, however, parallel the peaks in the T cell response, with the IgM-producing cell response in the spleen preceding the IgG-producing cell response (Fig. 1) (19). Antibody responses are of particular importance in viral infections not well controlled by T cells, such as poliovirus. Children with agammaglobulinemia succumb to the vaccine strain of poliovirus if not treated passively with antibody (28). For most infections antibody is thought primarily to play a role in limiting dissemination and to be useful in establishing immunity to reinfection. It is of note that, just as with T cells, there are polyclonal B cell responses to virus infections that are associated with spurious and autoimmune antibody production. These are discussed subsequently.

## PERSISTENT VIRAL INFECTIONS

Many viral infections are not completely cleared by the host response and develop into long-term persistent infections, which may occur in the form of chronic virus production or of discrete episodes of virus production interspersed with periods of latency. Two major factors are required for the establishment of a persistent infection: (1) the virus must escape eradication by the immune system, and (2) the virus must be sufficiently noncytopathic such that the host survives long enough to harbor the persistent infection. These obstacles are overcome by a variety of mechanisms.

### Escape from Immune Surveillance

An infectious agent may escape immune surveillance by being inherently nonimmunogenic, by being a beneficiary of immune tolerance, by being immunosuppressive, by sequestering itself from the immune response in immunologically privileged sites, by downregulating surface antigen expression, and by mutating to form escape variants (2,28). Putatively "nonimmunogenic" agents are the prions, or agents of the spongiform encephalopathies, such as scrapie, kuru, and Creutzfeldt-Jakob disease. Here, the infectious entity is associated with an evolutionarily conserved host prion protein (PrP), which fails to induce an immune response in its species of origin. The host fails to respond to the PrP because it is immunologically tolerant to this self protein (29). Immunologic tolerance is also seen with vertically transmitted viruses, particularly with retroviruses transmitted in the germ line. Congenital or neonatal infection usually results in a weak immune response to viruses. Children born with congenital rubella or CMV often shed virus for years, and there is a much higher incidence of persistent HBV infections in underdeveloped countries in which neonates are exposed. In most congenital infections, however, there is no complete or lasting tolerance. Classic experiments in the LCMV model have shown that congenitally or neonatally infected mice fail to generate a CTL response or clear the LCMV infection, but they do produce antiviral antibodies that mediate inflammatory lesions and a progressive degenerative disease (12).

Most systemic virus infections are only transiently immunosuppressive, but some infections, for reasons not yet clearly defined, establish a prolonged suppression. The best example is HIV and other lentivirus infections. It is speculated that such immunosuppression may be due to viral infection of lymphocytes, but it is likely that a variety of other factors, such as the production of inhibitory lymphokines, play a role.

Sequestration into immunologically privileged sites may allow a virus to escape surveillance. Many tissues have lumina that are exposed more to the outside world than to the immune system, and viruses that selectively bud into these lumina may be relatively resistant to immune attack. Examples of these sites are the salivary glands, which may harbor CMV, Epstein-Barr virus (EBV), or rabies virus infection, and the testes, which harbor CMV (30). Papillomavirus infections are nonproductive except at the very surface of the skin, where they are shed in high titers into an immunologically weak environment. Some cells have very low expression of MHC antigens, rendering them resistant to T cell-dependent surveillance. The brain may or may not be considered a privileged site, but it is clear that neuronal tissue in the brain expresses very low levels of MHC antigens, and persistent infections of neurons have been reported with measles, rubella, and various papovaviruses. Some viruses may render a tissue "immunologically privileged" by downregulating MHC antigen expression. The classic example is that of adenovirus-induced tumors in hamsters. Strains of adenovirus that downregulated class I MHC expression were more successful at forming tumors than strains that did not affect class I expression (27).

Downregulation of virally encoded cell surface antigen expression is a common feature of persistent virus infections and can be a consequence of the antiviral effects of IFN or of interference mediated by defective viruses. The immune system itself may render a site resistant to immune attack by modulating cell surface expression of viral antigens. Antiviral antibody can strip or "cap" off measles viral antigens from the cell surface, rendering the cell resistant to further immune attack (31).

Another means by which persistent viruses may escape immune surveillance is by mutation. In sheep infected with visna virus, neutralization antibody-resistant variants appear after each wave of neutralizing antibody is generated (32). The related HIV similarly has a high mutation rate in its envelope protein. Recent work in the mouse has shown that viruses can mutate to escape surveillance by CTL (33) and by NK cells (34).

### Limitations in Viral Cytopathology

In a persistent infection the virus infection must be sufficiently limited or noncytotoxic to prevent killing the host (30,35). Some infections, such as LCMV and HBV, are not very toxic to the infected cell, and most damage is done by immunologic attack mechanisms. Other viruses, such as HIV, have limited tropism and attack only part of the body's tissues. Some infections may be attenuated by constant production of interferon, which may occur in rubella infections, or by the generation of defective interfering viruses or of less cytopathic mutants. Other viruses establish a form of latency, in which the viral genome persists but little or no viral protein is produced. HSV-1 and 2 and VZV, for example, establish such latent infections in ganglia and are periodically reactivated and establish productive epidermal infections. Some virus infections of cells are not productive until the cell further differentiates. Examples of these are infections with the papillomaviruses, discussed earlier, and with CMV, whose replication in macrophages is stimulated after macrophage activation.

## MECHANISMS OF TISSUE INJURY AND DISEASE

Tissue injury and disease in virus infections can be caused by direct virus-induced CPE, by nonspecific inflammatory reactions resulting from virus-induced CPE, nonspecific virus-induced cytokines, specific immune attack against viral antigens and virus-infected cells, induction of autoimmunity, and induction of immunosuppression, which leads to infection by other agents (Table 1) (36,37).

### Virus-Induced CPE Leading to Cell Lysis

Viruses require host cell structures and macromolecular precursors for their replication, and to compete for these host cell resources, viruses have evolved

**Table 1** Virus-Induced Cytopathic Effect

- Cell membrane changes
  - Permeability changes
  - Syncytia formation
- Alterations in macromolecular synthesis
  - Transcription
    - Inhibition *or*
    - Activation of host cell RNA polymerase
  - Inhibition of translation
    - Resource competition between viral and host mRNA by
      - Abundance
      - Translational efficiency
    - Degradation of host cell mRNA (e.g., "cap snatching")
    - Alteration of host translation factors
  - DNA replication
    - Inhibition
      - Shortage of replication factors as a result of shut-down of host protein synthesis
      - Destruction of nascent DNA by nucleases
      - Altered location of the replication apparatus
    - Induction
      - Delivery of virus-encoded oncogenes
      - Stimulation of host protooncogenes
- Cytoskeletal damage
  - Precursor shortage
  - Depolymerization
  - Disruption
- Lysosomal discharge
- Chromosomal damage
  - Breakage, fragmentation, and pulverization
  - Apoptosis
- Inclusion bodies

a variety of mechanisms that result in preferential synthesis of viral products, often at the expense of host cell products. These mechanisms can involve inhibition of host cell macromolecular synthesis or alteration or destruction of cellular constituents. CPE refers to the cell injury that results from such a viral usurpation of cell function and architecture. Many viruses are *cytocidal* and cause *lysis* of the target, and the CPE in a target cell on the way to lysis frequently involves the appearance of inclusion bodies, membrane fusion, vacuolization, chromosomal aberrations, and cell enlargement, rounding, and lifting from the substrate. Associated with these events are alterations in RNA, DNA, and protein synthesis, plasma membrane permeability, and lysosomal integrity. These events are described here.

### Inclusion Bodies

Inclusion bodies are areas with altered histologic staining characteristics in virus-infected cells, and their presence can be used by pathologists to diagnose virus infections. The staining behavior, shape, and location of inclusion bodies within a cell are characteristic of particular viruses and often represent the location of viral replication and assembly. Inclusion bodies, which are actual viral "factories," include the HSV intranuclear inclusion, the poxvirus Guarnieri body, and the rabies virus Negri body. The HSV intranuclear inclusion, visible by light microscopy early as an hourglass shape and later in infection as an eosinophilic body, is termed a replication compartment. This inclusion is associated with viral DNA replication, transcription of late genes, and assembly of the virions. The microscopic characteristics of these inclusions are probably due in part to the displacement and compaction of chromatin.

### Cell Membrane Effects

The permeability of the plasma membrane of some virus-infected cells is altered, allowing intracellular components, such as ATP, $K^+$, $Mg^{2+}$, and cellular enzymes, to leak out while permitting normally excluded extracellular molecules, such as the viability dye trypan blue, to enter the cytoplasm (36). A variety of viruses, including encephalomyocarditis virus (EMCV), mengovirus, simian virus 40 (SV40), and Semliki Forest virus, increase the entry of large molecules, such as antibiotics and toxins, into infected cells. The mechanisms by which viruses alter membrane permeability are not clear, but viral membrane glycoproteins appear necessary for the membrane permeability changes seen in cells infected by the enveloped Newcastle disease and Semliki Forest viruses.

Increased levels of intracellular $Na^+$ have been described in cells infected by several of the picorna-, reo-, and togaviruses. Experiments with the togavirus Sindbis have indicated that the alterations in intracellular $Na^+$ and $K^+$ may be due to inhibition of the $Na^+$ pump (38). The translation of cellular mRNA is more sensitive to high intracellular $Na^+$ concentrations than is mRNA translation of some viruses; therefore, changes in membrane permeability or in the activity of the sodium pump that allows a net $Na^+$ influx may preferentially shut down host protein synthesis. The timing of the $Na^+$ influx and the shutoff of host protein synthesis correlates closely for some viruses, such as EMCV and Sindbis virus, but does not correlate well for a number of others (39,40).

*Syncytia* are multinucleated giant cells formed by plasma membrane fusion of two or more cells. Enveloped viruses, such as paramyxo- and herpesviruses, have envelope glycoproteins that promote the fusion of the virion envelope with the cell membrane. This is the normal mechanism of host cell penetration utilized by some viruses. Syncytia formation is likely a secondary effect of either (1) viral fusion proteins inserted into the plasma membrane of an infected cell, or (2) fusion proteins in the envelope of an extracellular virus spanning cell membranes. The formation of syncytia is a harbinger of lysis and a useful characteristic in diagnosing certain viral infections.

### Effects on Transcription

Viruses up- or downregulate host RNA polymerases depending on whether a host RNA polymerase is needed for replication. Some DNA viruses activate host RNA polymerases, which they then use for their own replication. The adenoviral E1A gene products activate several viral promotors and can control the transcription of specific cellular genes, such as heat-shock protein 70 and β-tubulin. E1A is not itself a DNA binding protein, but E1A directly or indirectly acts on DNA binding transcription factors that facilitate the ability of RNA polymerase to mediate transcription from the appropriate promoter. This activity of E1A products may involve phosphorylation of DNA binding proteins (41).

RNA viruses frequently inhibit cellular RNA polymerase, presumably because it acts as a competitor for nucleoside triphosphates. The inhibition of cell transcription mediated by vesicular stomatitis virus (VSV) requires viral transcription of a small leader RNA that binds to LA, a host protein that associates with an RNA polymerase III subunit. The binding of the VSV leader RNA to LA prevents the LA from associating with the RNA polymerase III subunit, thereby preventing activation of the enzyme (38). The abilities of VSV variants to synthesize leader RNA correlate with their abilities to shut down cellular transcription.

### Inhibition of Host Protein Synthesis

As with other aspects of virus-induced CPE, the effect of infection on host cell translation varies widely from virus to virus and ranges from complete inhibition to stimulation (37,38,41). Competition between viral and host mRNA is a common mechanism of shutoff of host protein synthesis. Viral mRNA may compete with host mRNA by simple abundance, as with reovirus, or by higher translational efficiency, as with influenza virus. Some viruses gain an additional advantage in translation by degrading host cell mRNA by diverse mechanisms. Influenza virus degrades some newly synthesized cellular mRNA by capturing the 5′ end of the host mRNA and ligating it to the viral mRNA by a process known as "cap snatching" (42). A hypothetical cellular nuclease, such as the latent endonuclease activated during IFN treatment of cells, has been suggested to degrade cellular RNA in EMCV infection (43). As mentioned earlier, the influx of $Na^+$ through virus-altered cell membranes may inhibit the translation of host mRNA without adversely affecting viral mRNA translation. Evidence in support of this mechanism has been presented for EMC and Sindbis viruses (39).

Poliovirus and other members of the picornavirus group have evolved a unique method for the preferential synthesis of viral proteins (44). Unlike eukaryotic mRNA, the 5′ end of poliovirus mRNA is uncapped and instead is attached to a viral protein. A cellular cap binding protein (CBP) facilitates the initiation of translation of capped mRNA. Poliovirus infection results in the cleavage of a subunit of the CBP, inhibiting the translation of the capped eukaryotic mRNA but not the uncapped poliovirus RNA. This altered specificity of the host translational apparatus allows preferential viral protein synthesis.

### Inhibition of Cell DNA Replication

Host cell DNA replication is commonly inhibited in virus-infected cells (38, 41). DNA viruses may inhibit cellular DNA replication as a means of competing for cellular polymerases, replication factors, nucleotide precursors, and other limited cell resources. Shutdown of host protein synthesis by both RNA and DNA viruses may result in a shortage of cellular factors necessary for host DNA synthesis. The margination of chromatin induced by herpesvirus infection interferes with cellular DNA replication and favors viral DNA synthesis. Vaccinia virus uses a more direct approach, carrying into the cell a single-strand–specific DNase that accumulates in the nucleus and is presumed to degrade nascent single-stranded cellular DNA. Many DNA viruses actually *stimulate* host DNA synthesis before eventually killing the cell. This can result in areas of intensified cell growth, or *hyperplasia*, which in more extreme forms can lead to cell transformation, as discussed later.

### Effects on the Cytoskeleton

The cytoskeleton is an intricate network of protein filaments involved in defining cell shape, movement, attachment, and intracellular transport. It is composed of actin microfilaments, microtubules, and intermediate filaments, all of which may be depolymerized or disrupted by virus infections (37,38). HSV, for example, causes depolymerization of actin microfilaments and microtubules in infected cells, whereas only intermediate filaments are disrupted in reovirus-infected cells. Vimentin-containing filaments, which are probably intermediate filaments, are present in reovirus inclusion bodies and may provide a framework for viral replication. Destruction or alteration of the cytoskeleton may be a direct effect of viral replication, as is likely the case with reovirus, but in general may be a result of the shutdown of host protein synthesis and subsequent shortage of cytoskeletal precursors.

### Lysosomal Discharge

The permeability of lysosomal membranes increases after many virus infections and is followed by release into the cytoplasm of lysosomal acid hydrolases, which include nucleases, proteases, and phospholipases. These degradative enzymes may be responsible for some virus-induced CPE, such as fragmentation of chromatin by lysosomal nucleases or breakdown of the plasma membrane by phospholipases, but it seems likely that lysosomal discharge is a secondary type of CPE rather than a primary cause of virus-induced cytopathology (37).

### DNA Strand Breaks

Chromosomal damage, described as chromatid breakage, fragmentation, and even pulverization, is common in virus-infected cells and, like lysosomal discharge, may represent secondary effects of other virus-inflicted damage to the cell (36,45). Chromosome breakage occurs in cells infected with a variety of viruses, but herpes, measles, and yellow fever viruses are notable for the frequency of this type of cytopathology. Typical features of herpesvirus CPE are chromosomal breakage and margination as well as nucleolar dislocation and fragmentation. *Pulverization* is a severe form of chromosome breakage that occurs when cells in different mitotic stages fuse, and early chromosomal condensation results in fragmentation of DNA from the cell in the earlier mitotic stage.

Most forms of virus-induced cell death have been reported to be due to necrosis of the target cell. Cells also have the capacity to undergo a programmed cell death, or *apoptosis*, which can be induced by NK cells, CTL, and regulatory cytokines (46,47). During apoptosis a nuclear disintegration precedes plasma membrane breakdown and the DNA degrades into oligomers of nucleosome-sized fragments. Recent work in our laboratory has indicated that mouse hepatitis virus, a coronavirus, stimulates an apoptosislike fragmentation of DNA in infected targets (Nishioka and Welsh, unpublished). Whether such a mechanism relates to the DNA strand breaks observed in other virus infections is not known.

## Virus-Induced Cell Dysfunction

Some viruses do not efficiently lyse cells but cause sublethal damage by interfering with specialized *luxury functions* of the cell not essential for viability or cell growth (35,48). The loss of these luxury functions, which may include inhibition of production of secreted substances, such as neurotransmitters, hormones, and cytokines, or the loss of killer function by lymphocytes, may not be essential for cell viability, but they may be absolute requirements for homeostasis or viability of the organism. The alteration of cell function in persistent infections with hard-to-detect viruses may be the cause of a variety of idiopathic human disorders involving the endocrine, immune, and nervous systems.

The term "luxury function" was first used to describe the reduction in the synthesis and degradation of acetylcholine in mouse neuroblastoma cells persistently infected with LCMV in vitro (49). The concentrations of acetylcholinesterase (ACHE) and of choline acetyltransferase (CAT) were significantly decreased, but total RNA synthesis, protein synthesis, and growth rate of the LCMV-infected neuroblastoma cells were comparable to those of the uninfected control cells. Mice persistently infected with LCMV had high titers of virus in brain tissue, evidence of viral replication in neurons, and altered brain levels of ACHE and CAT. A second example of LCMV influencing luxury functions in vivo is its ability to inhibit growth hormone production in suckling mice. LCMV establishes a persistent infection in the growth hormone-producing cells of the anterior pituitary gland and, without evidence of inflammation, cell necrosis, or cell dropout, causes a greatly reduced synthesis of growth hormone in these cells. The suckling mice suffer from a runting disease, which can be corrected by injections with growth hormone. The mechanism for these selective alterations in luxury functions is unclear, but similar findings have now been seen in a variety of other systems. For example, at permissive temperatures, various types of chick cells infected by temperature-sensitive mutants of Rous sarcoma virus lose their individual specialized functions, such as production of melanin, proteoglycans, or myosin, but then regain them at the restrictive temperature (50). Sublethal cellular dysfunction may also take place in human rhinovirus infections, as studies with organ cultures have shown that rhinoviruses cause a loss in the cilia activity of respiratory epithelium (45).

Virus-induced dysfunction of cells in the immune system can easily be demonstrated in vitro and may be of some significance in virus-induced immune suppression in vivo. Measles virus replicates in lymphocytes and, without evidence of CPE, causes depressed immunoglobulin synthesis by B cells. Measles virus, influenza virus, and CMV all cause sublethal infections of NK cells; influenza virus infection has no effect on NK cell activity, but measles virus and CMV inhibit NK cell-mediated lysis. Surprisingly, these viruses do not inhibit the antibody-directed cellular cytoxicity (ADCC) function of NK cells, attesting to the high selectivity of virus-induced cell dysfunction (51).

## Virus-Induced Cell Transformation

Many retroviruses and DNA viruses have the capacity to transform cells and directly or indirectly induce malignancies. Although many years passed before convincing connections were established between viral infections and human malignancies, examples now abound, including lymphomas and leukemias (EBV and human T cell leukemia virus, HTLV), Kaposi's sarcoma (HIV), cervical carcinoma (human papillomavirus, HPV), nasopharyngeal carcinoma (EBV), and hepatocellular carcinoma (HBV).

Cell transformation is a multistage phenomenon that results in the loss of normal cell growth control, which is regulated by a variety of cell surface, cytoplasmic, and nuclear proteins involved with growth factor-mediated signal transduction and transcriptional regulation (52). Mutations in these genes can result in cancer-causing genes, or *oncogenes*, which elicit cell transformation; the normal cell form of an oncogene is the *protooncogene*. A number of mechanisms are used by viruses to transform cells. Many retroviruses encode oncogenes that they deliver directly into the cell; for instance, the chicken retrovirus of Rous sarcoma carries the oncogene *src* (for sarcoma), which encodes a tyrosine kinase associated with signal transduction. Other viruses do not encode oncogenes per se but instead encode transcriptional regulatory proteins that stimulate cell growth and function to immortalize cells; examples of these include the SV40 T, the adenovirus E1A, and the HTLV-1 tax proteins. A third virus-induced mechanism of oncogenesis involves the mutation of the regulatory or structural regions of cellular protooncogenes. This mutation can be accomplished by the integration of viral genetic material into the host gene, a procedure known as *insertional mutagenesis*. The modification of the host epidermal growth factor receptor gene (c-*erbB*) into the truncated v-*erbB* oncogene is due to insertional mutagenesis by avian leukosis virus. In many lymphoma models, the transcription of host protooncogenes is enhanced by integration of the retroviral long terminal repeat (LTR) region (which regulates retroviral transcription) into the vicinity of the host protooncogene regulatory sequences. A fourth mechanism of transformation is by encoding a protein that modifies the function of a protooncogene. The polyoma middle T protein binds to the cellular *src* and modifies its function. The chromosomal translocation of the *myc* host protooncogene into the transcriptionally active area of antibody gene synthesis is found in some EBV-associated B cell lymphomas, such as Burkitt's lymphoma, but there is little indication that this and similar translocations found in avian retroviral systems are directly mediated by the virus. These tumor-associated translocations may occur randomly after cells have been immortalized by virus infections. Cellular "*anti-oncogene*" products, such as p53 and the retinoblastoma Rb nuclear phosphoproteins, inhibit rather than stimulate cell growth. These proteins may become inactivated by forming complexes with virus-encoded proteins, such as the SV40 T antigen, thereby facilitating the transformation process.

## Nonspecific Inflammatory Reactions

The killing of tissue by cytopathic viruses, like any form of cell killing, can result in nonspecific inflammatory reactions that may lead to systemic effects, such as fever and malaise, and in more severe forms metabolic disturbances and shock (2). These effects are associated with the release of a number of factors, including histamine, kinins, leukotrienes, complement breakdown products, and interleukin-1, otherwise known as "endogenous pyrogen." IL-1 enters the hypothalamus and binds to cells that regulate body temperature and secrete such substances as corticotropin releasing factor, which stimulates a cascade of events influencing energy storage and pituitary, adrenal, and sexual gland function. The result is fever, somnolence, malaise, anorexia, and decreased sexual function (53). This stress response may help the body direct its energy away from normal activities and toward fighting infection. IL-1 also binds to receptors on pain-perceiving neurons and, together with prostaglandins induced during infection, alters the sensitivity to pain messages produced by those neurons. Of particular significance to virus infections is the release of very high levels of IFN-$\alpha/\beta$ from living infected cells. IFN-$\alpha/\beta$ is likely to participate in the induction of many symptoms in virus infections, as patients treated with it experience fever and muscle aches. IFN-$\alpha/\beta$ also increases the frequencies of polarization waves in neurons and by this mechanism may contribute to neurologic symptoms in viral infections (13). TNF-$\alpha$, which is coordinately synthesized with IFN-$\alpha/\beta$, may also contribute to disease (21). TNF-$\alpha$ can kill cells by stimulating apoptosis, and it alters fat metabolism in adipocytes, leading to a wasting disease, or *cachexia*. Cachexia is a common occurrence in the acquired immunodeficiency syndrome (AIDS) and in patients with cancer. Cytokines released during the specific immune response may also lead to tissue injury and disease symptoms. IFN-$\gamma$ could potentially produce many of the same effects as IFN-$\alpha/\beta$, and IL-2 has been shown to be very toxic in treated patients by increasing vascular permeability.

## Immune Attack Against Viral Antigens

The viral life cycle usually involves expression of viral proteins or processed peptides on the surface of infected cells, thereby rendering these cells susceptible to attack by the immune system. Viral antigens are also shed into the blood and lymph, where they form circulating antigen-antibody complexes of pathologic consequence. Some degree of immunopathologic activity is found in most viral infections, and in some diseases it is of greater significance than direct virus-induced tissue injury (12,54).

Antibody-mediated immunopathologic injury can occur in several forms (54).

1. Viral antigen-antibody-complement complexes form in most infections and can become of particular pathologic consequence in persistent infections, such as chronic HBV infection. These complexes cause Arthus-like reactions (type III hypersensitivity reactions), and their accumulation in capillary beds and other small blood vessels causes arteritis and glomerulonephritis. Immune complexes are readily detectable in acute and persistent rubella infections and may account for the characteristic rash.
2. Antibody may bind to the surface of virus-infected cells, activate the complement cascade, and stimulate an inflammatory response.
3. Antibody may coat virus-infected cells and render them sensitive to direct lysis by complement, NK cells, monocyte-macrophages, or neutrophils. The significance of these type II hypersensitivity reactions in virus infections is not yet well established.
4. The host may develop an IgE (allergic) antibody response that triggers mast cells when exposed to antigens (type I hypersensitivity). This is not of great significance in most virus infections, but severe wheezing in children infected with respiratory syncytial virus has been correlated with an IgE response (54). It is of note that mast cell secretions are elevated in the presence of IFN, suggesting that viral infections could enhance the severity of allergic responses to nonviral antigens (55).

T-cell-dependent immunopathologic injury is attributed to direct cytotoxicity or to delayed (type IV) hypersensitivity (DTH) reactions associated with the infiltration of T cells and macrophages into tissue with subsequent release of toxic mediators. Both $CD4^+$ and $CD8^+$ T cells can mediate each type of reaction. The classic model for T cells in virus infection is the LCMV infection of mice. This relatively noncytopathic virus causes a persistent but benign infection in the immunosuppressed animal, but passive transfer of purified or cloned LCMV-specific $CD8^+$ T cells stimulates a lethal encephalitis in mice infected intracranially and a hepatitis in mice infected intraperitoneally; $CD8^+$ T cells also elicit a DTH-like reaction in various tissues and clear the infection (22,56,57). The hepatitis associated with acute HBV infection may also be associated with a T cell response (58).

## Induction of Autoimmunity

Autoimmunity is distinguished from virus-specific immunopathology in that the immune attack is directed against normal cell antigens. Antibodies to normal host antigens are frequently found after viral infections, including CMV, EBV, HBV, and HIV in the human. Exacerbations of multiple sclerosis, stimulation of type 1 diabetes resulting in antibodies to beta cells, and the Guillain-Barré syndrome involving autoimmunity to peripheral nervous tissue have all been reported following human viral infections (54). Numerous animal models attest to the ability of virus infections to trigger antibodies against normal antigens in the brain, liver, pancreas, and other tissue. Many mechanisms may be involved in the induction of autoimmunity.

1. Virus infections induce polyclonal B cells and T cells that do not cross-react with viral antigens with high affinity. This polyclonal stimulation may result from direct transformation and outgrowth of lymphocytes, as in B cells with EBV, from a polyclonal expansion due to the massive amounts of cytokine growth factors released during infection, from viral glycoproteins acting like lectin mitogens for B or T cells, or possibly from the stimulation of immune cells bearing low-affinity interactions with viral proteins or to virus-induced host antigens to which the host is not tolerant.
2. The infection of a cell by a virus may disrupt cells and release host antigens in a different form or into a different place in the body. For example, virus-induced CPE of brain tissue releases myelin into the bloodstream and induces anti-myelin antibody.
3. Viral and host proteins may have in common short sequences of amino acids (*molecular mimicry*), which in the context of a viral infection may be presented to the immune system in a different form or in juxtaposition with a viral sequence that may induce a potent helper T cell response (59). Mice made transgenic with a VSV protein, G, were tolerant to this protein and failed to generate an antibody response to it when immunized against it (60). When challenged with whole VSV, however, an antibody response was made against this protein. This argues that a virus infection can break the tolerance of the host to a given antigen.
4. It is hypothesized that an antiidiotype network of antibodies could be generated to create antibodies with specificity against host cell receptors for viruses. Here, an antibody to a virus attachment protein might resemble the host cell receptor. The idiotype on this antibody would then be seen as a foreign sequence and, according to the Jerne network theory, would stimulate an antiidiotype antibody response that might react with the host cell receptor (61).

## Virus-Induced Immune System Dysfunction

Viruses frequently suppress immune system functions, and this immunosuppression can contribute to a more prolonged course of disease or to secondary infections with bacteria, fungi, protozoa, or other viruses. The primary example of this in the human is the HIV infection, in which virus-induced immune suppression results in complications with numerous adventitious agents and many of the DNA viruses. Despite much research, the mechanism of virus-induced immunosuppression remains poorly understood and awaits further elucidation of the regulatory roles of different combinations of cytokines on the immune response. As outlined earlier, some viruses directly infect and either lyse or stimulate dysfunction of leukocytes, including macrophages, T cells, and NK cells, but usually only a small percentage of leukocytes are infected, arguing for more systemic mechanisms. Some systemic effects could be mediated by soluble viral proteins, such as the HIV envelope glycoprotein, which shuts down NK cell function at a postbinding step (62). Macrophages activated during virus infections or directly infected by such viruses as CMV may secrete prostaglandins or IL-1 inhibitors that mediate suppression (63). Lymphocytes isolated from virus-infected individuals frequently respond very poorly to mitogen stimulation, and recent studies have indicated that they fail to produce IL-2 when stimulated with lectins in vitro (64). This unresponsiveness is likely a function of lymphocyte anergy resulting from exposure to some other lymphokine in vivo, perhaps IL-2 itself, which has been shown in vitro to reduce the ability of T cells to secrete IL-2 when lectin stimulated (65). Other immunosuppressive lymphokines might be transforming growth factor $\beta$ and IL-10, which negatively act on many immune system functions (66,67). It is of interest that EBV encodes an immunosuppressive protein (BCRF1) that has 70% amino acid homology with IL-10 (67). Undoubtedly, different mechanisms of suppression may be of importance in different virus infections, and much work is needed to elucidate these processes.

## MULTIPLE MECHANISMS OF VIRAL DISEASES AND THEIR SEQUELAE

Most viral infections are clinically inapparent or present as acute diseases, sometimes ending in death but usually resolving without sequelae. In other cases lasting pathologic effects may be caused by persistent infection or by sequelae to the acute infection. These may involve neurologic, endocrinologic, immunologic, respiratory, cardiac, and other disturbances. Such disturbances can be caused by a variety of mechanisms. For example, animal models and human infections have provided evidence that demyelination may be caused by the cytocidal effects of viruses on neurons or on the myelin-producing oligodendrocytes, by an immune attack directed against viral antigens on neurons or oligodendrocytes, or by virus-induced humoral or cellular autoimmunity directed against these cells or to myelin (68). Virus-induced diabetes in animal models has been associated with direct virus-induced lysis of beta cells, immune T cell attack against viral antigens on beta cells, and the triggering of autoimmune diabetes in genetically predisposed animals (69). Some monoclonal antibodies directed against immunizing viruses cross-react with islet cell antigens (an example of molecular mimicry), and reduced insulin production has been noted in otherwise normal beta cells persistently infected in vivo with viruses (an example of reduced luxury function). Detailed examples of the mechanisms of diseases caused by specific viruses can be found in the other chapters of this book.

## REFERENCES

1. Tyler KL, Fields BN. Pathogenesis of viral infections. In: Fields BN, Knipe DM, eds. Virology. New York: Raven Press, 1990; 191–239.
2. White DO, Fenner FJ. Medical Virology. London: Academic Press, 1986; 119-216.
3. Gardner MB, Sullivan WF, Hinrichs SH. Pathology of virus infection. In: Rothschild H, Cohen JC, eds. Virology in medicine. New York: Oxford University Press, 1986; 65–86.
4. Bang F, Bang B, Foard M. Responses of upper respiratory tract mucosa to drugs and viral infections. Am Rev Respir Dis 1966; 93:5142–9.
5. Bass DM, Bodkin D, Dambrauskas R, Trier JS, Fields BN, Wolf JL. Intraluminal proteolytic activation plays an important role in replication of type 1 reovirus in the intestines of neonatal mice. J Virol 1990; 64:1830–3.
6. Forsgren M. The pathogenesis of congenital infections. In: Lycke E, Norrby E, eds. Textbook of medical virology. Kent, England:Butterworth, 1983; 135–43.
7. Cooper NR, Welsh RM. Antibody and complement dependent viral neutralization. Springer Semin Immunopathol 1979; 2:285–310.
8. Scheid A, Choppin PW. Protease activation mutants of Sendai virus: activation of biological properties of specific protease. Virology 1976; 69:265–77.
9. Haller O. Inborn resistance of mice to orthomyxoviruses. Curr Top Microbiol Immunol 1981; 92:25–52.
10. Mims CA. Aspects of the pathogenesis of virus diseases. Bacteriol Rev 1964; 28:30–71.
11. Fenner F. Mousepox (infectious ectromelia of mice): a review. J Immunol 1964; 63:341–73.
12. Buchmeier MJ, Welsh RM, Dutko FJ, Oldstone MBA. The virology and immunobiology of lymphocytic choriomeningitis virus infection. Adv Immunol 1980; 30:275–331.
13. Welsh RM. Natural killer cells and interferon. Crit Rev Immunol 1984; 5:55–93.
14. Welsh RM, Yang H, Bukowski JF. The role of interferon in the regulation of virus infections by cytotoxic lymphocytes. Bioessays 1988; 8:10–3.
15. Bro-Jorgensen K. The interplay between lymphocytic choriomeningitis virus, immune function, and hemopoiesis in mice. Adv Virus Res 1978; 22:327–69.
16. Lehmann-Grube F. Role of mononuclear phagocytes in the control of lymphocytic choriomeningitis virus infection of mice. In: Lopez C, ed. Washington DC: American Society for Microbiology 1988; 105–24.
17. Kasaian MT, Biron CA. The activation of IL-2 transcription in L3T4$^+$ and LYT-2$^+$ lymphocytes during virus infection in vivo. J Immunol 1989; 142:1287–92.

18. Gessner A, Moskophidis D, Lehmann-Grube F. Enumeration of single IFN-$\gamma$-producing cells in mice during viral and bacterial infection. J Immunol 1989; 142:1293–8.
19. Moskophidis D, Lehmann-Grube F. The immune response of the mouse to lymphocytic choriomeningitis virus. IV. Enumeration of antibody-producing cells in spleens during acute and persistent infection. J Immunol 1984; 133:3366–70.
20. Goldfield AE, Maniatis T. Coordinate viral induction of tumor necrosis factor $\alpha$ and $\beta$ in human B cells and monocytes. Proc Natl Acad Sci U S A 1989; 86: 1490–4.
21. Rosenblum MG, Donato NJ. Tumor necrosis factor $\alpha$: a multifaceted peptide hormone. Crit Rev Immunol 1989; 9:21–44.
22. Welsh RM. Regulation and role of large granular lymphocytes in arenavirus infections. Curr Top Microbiol Immunol 1987; 134:185–209.
23. Thomsen AR, Pisa P, Bro-Jorgensen K, Kiessling R. Mechanisms of lymphocytic choriomeningitis virus-induced hemopoietic dysfunction. J Virol 1986; 59:428–33.
24. Allison AC. Role of monocytes, macrophages, Langerhans cells, and follicular dendritic cells in persistent virus infections. In: Lopez C, ed. Washington DC: American Society for Microbiology, 1988; 18–38.
25. Ljunggren HG, Karre K. In search of the 'missing self': MHC molecules and NK cell recognition. Immunol Today 1990; 11:237–44.
26. Trinchieri G, Santoli D. Antiviral activity induced by culturing lymphocytes with tumor derived or virus-transformed cells. Enhancement of natural killer activity by interferon and antagonistic inhibition of susceptibility of target cells to lysis. J Exp Med 1978; 147:1314–33.
27. Schrier PI, Bernards R, Vaessen RTM, Houweling A, van der Eb AJ. Expression of class I major histocompatibility antigens switched off by highly oncogenic adenovirus 12 in transformed rat cells. Nature 1983; 305:771–5.
28. Wright PF, Hatch MH, Kasselberg AG, Lowry SP, Wadlington WB, Karzon DT. Vaccine-associated poliomyelitis in a child with sex-linked agammaglobulinemia. J Pediatr 1977; 91:408–12.
29. Prusiner SB. Molecular structure, biology, and genetics of prions. Adv Virus Res 1988; 35:83–136.
30. Mims CA. Immunobiology and pathogenesis of persistent virus infections. In: Lopez C, ed. Immunology and pathogenesis of persistent virus infections. Washington DC: American Society for Microbiology, 1988; 3–17.
31. Joseph BS, Oldstone MBA. Immunologic injury in measles virus infection. II. Suppression of immune injury through antigenic modulation. J Exp Med 1975; 142:864–76.
32. Narayan O, Clements JE. Lentiviruses. In: Fields BN, Knipe DM, eds. Virology. New York: Raven Press, 1990; 1571–89.
33. Pircher H, Moskophidis D, Rohrer U, Burki K, Hengartner H, Zinkernagel RM. Viral escape by selection of cytotoxic T cell resistant virus variants in vivo. Nature 1990; 346:629–32.

34. Welsh RM, Brubaker JO, Vargas-Cortes M, O'Donnell CL. Natural killer (NK) cell response to virus infections in mice with severe combined immunodeficiency. The stimulation of NK cells and the NK cell-dependent control of virus infections occur independently of T and B cell function. J Exp Med 1991; 173:1053-1063.
35. Oldstone MBA. Viral persistence. Cell 1989; 56:517–20.
36. Fenner F, McAuslan BR, Mims CA, Sambrook J, White DO. The biology of animal viruses. New York: Academic Press, 1974; 341–3.
37. Wagner RR. Cytopathic effects of viruses: a general survey. In Fraenkel-Conrat H, Wagner RR, eds. Comprehensive virology, vol. 19. Viral cytopathology, cellular macromolecular synthesis and cytocidal viruses. New York: Plenum Press, 1984; 21–58.
38. Knipe DM. Virus-host-cell interactions. In: Fields BN, Knipe DM, eds. Virology. New York: Raven Press, 1990; 293–316.
39. Kozak M. Regulation of protein synthesis in virus-infected animal cells. Adv Virus Res 1986; 31:229–92.
40. Carrasco L. The inhibition of cell functions after viral infection. A proposed general mechanism. FEBS Lett 1977; 76:11–5.
41. Fernandez-Tomas C. Virus-directed suppression of host transcription. In: Mechanisms of viral toxicity in animal cells. Boca Raton, FL: CRC Press, 1987; 38–9.
42. Plotch SJ, Bouloy M, Ulmanen I, Krug RM. A unique cap(m7GpppXm)-dependent influenza virion endonuclease cleaves capped RNAs to generate the primers that initiate viral RNA transcription. Cell 1981; 23:847–58.
43. Silverman RH, Cayley PJ, Knight M, Gilbert CS, Kerr IM. Control of the ppp (A2'p)nA system in HeLa cells: effects of interferon and virus infection. Eur J Biochem 1982; 124:131–8.
44. Sonenberg N. Regulation of translation by poliovirus. Adv Virus Res 1987; 33: 175–204.
45. Lycke E, Norrby E. Virus-induced changes of cell structures and functions. In: Lycke E, Norrby E, eds. Textbook of medical virology. Kent, England: Butterworth, 1983; 93–104.
46. Arends RG, Morris RG, Wyllie AH. Apoptosis: the role of the endonuclease. Am J Pathol 1990; 136:593–608.
47. Martz E, Howell DM. CTL: virus-control cells first and cytolytic cells second? Immunol Today 1989; 10:79–86.
48. Oldstone MBA. Virus can alter cell function without causing cell pathology: disordered function leads to imbalance of homeostasis and disease. In: Notkins AL, Oldstone MBA, eds. Concepts in viral pathogenesis. New York: Springer-Verlag, 1984; 269–76.
49. Oldstone MBA, Holmstoen J, Welsh RM. Alterations of acetylcholine enzymes in neuroblastoma cells persistently infected with lymphocytic choriomeningitis virus. J Cell Physiol 1977; 91:459–72.
50. Holtzer H, Pacifici M, Tapscott S, Bennett G, Payette R, Dlugosz A. Lineages in cell differentiation and in cell transformation. In: Revoltella RP, Pontieri

GM, Basilico C, Rovera G, Gallo RC, Subak-Sharpe JH, eds. Expression of differentiated functions in cancer cells. New York: Raven Press, 1982; 169–80.
51. McChesney MB, Oldstone MBA. Viruses perturb lymphocyte functions: selected principles characterizing virus-induced immunosuppression. Annu Rev Immunol 1987; 5:279–304.
52. Benjamin T, Vogt PK. Cell transformation by viruses. In: Fields BN, Knipe DM, eds. Virology. New York: Raven Press, 1990; 317-367.
53. Sapolsky RM. Why you feel crummy when you're sick. Discover 1990; July:66–70.
54. Mims CA. Immunopathology in virus disease. Philos Trans R Soc Lond [Biol] 1983; 303:189–98.
55. Ida S, Hooks JJ, Siraganian RP, Notkins AL. Enhancement of IgE-mediated histamine release from human basophils by viruses: role of interferon. J Exp Med 1977; 145:892–906.
56. Allan JE, Dixon JE, Doherty PC. Nature of the inflammatory process in the central nevous system of mice infected with lymphocytic choriomeningitis virus. Curr Top Microbiol Immunol 1987; 134:131–43.
57. Zinkernagel RM, Haenseler E, Leist T, et al. T cell-mediated hepatitis in mice infected with lymphocytic choriomeningitis virus. Liver cell destruction of H-2 class I-restricted virus-specific cytotoxic T cells as a physiological correlate of the $^{51}Cr$-release assay? J Exp Med 1986; 164:1075–92.
58. Hollinger FB. Hepatitis B virus. In: Fields BN, Knipe DM, eds. Virology. New York: Raven Press, 1990; 2171–236.
59. Fujinami RS, Oldstone MBA, Wroblewska Z, Frankel ME, Koprowski H. Molecular mimicry in virus infection: crossreaction of measles virus phosphoprotein or of herpes simplex virus protein with human intermediate filaments. Proc Natl Acad Sci U S A 1983; 80:2346–50.
60. Zinkernagel RM, Cooper S, Chambers J, Lazzarini RA, Hengartner H, Arnheiter H. Virus-induced autoantibody response to a transgenic viral antigen. Nature 1990; 345:68–71.
61. Jerne NK. Idiotype networks and other preconceived ideas. Immunol Rev 1984; 79:5–24.
62. Cauda R, Tumbarello M, Ortona L, Kanda P, Kennedy RC, Chanh TC. Inhibition of normal human natural killer cell activity by human immunodeficiency virus synthetic transmembrane peptides. Cell Immunol 1988; 115:57–65.
63. Kapasi K, Rice GPA. Cytomegalovirus infection of peripheral blood mononuclear cells: effects on interleukin-1 and -2 production and responsiveness. J Virol 1988; 62:3603–7.
64. Saron MF, Shidani B, Nahori MA, Guillon JC, Truffa-Bachi P. Lymphocytic choriomeningitis virus-induced immunodepression: inherent defect of B and T lymphocytes. J Virol 1990; 64:4076–83.
65. Schell SR, Fitch FW. Pretreatment of cloned helper T lymphocytes with IL-2 induces unresponsiveness to antigen and concanavalin A, associated with decreased inositol phosphate and diacylglycerol production. J Immunol 1989; 143: 1499–505.
66. Balkwill FR, Burke F. The cytokine network. Immunol Today 1989; 10:299–304.

67. Hsu DH, Malefyt R de W, Fiorentino DF, et al. Expression of interleukin-10 activity by Epstein-Barr virus protein BCRF1. Science 1990; 250:830–2.
68. Lampert PW, Rodriguez M. Virus-induced demyelination. In: Notkins AL, Oldstone MBA, eds. Concepts of viral pathogenesis. New York: Springer-Verlag, 1984; 260–8.
69. Notkins AL, Yoon J-W. Virus-induced diabetes mellitus. In: Notkins AL, Oldstone MBA, eds. Concepts of viral pathogenesis. New York: Springer-Verlag, 1984; 241–7.

# 2

# Immune Response to Viral Infection

**Caroline I. B. Kurtz and Robert S. Fujinami**

*University of Utah School of Medicine*
*Salt Lake City, Utah*

## INTRODUCTION

The vertebrate immune system consists of a complex assemblage of defense mechanisms designed to protect the host from microbes constantly encountered in its environment. This system is highly redundant, providing multiple mechanisms to accomplish the elimination of bacteria, parasites, fungi, and viruses. The immune system can be divided into two broad categories known as nonspecific and specific immunity.

Nonspecific immunity, also described as innate, natural, or nonadaptive immunity, consists of systems that can be activated rapidly (within a few hours to a few days) following exposure to a pathogen but that cannot distinguish among or react specifically with different types of microbial pathogens. These systems probably represent the most primitive mechanisms of immunity and are present in some simple, invertebrate life forms as well as vertebrates. They include the complement system, interferons, phagocytic cells, and natural killer cells.

Specific immunity, also described as inducible or adaptive immunity, provides the host with both humoral and cellular mechanisms capable of recognizing and eliminating myriad unique microbial pathogens. Specific immunity is not constitutively present in the host but is induced by exposure to a pathogen. For this reason, specific immunity takes longer to develop compared with nonspecific immunity. It may take 1–2 weeks before specific immune responses can peak in effectiveness. However, the specific immune response has the capacity of memory. Upon second exposure to a pathogen, the specific immune system reacts both more rapidly and with greater affinity and intensity to eliminate the invading microbe. Specific immunity is mediated by B and T lymphocytes.

Viruses present a special challenge to the vertebrate immune system. They are obligate intracellular parasites utilizing natural cell membrane structures to gain entry into their target cells. Once inside they are shielded from a potentially harsh extracellular environment that might destroy some pathogens. They monopolize the host cell's metabolic machinery and either interfere with normal cellular function or destroy the cell when their replication cycle is complete. Many viruses have evolved strategies to avoid the host's immune mechanisms as well. Antigenic variation is a common strategy of viral evasion. By constantly changing the structure of their outer coat proteins, viruses can elude specific immune memory cells long enough to establish reinfection of a host. Finally, many viruses infect and destroy cells of the immune system itself, compromising the host's capacity to mount a specific immune response. Given the capacity of viruses to replicate in tremendous numbers and to evolve rapidly, it is testimony to the sophistication of the vertebrate immune system that most viral infections are kept in check.

This chapter describes in detail both the nonspecific and specific immune responses that work together to eliminate viral infections. Much of our knowledge of the immune response has come from studies in mammals, particularly humans and rodents. Thus much of the work cited in this chapter refers to studies that have been done in humans or murine model systems. For each mechanism of immunity that mammals have developed, an example of a virus that has evolved a strategy to overcome this mechanism can be found. Collectively however, very few viruses can overcome all the immune mechanisms. This chapter emphasizes the successes and relative importance of the different mechanisms of immune protection rather than the strategies viruses have developed to evade the immune response.

## NONSPECIFIC IMMUNITY TO VIRAL INFECTION

The generation of an antiviral immune response during viral infection can often take 1–2 weeks to peak in effectiveness. If this were the only mechanism of protection from infection, the host would be extremely vulnerable, since viral infection could proceed unchecked for many days before a specific immune response is mounted. However, many non-antigen-specific defense mechanisms are available to the host that can be mobilized rapidly to slow dissemination of virus while antigen specific immune responses are being generated. These include the complement system and the production of antiviral mediators, such as interferons, phagocytic cells, and natural killer cells.

## Complement

Complement is a series of over 20 serum glycoproteins involved in the natural defense against microbial pathogens. Through direct lysis of pathogens, opsonization, chemotaxis, and induction of inflammation, the complement system helps to control microbial infections (1). Complement is activated through two distinct mechanisms known as the classical and alternative pathways (detailed in Fig. 1). These pathways share a common terminal pathway that results in the formation of a structure known as the membrane attack complex on the surface of cells. Activation through either pathway involves the formation of a central enzyme known as the C3 convertase. In the classical pathway the C3 convertase is composed of complement proteins C2 and C4; in the alternative pathway, it is composed of C3 and factor B. In either case, this enzyme cleaves a peptide from the C3 molecule, which leads to destabilization of a thiol-ester bond found within C3 and exposure of a reactive acyl group. This acyl group rapidly reacts with the nearest nucleophilic group possible, which is most often a water molecule but can occasionally be an amino or hydroxyl group present on the microbial surface under attack. The C3 convertase can bind additional molecules of C3 and form an enzyme known as a C5 convertase. This enzyme cleaves C5 into C5a and C5b. C5a is a potent chemotactic agent, drawing mononuclear and polymorphonuclear cells to the site of activation. C5b, when generated on a membrane surface, is the cornerstone for the construction of a cytolytic pore structure known as the membrane attack complex. When many of these are deposited on a cell membrane, the normal cellular repair mechanisms are overcome and the cell dies as a result of osmotic lysis or disruption of the lipid bilayer (2).

The classical and alternative pathways are activated through different mechanisms. Antigen-antibody complexes and some viruses are capable of activating the classical pathway (1). The alternative pathway is activated by Gram-negative bacteria, yeast zymosan, viruses, virally infected cells, parasites, and polyanionic substances. There is also a slow rate of activation of the alternative pathway by spontaneous hydrolysis of the thiol-ester bond in C3. The hydrolyzed C3 can interact with alternative pathway factor B to form a C3 convertase.

An intact complement system has been shown to be a vital defense mechanism during viral infection (1). There are many reports in the literature of complement lysing viruses in vitro or enhancing the neutralization of virus by antibody. Complement also has been shown to play a role in defense against viral infections in vivo. When infected with influenza virus, decomplemented

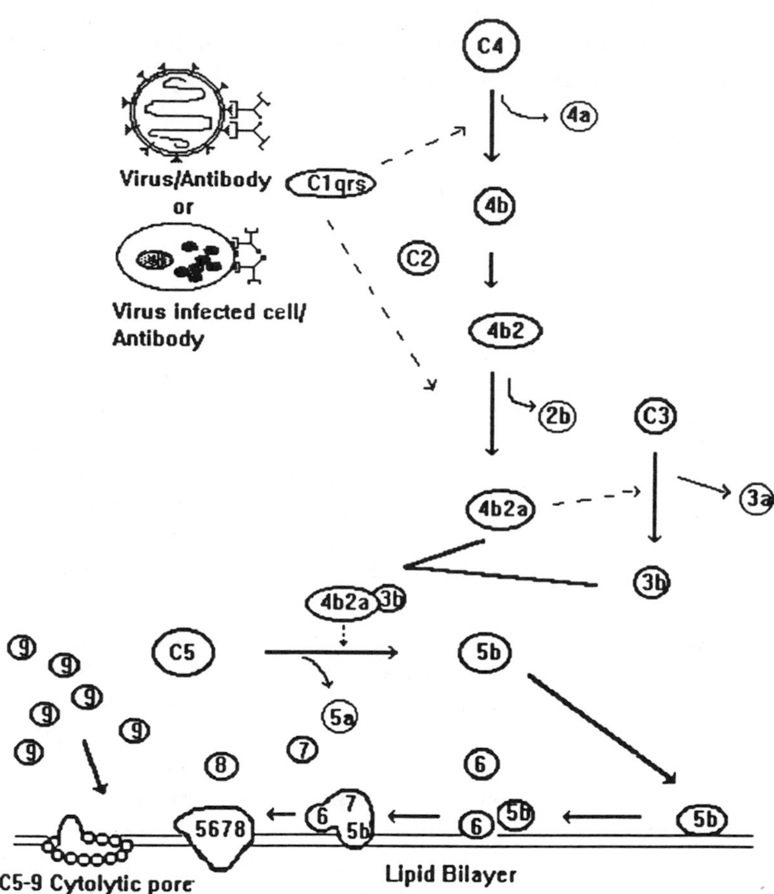


**Figure 1A** Classical pathway of complement activation. Antigen-antibody complexes, such as antibody-bound virus complexes, some viruses alone, and virus-infected cells are capable of initiating the classic pathway of complement activation. C1qrs cleaves peptides from C4 and C2, resulting in formation of the C3 convertase C4b2a. C3b can bind to the C4b2a complex to form the C5 convertase C4b2a3b. The C5 convertase cleaves C5 into C5a and C5b. C5b associates with a lipid bilayer and, in conjunction with C6, C7, C8, and C9, forms a cytolytic pore structure, causing destruction of the viral envelope or virally infected cell.

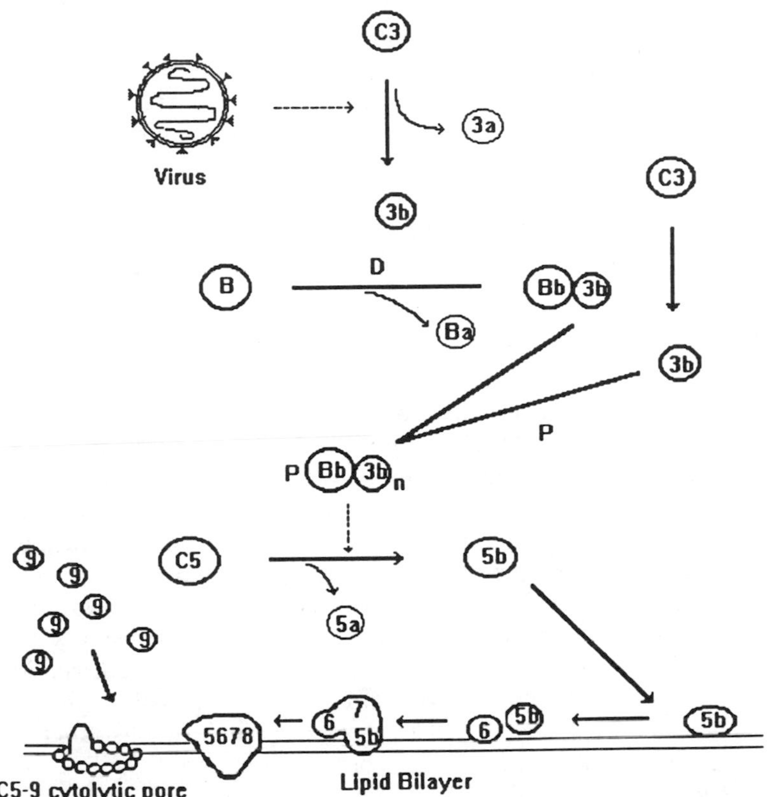


**Figure 1B** Alternative pathway of complement activation. Viruses can activate the alternative pathway. This pathway is initiated when C3 is cleaved into C3b and C3a. C3b binds to factor B, and in the presence of factor D the peptide Ba is released, resulting in the formation of the C3 convertase C3bBb. C3bBb can cleave more C3 into C3b. Complexes of C3bBb are stabilized by properdin, P. When multiple molecules of C3b associate with C3bBb, a C5 convertase is formed. The C5 convertase cleaves C5 into C5a and C5b. C5b associates with a lipid bilayer and, in conjunction with C6, C7, C8, and C9, forms a cytolytic pore structure, causing lysis or neutralization of the virus.

mice or C5-deficient mice were found to have a prolonged viral infection, increased morbidity and mortality, and increased pulmonary consolidation compared with infected littermates having normal levels of complement (3). Similarly, mice depleted of complement and infected with Sindbis virus demonstrated prolonged viremia and poor viral clearance (4). Complement can aid in the elimination of a viral infection by several means: directly lysis of virus; destruction of antibody-coated virus or virally infected cells; steric blockade of attachment of virus to its host cell; attraction of inflammatory cells into the site of infection; and enhanced uptake of virus by phagocytic cells (Table 1).

### Direct Virolysis

Pillemar first showed that infectivity of Newcastle disease virus was blocked by activation of the alternative pathway in the absence of serum antibody (1). More recently it was found that lymphocytic choriomeningitis virus could also be inactivated by the alternative pathway of complement (1). RNA tumor viruses, such as murine leukemia virus, are lysed by activation of the classical pathway in the absence of antibody. These viruses directly bind complement component C1q and initiate the complement cascade. Sindbis virus can directly activate both the classic and alternative pathways of complement.

Other viruses are neutralized by complement in the presence of virus-specific antibodies. Neutralization can be accomplished either by disruption of the virion integrity or by blocking viral attachment or uncoating, preventing infection. Complement-mediated virolysis has been demonstrated for enveloped viruses, such as avian infectious bronchitis virus and Sindbis virus (1). Other viruses can be neutralized without virolysis. Herpes simplex virus requires complement for neutralization with antiviral IgM, and complement components C1–3 but not C5–7 enhance neutralization of polyomavirus (1).

**Table 1** Role of Complement in Immunity to Viral Infection

| Mechanism | Pathway | Example | References |
|---|---|---|---|
| Direct virolysis | Alternative | Sindbis virus | 4, 5 |
| | Classical | RNA tumor virus | |
| Lysis of infected cells | Alternative | Measles virus | 6, 7 |
| Steric hindrance | Classical<br>Alternative | Avian IBV, EAV | 1, 8, 9 |
| Chemotaxis | Classical<br>Alternative | HSV | 1, 10 |
| Phagocytosis | Classical<br>Alternative | HSV | 11, 12 |

### Destruction of Virally Infected Cells by Complement

Numerous examples of lysis of virally infected cells by complement have been reviewed (1,13). Of these, the studies employing homologous systems (keeping within the same species for the virally infected cells, serum and complement) have the most relevance in vivo. Many studies have been done with virally infected human cells and human serum. Cells infected in vitro with HSV types 1 and 2, influenza A, parainfluenza 1–4, mumps, and measles viruses can all be lysed by complement (see Appendix for definition of abbreviations). Lysis of virally infected cells in vitro requires that the infected cell express viral antigen at the cell surface and requires IgG specific for the virus and an intact alternative pathway of complement activation. Surprisingly, despite the requirements for antibody, the classical pathway is not required for lysis of virally infected cells in vitro (7,13).

### Chemotaxis and Phagocytosis

Activation of either the classical or alternative pathway of complement activation leads to the release of inflammatory mediators (Fig. 1). C5a is a potent chemotactic agent, drawing neutrophils into the site of infection. Neutrophils have been demonstrated to lyse vaccinia virus and HSV-infected cells in vitro (10,11). Complement fragments can enhance the localization of leukocytes to the site of infection. C3a, C4a, and C5a, also known as the anaphylotoxins, bind to smooth muscle, inducing contraction and increasing vascular permeability. The infiltration of cells into a site of infection can help to wall off the infection and limit its spread to other areas. Complement deposition on the surface of a virus may help mediate its uptake by mononuclear cells and macrophages, which bear C3 receptors. Virus-antibody complexes that activate complement can be more effectively cleared from the circulation by erythrocytes, which bear the complement receptor CR1.

## Interferon

Interferon was first discovered over 30 years ago as a substance secreted by chick egg chorioallantoic membrane infected with heat-inactivated influenza virus (14). This secreted substance was able to protect chorioallantoic membrane fragments from infection with influenza virus. Since its discovery, much has been learned about the biochemical nature of IFN and its mechanism of action. IFN is a family of proteins produced during viral infection. IFN can be classified as either type 1 or type 2. Type 1 IFN, known as $\alpha$ and $\beta$, are produced by virally infected cells. Type 2 IFN, known as IFN-$\gamma$, is produced by activated T cells and natural killer cells. In humans there are 20 $\alpha$ genes and single $\beta$ and $\gamma$ genes. The type 1 and 2 IFN differ in their cell surface receptors and biologic roles.

IFN acts by binding species-specific cell surface receptors and inducing signals that lead to the production of specific proteins, known as interferon-regulated proteins. Interferon-regulated proteins have diverse biologic effects, including induction of an antiviral state, inhibition of cell growth, immunomodulation, and regulation of oncogene expression (15–17). Several interferon-regulated proteins have been characterized and are described here.

### Mx Proteins

Expression of Mx proteins is induced in response to INF-$\alpha$ or $\beta$ during orthomyxovirus infection (18). Humans, rats, mice, pigs, and horses all produce Mx proteins during influenza virus infection in response to type 1 IFN. The murine Mx protein, Mx-1, has been characterized most extensively. It is a 72 kD protein encoded by a gene located on chromosome 16. Mx-1 expression can by itself confer resistance to influenza viruses but does not affect the replication of other viruses (15). The mechanism of action of Mx proteins is not known. Recently, Mx-1 was characterized as a minor histocompatibility antigen (19). It has been suggested that the Mx proteins act by interfering with normal cell-sorting mechanisms and disrupting the production and assembly of virions (15).

### 2′,5′-Oligoadenylate Synthetase

In the presence of RNA viruses, IFN can induce an enzyme pathway known as the 2′,5′-oligodenylate synthetase pathway. This pathway is composed of three enzymes that lead to the degradation of viral RNA. The first enzyme, 2′,5′-oligoadenylade synthetase, catalyzes the synthesis of a polyadenosine of the structure ppp(A2′p5′)$_n$A with $n > 2$, abbreviated 2,5A. This enzyme becomes activated in the presence of double-stranded RNA. The 2′,5′-oligonucleotides activates an endoribonuclease that cleaves single-stranged RNA at the sequence UpXp (15). The final enzyme in the pathway is 2′,5′-phosphodiesterase, which degrades the 2,5A into AMP and ATP. This enzyme system selectively protects cells from infection by picornaviruses but not by other families of animal viruses (20).

### P1/elf-2 Protein Kinase

The $\alpha$ and $\beta$ IFN in the presence of double-stranded or single-stranded viral RNA, can also trigger a viral protection system that works by inhibiting protein synthesis. IFN can induce the expression of an RNA-dependent protein kinase known as P1/elf-2 protein kinase (21). This kinase phosphorylates the $\alpha$ subunit of elf-2, an initiation factor involved in protein synthesis. When elf-2 is phosphorylated, the initiation step of protein synthesis is inhibited. This kinase is believed to be the mechanism of an IFN-induced antiviral state, but a number of viruses have also evolved strategies to block the action of this kinase (15). Adenovirus and human immunodeficiency virus both produce RNA molecules capable of blocking the activity of this kinase (15).

### Major Histocompatibility Complex Antigens

MHC antigens are polymorphic cell surface glycoproteins that are vital in the recognition of self and nonself by the immune system. These molecules present antigen to T cells, and they provide one means by which a virally infected cell can be recognized and eliminated. Recognition and destruction of a virally infected cell requires a certain density of cell surface MHC molecules. Some cell types, such as those found in the central nervous system, express very low levels of these molecules. The $\alpha$, $\beta$, and $\gamma$ IFN induce an upregulation of cell surface expression of class I MHC molecules (22). IFN-$\gamma$ can also upregulate class II MHC molecules. Induction of class I and class II MHC molecules by IFN may enhance the cellular immune response to viruses by increasing the probability of recognition of viral antigen by T cells.

### Immunomodulatory Actions of IFN

IFN-$\gamma$ has diverse effects on the immune response. IFN-$\gamma$ is produced by activated T cells in response to antigenic stimulation. In turn, the cytotoxic activities of T cells and NK cells are both enhanced by IFN-$\gamma$ (23). IFN-$\gamma$ can promote maturation of B cells (17). Macrophages are activated by IFN-$\gamma$, resulting in enhanced phagocytosis, microbicidal activity, cytotoxicity, and release of IL-1 (24,25). IL-1 has many effects on nonspecific and specific immune responses, including activation of growth and differentiation of T and B cells, induction of inflammatory mediators, such as prostaglandins, activation of neutrophils, and induction of a fever response. Thus, release of IFN-$\gamma$ can trigger a cascade of responses that aid in the clearance of viruses.

## Phagocytic Cells

Macrophages and neutrophils mediate nonspecific defense mechanisms that aid in the destruction of virus and clearance of viral infections. These phagocytic cells contribute to the nonspecific defense against viral infections by four distinct mechanisms (Table 2).

1. They can engulf or endocytose antibody and/or complement-coated viral particles and destroy them internally.
2. Phagocytic cells, particularly macrophages, produce a variety of inflammatory mediators with antiviral effects.
3. Macrophages and neutrophils can mediate antibody-dependent cellular cytotoxicity.

**Table 2** Role of Phagocytic Cells in Immunity to Viral Infection

| Mechanism | Cells | Example | References |
|---|---|---|---|
| Phagocytosis | Monocytes<br>Macrophages<br>Neutrophils | Vaccinia virus, HSV | 11, 12 |
| Mediators | Monocytes<br>Macrophages<br>Neutrophils | HSV-2 | 26–28 |
| Antibody-dependent cellular cytotoxicity | Macrophages<br>Neutrophils | HSV-2, HIV, Sindbis, Semliki Forest virus | 28–31 |
| Antigen presentation | Monocytes<br>Macrophages | Influenza virus, LCMV | 32–34 |

4. Finally, macrophages can enhance the cellular immune response to viruses by presenting viral peptides to T cells in the context of class I and class II MHC molecules.

### Phagocytosis

Both macrophages and neutrophils have Fc receptors for IgG (FcRI, FcRII, and FcRIII on human cells), which mediate the uptake of antibody-coated virus particles. Vaccinia virus is phagocytosed by macrophages and neutrophils in the presence of serum. Although phagocytes are not traditionally associated with viral infections, West et al. demonstrated that in the presence of serum vaccinia virus can be phagocytosed by human neutrophils, and virus particles were seen by electron microscopy to be localized in phagolysosomes (11). The loss of clarity of virion structure and the absence of detectable viral assembly complexes within the cytoplasm suggested that virus was being degraded. Viral titers measured by a pox-forming assay declined during the first 5 h of infection, but they rose again by 6 h. It is not known whether this rise in viral titer was a result of viral replication within neutrophils or within another cell type contaminating the neutrophil preparation in this study.

In addition to uptake by Fc receptors, neutrophils, and macrophages express complement receptors CR1 and CR3. These receptors can mediate endocytosis of C3-coated virus in neutrophils. Resting macrophages can bind C3-coated particles but must be activated for phagocytosis to occur through these receptors (24). A number of viruses can activate complement directly, leading to C3 deposition of their cell surface. These viruses may be susceptible to complement receptor-mediated phagocytosis.

### Mediators

Macrophages produce a variety of mediators that may enhance both specific and nonspecific defenses against virus, including IFN-$\alpha$ and IFN-$\beta$, IL-1, neutral proteases, arachidonic acid metabolites, and reactive oxygen species produced during an oxidative burst (24). IFN are important in establishing an antiviral state, as described earlier. IL-1 is an important stimulator of B and T cells and can induce prostaglandin release, acute-phase response proteins, and fever (35). During microbial infection, macrophages may undergo an oxidative burst, leading to the production of a variety of toxic oxygen species. These include such molecules as hydrogen peroxide, superoxide anion, and singlet oxygen (24). These molecules can destroy intracellular parasites present in phagolysosomes or, if released into the extracellular milieu, can contribute to the pathology associated with viral infections (27). During HSV-2 infection, $\alpha$ and $\beta$ IFN have been shown to stimulate an oxidative burst in macrophages both in vivo and in vitro (26). Macrophages from HSV-2-resistant mice (C57B6) are more readily primed for an oxidative burst in response to IFN than macrophages from HSV-2-sensitive (Balb/c) mice. This observation suggests a possible role for oxidative burst metabolites in defense against viral infections.

### Antibody-Dependent Cellular Cytotoxicity

Macrophages and neutrophils can destroy virally infected cells through ADCC. Macrophages, neutrophils, and NK cells are all capable of ADCC. The specific mechanism of ADCC-mediated killing by NK cells may be different from that of macrophages and neutrophils. In general, killing by ADCC requires two steps. The first is cross-linking of the effector cell with the virally infected target. Antibodies specific for cell surface viral antigens can cross-link targets to effector cells via Fc receptors for IgG found on the surface of macrophages and neutrophils. The second step involves triggering of the lytic mechanism. Engagement of Fc receptors stimulates degranulation and an oxidative burst, leading to the release of large amounts of reactive oxygen molecules like hydrogen peroxide and oxygen radicals. These molecules can lyse cells by reacting with unsaturated lipid molecules on the target cell membrane and disrupting the lipid bilayer. Granule enzymes, such as neutral proteases and lysozyme, can damage target cells. Neutrophils release cationic peptides called defensins, which have been demonstrated to lyse herpesvirus as well as human and murine target cells (28). These molecules are released in a directed fashion into the space between the effector and target cell, minimizing innocent bystander killing (28). ADCC has been demonstrated to play a role in several viral infections. Acquired immunodeficiency syndrome and AIDS-related complex patients produce antibodies that can induce killing of HIV-infected targets in ADCC assays in vitro (29,30). Asymptomatic but HIV-seropositive patients had higher titers of ADCC antibodies than patients who had become symptomatic with AIDS or ARC, suggesting that ADCC killing of HIV-infected cells in vivo is the mechanism of the prolonged asymptomatic period associated with this disease. ADCC may also play a role in immunity to alphavirus infection. Serum from Sindbis virus-hyperimmunized mice can protect mice from challenge with Semliki Forest virus infection (31). This protection was dependent on macrophages, and the serum had ADCC activity in vitro. Thus, in the presence of specific antiviral IgG antibodies, ADCC can be a mechanism of clearance for virally infected cells.

**Antigen Presentation**

Both cytotoxic and helper T cells play an important role in the defense against viral pathogens. They provide help for humoral immune responses, directly lyse infected cells, and produce IFN-$\gamma$. To become activated and respond to virus, T cells must be provided with the appropriate signals. The most important of these signals is the presentation of foreign antigen to the T cell receptor. The T cell receptor recognizes antigen only as peptide associated with MHC molecules. T helper cells recognize antigen as peptides bound to class II MHC molecules, and cytotoxic T cells recognize antigen as peptides bound to class I MHC molecules. Macrophages express both class I and class II MHC molecules. Traditionally, antigen presentation through class I and class II MHC molecules has been believed to occur through different mechanisms. Antigen entering an antigen-presenting cell through phagocytosis or endocytosis enters the class II pathway of antigen presentation, but presentation through class I molecules requires either endogenous expression of that antigen or production of antigen in the cytoplasm. Because of the phagocytic nature and expression of class II MHC molecules, macrophages are excellent antigen-presenting cells for helper T cells but have been believed to be less effective in priming cytotoxic T cells unless directly infected with virus. It was demonstrated recently, however, that in vivo depletion of macrophages completely abrogated the cytotoxic T cell response to influenza virus, and adoptive transfer of macrophages could restore the CTL response to influenza virus (32). To determine if macrophages are capable of processing and presenting extracellular antigen through the class I pathway of antigen presentation in vivo, Debrick et al. inoculated mice with cellular debris from an ovalbumin-expressing tumor cell line and assayed for the induction of OVA-specific CTL (32). These mice mounted a CTL response to OVA that could be abrogated by depleted of macrophages in vivo with carrageenan. CTL responses to OVA could be restored by infusion of syngeneic macrophages. The CTL response was shown to be MHC restricted and required cognate interaction between the macrophages and the OVA-specific CTL. These observations suggest that macrophages play an important role in the induction of CTL to extracellular antigens and may be important for the induction of antiviral CTL to antigens that have been released from virally infected cells.

## NK Cells

NK cells are bone marrow-derived cells that have the morphology of large granular lymphocytes. These cells are capable of mediating nonspecific killing of both tumor cells and virally infected cells. NK cells are distinct from CTL in that they lack T cell receptors, do not express T cell, markers such as CD3 and CD8, and do not require MHC restriction to kill target cells. NK cells vary in morphology and phenotype, but some characteristic markers have been identified. NK cells express the markers NK1.1 and NK2.1, asialo-gM1, and Fc receptors for IgG (36). NK cells are induced early during viral infection and can peak in numbers and activity at around 3 days postinfection, and then they decline by day 7 when CTL activity is rising (37). Some similarities between NK cells and CTL include their activation by IL-2 and IFN-$\gamma$ and their granule exocytosis and release of perforins when triggered to kill. NK cells can kill either by direct recognition of targets or by ADCC.

### Target Cell Recognition by NK Cells

Neither the NK receptor nor its ligand on the target cell surface has been identified. NK cells have diverse capacities, including recognition of virally infected cells, tumor cells, certain bacteria, and antibody-coated target cells (38). It may be that NK cells have multiple recognition systems for identifying these diverse target cell phenotypes.

One hypothesis has been that NK cells recognize targets based on their expression of class I MHC molecules (39). There is an inverse correlation between NK susceptibility and class I MHC expression. In vivo it has been observed that lymphomas expressing low levels of class I were more readily rejected than their wild-type counterparts, and this rejection was abrogated by depletion of NK cells with the antibody NK1.1 (5). In vitro class I MHC low or deficient cell lines RBC-5 and YAC-1 are sensitive to NK-mediated killing. Reconstitution of class I MHC expression in both human and mouse NK susceptible cell lines reduces their sensitivity to killing (40–42). Class I expression does not always correlate with NK cell susceptibility, however. Some cell lines with high class I expression are susceptible to NK killing, and some class I low lines are NK cell resistant (39). Clearly multiple factors can determine whether a cell is susceptible or resistant to NK cell-mediated lysis.

The recognition structure involved in ADCC is the Fc portion of IgG molecules. NK cells express a single form of Fc receptor $\gamma$. In humans this molecule is FcRIII (CD16), a low-affinity receptor for monomeric IgG. A homologous protein is expressed by murine NK cells designated FcRII. Antibodies to these Fc receptors block NK cell-mediated ADCC (38,43). Binding to FcRIII stimulates phosphoinositide metabolism, leading to release of inositol phosphate molecules, such as $IP^3$ and $IP^4$. These molecules induce the release of $Ca^{2+}$ from intracellular stores (38,44). These signals lead to activation of NK cells and target cell lysis.

The leukocyte adhesion molecule CD11/CD18 family also plays a role in NK cell killing. An inherited deficiency of these molecules, LAD, in the human leads to defective CTL and NK cell-mediated killing (38). Antibodies to CD11a (LFA-1) are also capable of blocking NK cell killing. These molecules play an important role in stabilizing effector-target conjugates necessary for activation and delivery of the lethal hit.

**Mechanism of NK Cell Killing**

NK cell killing occurs in three independent stages: (1) NK cell recognition of and binding to its target; (2) programming for lysis; and (3) delivery of a lethal hit. The binding of NK cells to their appropriate target involves cell membrane proteins and is blocked by proteases (38,45). It also requires $Mg^{2+}$ but is temperature independent, occurring equally well at 4 as at 37 °C. Programming for lysis requires $Ca^{2+}$-dependent cellular changes, including polarization of granules toward the target membrane, and degranulation. This step is temperature dependent (it does not occur at 4 °C) and is enhanced by IFN-$\gamma$ treatment. Delivery of the lethal hit is independent of the cytotoxic effector cell and is sensitive to proteases. Lysis of the target cell is believed to be mediated through the degranulation and release of cytotoxic factors by the NK cell (45). Some of the molecules that are found in NK granules and may play a role in NK killing are NK cytotoxic factor, perforin, and serine esterases. Lymphokines also play a role in NK activity and killing. Some of the molecules involved in NK cell-mediated killing have been identified and are described here.

A soluble factor released from NK cells during lectin stimulation was first identified by Wright and Bonavida (46). This factor was demonstrated to lyse NK-sensitive but not insensitive targets, was greater than 12,000 kD, and was heat labile. The factor has been designated NK cytotoxic factor. NKCF differs from other NK cell killing mechanisms in that it has slow kinetics of killing. Killing required an incubation period of up to 40 h to achieve target cell lysis. NKCF has been identified in supernatants from a rat NK/LGL tumor cell line. Monoclonal antibodies can neutralize this NKCF and human NKCF, but they do not neutralize tumor necrosis factor, demonstrating that these have separate activities.

Following NK cell interaction, target cells have tubular lesions on the membrane similar to those resulting from complement activation but larger, 15 nm in diameter compared with only 10 nm for complement C9 lesions (38, 45). Perforin is stored in NK granules and can be rapidly released during NK cell activation. Perforin forms a porelike structure on the surface of the target cell and is believed to mediate killing by colloid osmotic lysis (45).

Protease inhibitors have been found to be capable of blocking NK cell killing when added after conjugate formation has occurred (38). Serine esterases have been identified in CTL, and transcripts for these proteases have been demonstrated in NK cells (38). Trypsin and chymostrypsinlike protease activity has been demonstrated in NK granules. Proteases may be directly cytotoxic for target cells, or they may activate another cytotoxic factor stored in granules and released during activation.

NK cells have been reported to produce a variety of different lymphokines. Activation through IL-2 or CD16 induces human NK cells to produce IFN-$\gamma$, TNF, lymphotoxin, granulocyte-macrophage colony-stimulating factor, and colony-stimulating factor 1 (38). Exposure to endotoxin induces NK cells to produce IL-1$\alpha$ and $\beta$, TNF, and IL-6 (38). IFN-$\gamma$ activates NK cells and can alter the susceptibility of targets to NK-mediated killing (23). Killing of virally infected targets is enhanced by IFN-$\gamma$, but uninfected cells are protected by IFN-$\gamma$ (39). TNF and LT also play a role in NK cell-mediated cytotoxicity. Paya et al. observed that human NK cells secrete LT and TNF and that killing of vesicular stomatitis virus-infected cells by NK cells could be inhibited by antibodies specific for TNF and LT (47). Furthermore, purified recombinant TNF was able to mimic the NK cytotoxicity of VSV, cytomegalovirus, Theiler's murine encephalomyelitis virus, and HSV-infected cells (38). Thus, production of lymphokines by NK cells during an immune response can directly and indirectly enhance killing of virally infected cells.

### Role of NK Cells During Viral Infection

An important role for NK cells during viral infection is suggested by several observations. Individuals with defects in NK cell development or activity have markedly increased viral infections (48). During experimental viral infection in mice with LCMV, bone marrow NK cell blastogenesis is induced and NK cells reach high numbers in the blood and infected tissues (37). NK cells also play an important role in resistance to tumor cells induced by oncogenic viruses (36,38). Enhanced NK activity has been demonstrated during a number of human and murine viral infections. In humans, NK cells have been demonstrated to lyse autologous HSV-infected lymphoblastoid cell lines in vitro (49). NK cells may play a role in the development of early gray matter disease in mice infected with TMEV. NK-deficient strains or strains depleted of NK cells show enhanced gray matter inflammation and higher viral titers in the CNS during the early phase of disease (50). During coxsackievirus B3 infection in mice, viral titers in cardiac tissue and myocyte degeneration are increased by depletion of NK cells (51). Increased viral titers have been observed in mice depleted of NK cells during HSV, vaccinia virus, hepatitis virus, and cytomegalovirus infections as well (38,49,52). These observations suggest that NK cells are an important first line of defense in controlling the level of viral infection and dissemination.

## ANTIGEN-SPECIFIC IMMUNE RESPONSES TO VIRAL INFECTION

B and T lymphocytes can generate highly specific immune responses during viral infection. These responses play an important role in viral clearance. B and T cell responses are also capable of providing long-lasting immunity to reinfection by the generation of memory cells that respond rapidly to a second exposure to viral antigens. Specific immunity can be divided into two categories. B cells are responsible for an antigen-specific humoral immune response. T cells mediate antigen-specific cellular immune responses, such as providing help for B lymphocyte activation, mediating delayed-type hypersensitivity responses, and mediating the cytotoxicity of virally infected cells.

### Humoral Immune Response

The activation of B cells and production of antibody have important roles in the protective immune response to viral infection. Infection by many types of viruses induces the production of virus-specific protective antibodies. Antibody has three important roles during viral infection: virus neutralization, ADCC, and complement-mediated lysis of virus and virally infected cells.

#### B Cell Development and Antibody Production

B cells are derived from hematopoietic stem cells found in bone marrow (Fig. 2) (53). During development, stem cells undergo rearrangement of their immunoglobulin genes and become committed to the B cell lineage. Every precursor, or pre-B cell, undergoes a unique rearrangement of heavy- and light-chain variable-region genes. This genomic rearrangement establishes the immunoglobulin specificity for a B cell and all its progeny. The immunoglobulin molecule is composed of two heavy and two light chains held together by disulfide bonds. Heavy-chain genes are derived by rearrangement and combination of polymorphic variable V, diversity D, and joining J gene segments with conserved constant-region C gene segments. Immunoglobulin light-chain genes are derived by combination of polymorphic V and J gene segments with conserved C gene segments.

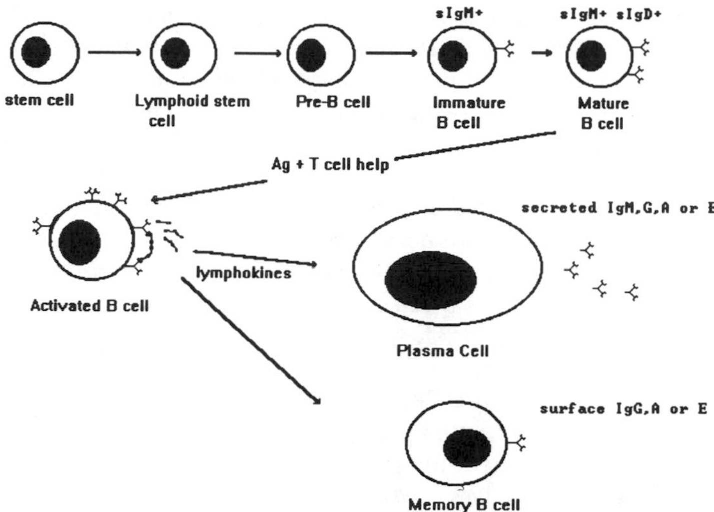


**Figure 2** B cell development. B cells are derived from hematopoietic stem cells found in the bone marrow and fetal liver. During development, stem cells become committed to a B cell lineage. In pre-B cells, immunoglobulin gene rearrangement begins first in the light-chain genes and then in the heavy-chain genes. Immature B cells express IgM on their surface. Mature B cells express both IgM and IgD. Following antigen or mitogen stimulation, B cells become activated. B cells enter a proliferating phase and continue to divide. T cell signals can induce proliferating B cells to stop dividing. Heavy-chain class switching occurs, allowing the expression of IgG, IgA, or IgE and the development to antibody-secreting plasma cells or memory B cells.

There are five mechanisms that contribute to the generation of diversity among immunoglobulin genes. First, many V, D, and J genes are encoded in the heavy- and light-chain immunoglobulin loci. Second, these gene segments can be combined differently, creating many possible immunoglobulin genes. Third, the rearrangement of V, D, and J gene segments can be imprecise, creating diversity at the VD and DJ or VJ junctions. Fourth, after immunoglobulin gene rearrangement has been completed somatic mutations can occur, adding diversity. Finally, the varied combinations of heavy-chain genes with light-chain genes generates additional antigen specificities. The murine immunoglobulin repertoire has been estimated to have the potential of $10^{11}$ different immunoglobulin specificities (54)!

Immature B cells express IgM molecules on the cell surface (Fig. 2). Antigen activates specific B cells to produce complementary antibody by binding to cell surface immunoglobulin. As they mature, B cells also express surface IgD. There are three stages involved in the maturation of B cells to the antibody secreting stage: activation, proliferation, and differentiation

(53). Activation of B cells is accomplished by the binding of an antigen, such as a virus or viral protein, to cell surface immunoglobulin molecules. Cross-linking of surface immunoglobulin by antigen stimulates a multitude of intracellular events, including elevation of intracellular $Ca^{2+}$ levels, phosphoinositide metabolism, release of diacylglycerol, activation of protein kinase C, and transcription of the cellular oncogenes c-*fos* and c-*myc*. These intracellular signals induce a change in the activation state of the B cell. During the activation stage, B cells move from a resting $G_0$ state to the $G_1$ phase of the cell cycle. They also become more responsive to T cell factors. The T cell-derived lymphokine IL-4 enhances B cell activation and promotes entry of B cells into *S* phase of the cell cycle. The proliferation stage of B cell maturation expands clones of antigen-reactive B cells.

Proliferation by B cells requires interaction with T helper cells. For T cells to provide B cells with the factors needed to induce proliferation, they must also become activated. Activation of $CD4^+$ T cells requires presentation of antigen in the context of class II MHC molecules. Monocytes, macrophages, and B cells are all effective antigen-presenting cells. Antigen presentation leads to T cell activation and the production of specific lymphokines that induce B cell maturation. T cell-derived IL-4, IL-5, and IFN-$\gamma$ all induce B cell proliferation. Differentiation of B cells to the antibody-secreting plasma cells also requires T cell-derived factors. Following extensive proliferation, B cells stop dividing and differentiate into antibody-secreting cells. Isotype switching from IgM production to IgG, IgA, or IgE production also occurs during this stage (Fig. 2). T cell-derived lymphokines signal B cell maturation and isotope switching. IL-5 and IL-6 are both able to induce B cell differentiation to immunoglobulin secretion. The presence of a particular lymphokine can influence class switching to a particular immunoglobulin isotype as well. IL-4 induces switching to $IgG_1$ or IgE synthesis; IL-5 induces IgA synthesis, and IFN-$\gamma$ induces $IgG_{2b}$ or $IgG_3$ synthesis.

The primary antibody response peaks about 7 days following exposure to antigen. This response consists of immunoglobulins or primarily the IgM isotype, with lower levels of IgG and other isotypes. Memory B cells are generated during this stage. A large number of clones with varying antigen specificities are activated, resulting in an overall antibody response that may have low affinity for a particular antigen. Upon second exposure to the antigen, however, memory B cells are more rapidly activated. IgG titers are higher and have greater affinity for antigen. This process is known as affinity maturation. Affinity maturation can result in a more rapid and specific protective antibody response during second exposure to a pathogen, such as a virus.

### Neutralization

For a virus to establish an infection in a susceptible host it must be able to bind to specific target cells, penetrate the cell membrane, and uncoat within the cell. Antibodies that interfere with any of these stages neutralize infection. Most commonly, antibodies block attachment of virus to specific cellular receptors by binding to antigenic determinants on the viral capsid. Many viral infections are known to induce neutralizing antibodies. Neutralizing antibodies produced during rabies virus, influenza virus, and rhinovirus infections play an important role in the host's recovery from disease, as well as protection of the host from reinfection. Perhaps the most prominent example of a virus that induces protective neutralizing antibody is poliovirus. Poliovirus is an enterovirus known for its capacity to cause gastrointestinal and neurologic disease in the human. Infection with poliovirus induces high titers of neutralizing antibodies that may persist for life. The importance of an antibody response during enterovirus infection is illustrated in patients with defects in B cell immunity. Hypogammaglobulinemic or agammaglobulinemic patients may have severe or fatal infections with enteroviruses (55).

Neutralizing antibodies to poliovirus are directed at VP1, VP2, and VP3, the structural proteins composing the viral capsid. The antigenic structures vary slightly among the three major strains of poliovirus. Three major neutralization sites have been identified (56). Site 1 is located at amino acids 80–100 of VP1 in strains 2 and 3. Site 2 is located in VP1 from amino acids 220–222 and VP2 from amino acids 169 to 170 only in strain 1. Strain 3 has only the VP2 portion of site 2 as an immunodominant epitope. Site 3 is located in VP1 from amino acids 286 to 290 and in VP3 from amino acids 58 to 59. Infectious virus is more effective at inducing neutralizing antibodies. Successful vaccination against poliovirus requires that the vaccine induce high titers of neutralizing antibody to all three strains of poliovirus. Two vaccination strategies are the inactivated virus (Salk) vaccine and the live attenuated virus (Sabin) vaccine. Both vaccines induce neutralizing antibodies to the three serotypes of poliovirus. The Salk vaccine consists of formalin-inactivated poliovirus of all three serotypes, and this vaccine has the advantage of safety: inactivated virus is not infective, and therefore it does not present a risk to unvaccinated individuals in the population. The Salk vaccine has had widespread use in Europe. The disadvantage of the Salk vaccine is that booster immunizations are required to maintain immunity, and the inactivated vaccine does not induce intestinal and secretory immunity, which could provide a first line of defense against wild-type strains of poliovirus. The Sabin vaccine utilizes live attenuated viruses of all three serotypes and is administered orally. It induces both intestinal and secretory neutralizing antibody as well as serum neutralizing antibody, and protection typically persists for a lifetime. The risk of the Sabin vaccine is that live virus can revert to a more virulent form and may cause disease. Some cases of polio have been associated with the live virus vaccine, but the incidence of vaccine-related polio among nonimmunodeficient individuals is very low (<1:1 million) (55). The Sabin vaccine is the polio vaccine given in the United States.

### ADCC

During viral infection, viral glycoproteins can be transported to the cell membrane of infected cells. These viral antigens can induce the production of a humoral immune response to virus, or they can combine with already formed antiviral antibodies. When antiviral antibodies of the IgG subclass bind to infected cells, the infected cells can be destroyed by ADCC. Since viral antigens are expressed on the cell membrane before release of viral progeny, this mechanism of protection represents an important host defense by limiting the spread of virus throughout the host. Monocytes, macrophages, neutrophils, and NK cells all express Fc receptors for IgG and can mediate killing of antibody-coated target cells by ADCC. ADCC is believed to be an important mechanism of protection during HSV infection. HSV infection is particularly damaging and can be fatal to immunocompromised individuals or neonates who have an immature immune system. NK cells and mononuclear cells, which are important for ADCC, are both present in lower levels in the neonate compared with the adult. Adults infected with HSV produce high titers of neutralizing and ADCC-mediating antibodies, which are associated with protection from disease (57,58). These antibodies can be transferred across the placenta to the fetus. HSV-infected infants having high titers of passively transferred antibodies capable of mediating ADCC are more frequently asymptomatic, and they have a lower incidence of disseminated disease (57–59). Certain antibody isotypes are more effective in mediating ADCC than others. This is due to the binding properties of the Fc receptors found on the surface of the cells mediating ADCC. NK cells have only one type of Fc receptor. In humans this is the CD16 molecule. This Fc receptor binds $IgG_1$ most effectively. Analysis of sera from HSV-1-infected human donors revealed that ADCC activity was concentrated in the $IgG_1$ and $IgG_3$ fractions (60). In mice the predominant NK cell Fc receptor is specific for $IgG_{2b}$. Mice infected with HSV produce high titers of $IgG_1$, $IgG_{2a}$, and $IgG_{2b}$. $IgG_{2a}$ and $IgG_{2b}$ have been found to be important mediators of ADCC in mice (61). ADCC may therefore be an important mechanism of protection of adults and neonates from symptomatic HSV infection.

### Complement-Mediated Destruction of Virally Infected Cells

Virally infected cells expressing cell surface viral antigens are also subject to destruction through complement activation. Antigen-antibody complexes activate the classical pathway of complement and can lead to the deposition of cytolytic pores on the surface of the virally infected cells. Certain immunoglobulin isotypes are more efficient at activating the complement cascade than others: $IgG_{1,2,3}$ and IgM immune complexes are more efficient than $IgG_4$, IgA, or IgE. Although the alternative pathway does not generally require antigen-antibody complexes to be activated, the lysis of cells infected with a variety of RNA and DNA viruses by antibody requires an intact alternative pathway of complement. Lysis of measles virus-infected cells by homologous serum requires the presence of an intact alternative pathway (6,7). Removal of the alternative pathway components, factor B, factor D, or properdin, reduces the lysis of measles virus-infected cells by homologous serum by as much as 80%. Reconstitution of these factors restores lysis activity. Removal of classical pathway components C2 or C4, however, does not block lysis of measles virus-infected cells by antibody plus complement. Cells infected with mumps virus, influenza A virus, and HSV-1 and HSV-2 are also lysed by antibody plus complement and require an intact alternative pathway for destruction (1,7). Antibody seems to be required for lysis of virally infected cells by complement since virally infected cells alone are not very efficient at activating either complement cascade (7). C4 is deposited on the surface of measles virus-infected cells in the presence of serum with or without an intact alternative pathway, indicating that the classical pathway is activated by virally infected cells (7). It may be that the classical pathway is important for initiation of the cascade on virally infected cell membranes, but the alternative pathway allows amplification of the pathway to the levels needed to achieve lysis.

Antibody can also play a role in direct lysis of enveloped viruses. Avian IBV, Sindbis virus, LCMV, and equine arteritis virus can be lysed by specific antibody plus complement (7). Antibody can also enhance virus neutralization by coating viruses and allowing cell recognition by Fc receptors on the surface of phagocytic cells and subsequent destruction.

### Natural Antibodies

Before infection with virus, a host can have low titers of circulating antibody that cross-react with multiple antigens, including viral antigens. These polyreactive antibodies have been termed natural antibodies since they do not arise as a result of antigen stimulation. During the early stage of infection and before the development of specific immune responses, these antibodies may help to neutralize virus and limit its spread. They may also be very important in the initiation of specific immune responses by enhancing uptake of virus by antigen-presenting cells through Fc receptors. Natural antibodies have been described in mice and humans with autoimmune diseases, but they are also present in healthy mice and humans (62–64). A subset of B cells known as CD5$^+$ in humans and Ly1$^+$ in mice is responsible for producing these polyreactive antibodies. These cells represent an immature subset of B cells and constitute about 25% of circulating and splenic B cells in the adult (62). The antibodies they produce are primarily of the IgM subclass, but IgG and IgA polyreactive antibodies have also been identified. Polyreactive antibodies have a distribution of usage of V-region segments biased toward certain V heavy-chain ($V_h$) regions. In humans, $V_h$III and $V_h$IV gene segments are expressed twice as frequently in polyreactive antibodies as expected from their numeric representation among $V_h$ genes (61). It has been hypothesized that natural antibodies are polyreactive because they do not undergo somatic hypermutation, which leads to affinity maturation. It has also been observed that the antibody combining site is larger than normal and may therefore be able to accommodate more than one type of ligand. Natural antibodies have been found to react with normal cellular antigens, nuclear antigens, bacterial polysaccharides, and viruses, including rabies virus, HSV, and HIV (62,64).

## T Cell Response

T cells play a central role in the immune response to viral infection. They provide help for humoral immune responses, produce IFN-$\gamma$, and mediate lysis of virally infected cells. T cells are derived from hematopoietic stem cells found in the bone marrow. During development stem cells committed to the T cell lineage leave the bone marrow and mature in the thymus (Fig. 3). T cells recognize antigen by expression of polymorphic T cell receptors. T cell receptors are composed of polymorphic $\alpha$ and $\beta$ chains. T cell receptor genes are similar to immunoglobulin genes in that they undergo rearrangement of the variable gene V, diversity D, and joining J gene segments to generate unique antigen specificities. There are four mechanisms that contribute to the vast diversity in T cell receptors. First, there are multiple germ line V, D, and J gene segments that can be combined during T cell receptor gene rearrangement. Second, these multiple gene segments can be arranged in different combinations of V and J for the $\alpha$ chain and V, D, and J for the $\beta$ chain. Third, joining of V, D, and J gene segments is imprecise, creating nucleotide diversity at the junctions of segments, and random insertion of nucleotides can also occur at these junctions during rearrangement in a process known as N-region diversification. Finally, the random combination of different $\alpha$ and $\beta$ chains adds additional diversity to the T cell repertoire. It has been estimated that the murine T cell repertoire can generate $10^{16}$ different $\alpha\beta$ T cell receptors (54).

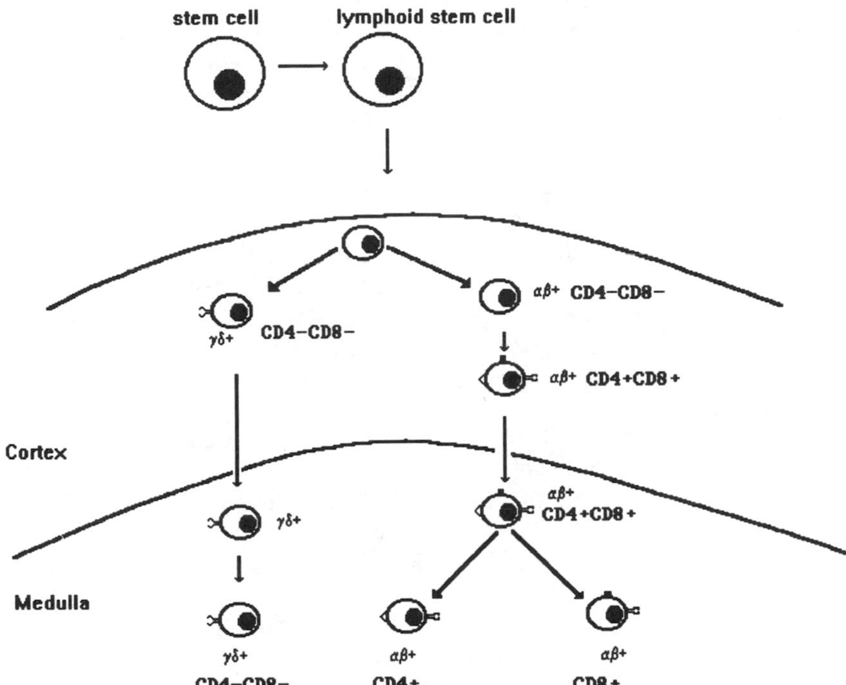


**Figure 3** T cell development. T cells are derived from hematopoietic stem cells found in the bone marrow or fetal liver. During development stem cells become committed to the lymphoid lineage and migrate to the thymus. The thymus has two structural compartments, known as the cortex and the medulla. Most immature T cells are found in the cortex, and the more mature T cells are found in the medulla. It is believed that during maturation stem cells first enter the cortex of the thymus. Here they rearrange T receptor genes and become committed to expression of either $\alpha\beta$ or $\gamma\delta$ T cell receptors. The $\alpha\beta$ T cells also begin to express both $CD4^+$ and $CD8^+$ markers, T cells migrate to the medulla and lose expression of either $CD4^+$ or $CD8^+$ T cells to become either $CD4^+$ or $CD8^+$ T cells. From the medulla, mature T cells enter the periphery. During development in the thymus, both positive and negative selection is believed to occur such that clones of T cells emigrating from the thymus have affinity for self class I or class II MHC molecules but are not autoreactive.

During maturation in the thymus, T cell clones are selected that have affinity for class I or class II MHC antigens. Mature T cells can only recognize processed antigen presented as peptides bound to class I or class II MHC molecules.

The majority of mature T cells can be divided into two broad categories, based on cell surface phenotype subsets called $CD4^+$ and $CD8^+$. These subsets correlate with functional characteristics as well as the mode of antigen recognition. $CD4^+$ T cells recognize antigen presented on class II MHC molecules. They are often mediators of help for humoral immune responses and CTL responses and are associated with delayed-type hypersensitivity. $CD8^+$ T cells recognize antigen presented on class I MHC molecules and are generally the mediators of CTL responses or suppression.

### Antigen Presentation

During maturation of T cells in the thymus, T cell clones are selected that have affinity for MHC antigens. $CD4^+$ T cell clones are selected for affinity to class II MHC molecules, and $CD8^+$ T cell clones are selected for affinity to class I MHC molecules. Therefore, mature $CD4^+$ T cells leaving the thymus recognize antigen as peptides presented by self class II MHC molecules, and $CD8^+$ T cells recognize antigen as peptides presented by self class I MHC molecules. Allo-MHC recognition by T cells is believed to occur when foreign MHC molecules resemble self MHC plus antigen.

Presentation through class I MHC and class II MHC molecules occurs through distinct intracellular pathways. Antigens taken into a cell through receptor-mediated endocytosis or phagocytosis enter the class II pathway. These antigens follow a pathway from endocytic vesicles to lysosomes, where they are degraded by proteases into peptide fragments. Newly formed class II molecules leave the Golgi apparatus in vesicles that fuse with lysosomes or lysosomelike vesicles (65). In this post-Golgi compartment, class II molecules bind the peptide fragments of processed antigens, and the complexes are then transported to the cell membrane (65). Antigens entering the endocytic or phagocytic pathways generally do not become presented by class I MHC molecules. Presentation through class I molecules usually requires that the antigen is synthesized within the antigen-presenting cell. Viral antigens are often very effectively presented by class I MHC molecules of the infected cell. Artificial introduction of antigen directly into the cytoplasm of a cell also allows it to be presented by class I MHC molecules (66).

Class I MHC molecules must associate with peptide to maintain stability and be transported to the cell surface. X-ray crystallography of class I molecules has revealed that peptides are present constitutively in the cleft of cell surface class I molecules (67). Studies with mutant cell lines that fail to express class I MHC molecules have been helpful in elucidating the mechanism of class I molecule assembly and antigen presentation. The murine mutant cell line RMA-S expresses only low levels of class I molecules on the cell surface compared with its parent line RMA and fails to present influenza virus peptides to CTL (33). Genetic analysis of this cell line has revealed that its defect maps to a gene encoded in the class II region of the MHC (68). This gene, designated HAM-1, is homologous to a family of ATP-dependent transmembrane transporter genes. These genes are responsible for multidrug resistance in prokaryotes, yeast, and mammalian cells, and their products can transport a wide range of substances across membranes, including peptides (69). HAM-1 is linked to a second gene, HAM-2, also homologous with peptide transporters. Peptide transporter genes have been identified in the human and rat class II MHC region as well (69–71). These transporter genes are believed to be expressed on the endoplasmic reticulum and function to transport cytoplasmic peptides into the lumen of the ER where they can associate with newly formed class I MHC molecules. Also found in this region are two genes encoding polymorphic proteins that are part of a cytoplasmic protein complex known as a proteosome. Proteosomes are cytoplasmic protein complexes that have protease activity (68,72). Proteosomes may be important in the degradation of cytoplasmic proteins and delivery of peptides to the peptide transporter molecules. The current model of antigen presentation through the class I pathway is that cytoplasmic proteins are degraded by proteases found in proteosomes and are then transported as peptides across the ER by an MHC-encoded peptide transporter molecule. Inside the lumen of the ER, peptides then bind to newly formed class I MHC molecules, stabilizing them and allowing their transport to the cell surface where they can activate class I restricted CTL.

### Helper T Cell Response to Virus

$CD4^+$ T cells have at least three possible roles during viral infection. First, they are essential in providing help to B cells in the generation of an antibody response, a function particularly important for viral infections in which humoral immune responses are the primary mechanism of immunity. Second, $CD4^+$ T cells can mediate DTH responses. Generation of lymphokines by DTH T cells can draw macrophages into the site of infection in large numbers. These macrophages become activated and can mediate phagocytosis, release of toxic oxygen molecules, production of inflammatory mediators and lymphokines, such as IL-1 and TNF, and direct cytotoxicity against infected cells, viruses, tumor cells, bacteria, or allografts (24). DTH responses can also lead to bystander damage of surrounding normal tissue. Third, $CD4^+$ T cells can provide help to $CD8^+$ T cells required for cytotoxic responses against virally infected cell. However, not all $CD8^+$ T cell responses to viral infection require the presence of $CD4^+$ T cell-mediated help: CTL responses to ectromelia virus and LCMV can occur in the absence of $CD4^+$ T cells (73–75).

$CD4^+$ T cells have been shown to protect against viral disease by cell depletion studies and adoptive transfer of cloned T cells. The murine picornavirus, TMEV, induces a biphasic disease in susceptible strains of mice (76). The early phase (acute phase) is characterized by infection of neurons in the brain and spinal cord (76). Mice surviving the acute phase progress to a chronic disease, with infection of glial cells and demyelination of the brain and spinal cord white matter. Depletion of $CD4^+$ T cells before or early during infection results in a high frequency of fatal encephalitis (77,78). Undepleted mice or $CD8^+$-depleted mice survive the acute phase of the disease but develop a chronic demyelinating disease. Mice depleted of $CD4^+$ T cells fail to generate an antibody response to virus. This observation suggests that a $CD4^+$ T cell-dependent antibody response may provide protection to neurons in the early stages of infection with TMEV. Similarly, the JHM strain of mouse hepatitis virus can cause a fatal encephalitis in mice. Adoptive transfer of primed mouse splenocytes can protect mice from a lethal infection (79). Two groups have demonstrated that cloned $CD4^+$ T cells can protect mice from lethal infection (80,81). One group demonstrated that the antigen specificity of the protective cells was directed against the spike protein or the nucleocapsid protein. These clones were not acting through stimulation of cytotoxic effector cells, since $CD8^+$ T cell depletion did not abrogate their protective capacity (80). An independent group demonstrated that the $CD4^+$ clones responsible for the protection from hepatitis-induced lethal encephalitis have the functional characteristics of a DTH-mediating T cell (81).

### CTL Response to Virus

Cytotoxicity of virally infected cells is mediated primarily by the $CD8^+$ subset of T cells. These T cells recognize viral peptides presented by class I MHC molecules on the surface of infected cells (82). There have been some reports of $CD4^+$ T cells that possess cytotoxic activity, but these represent a small fraction of CTL responses. Viruses are very effective activators of CTL responses. During viral infection, new viral proteins are synthesized in the infected cell. Some of these proteins are also degraded intracellularly and can enter the class I pathway of antigen presentation. Since most cell types express class I MHC molecules, the majority of infected cells can be destroyed by CTL, aiding in the limitation of spread and clearance of virus from the host. CTL activity becomes measurable 1–2 weeks after infection and often correlates with viral clearance. Adoptive transfer experiments with cloned CTL have demonstrated their efficacy in resolving viral infections (82,83,84). CTL are generated during infection with a variety of RNA and DNA viruses, including influenza virus, vaccinia virus, LCMV, and coxsackievirus B3 infection. CTL can also be responsible for some of the pathology associated with severe viral infections.

**Recognition**

In addition to recent studies on the pathways of antigen presentation, studies of the CTL response to influenza virus have been very important in developing the current models of CTL recognition. Zinkernagel and Doherty first observed that CTL-mediated killing of virally infected cells required histocompatibility between the CTL and the infected target cell (85). Histocompatibility mapped to a set of genes designated the MHC. $CD8^+$ CTL had to share histocompatibility with a specific subset of MHC genes designated class I MHC molecules. Class I molecules are cell surface glycoproteins composed of two chains, a polymorphic transmembrane heavy chain and a conserved light chain, $\beta_2$-microglobulin, which is associated noncovalently with the extracellular domains of the heavy chain. More recently, the T cell antigen recognition molecule, the T cell receptor, was described. The T cell receptor was found to be composed of $\alpha$ and $\beta$ chains that had polymorphic amino termini. The T cell receptor belongs to the same family of genes as immunoglobulin, and polymorphisms are generated by germ line rearrangement of variable-region genes. T cell receptors recognize antigen and MHC molecules as a unit.

During influenza virus infection, viral hemagglutinin and neuraminidase proteins become inserted in the membrane of the infected cell. When virion assembly is complete, influenza viruses bud from the membrane of the infected cell, taking a lipid envelope containing the hemagglutinin and neuraminidase proteins with them. Influenza virus-specific CTL were once thought to recognize native viral proteins inserted in the membrane of infected cells (86). However, studies with strains of influenza virus that differed mainly in their nucleoprotein gene sequences, not in their hemagglutinin or neuraminidase genes, produced results that conflicted with this model. CTL generated against one strain of virus could not kill target cells infected with the second strain of virus. This observation suggested that nucleoprotein rather than neuraminidase or hemagglutinin was the target antigen. However, nucleoprotein did not contain a transmembrane domain necessary for expression on the surface, nor could it be detected on the surface of infected cells. Proof that influenza virus-specific CTL could recognize nucleoprotein was provided by transfection of target cells with the gene encoding nucleoprotein: these target cells could be killed by influenza virus-specific CTL. Since nucleoprotein could not be inserted into cell membranes and was not detectable in native form on the cell surface, it was hypothesized that it was present on the cell surface in a denatured form and that CTL actually recognized fragmented antigen. Townsend et al. treated target cells with nucleoprotein synthetic peptides and assayed for their capacity to be lysed by influenza-specific CTL: CTL lysed the nucleoprotein-sensitized targets, demonstrating that CTL can recognize denatured antigen at the cell surface (34). Studies of the assembly, structure, and expression of class I MHC molecules provided evidence that the degraded antigens were actually short peptides bound directly to class I MHC molecules (34,67).

**Mechanism of Killing**

CTL have many similarities in their mechanism of killing to NK cells. Like NK cell-mediated killing, CTL-mediated killing involves three stages: binding of the effector cell to the target, programming for lysis, and delivery of the lethal hit. The binding stage of CTL-mediated killing involves the interaction between an antigen-specific T cell receptor and antigen presented on class I MHC molecules of the target cell. Formation of target cell CTL conjugates requires the presence of $Mg^{2+}$. In addition to T cell receptor-antigen-MHC interactions, there are a variety of other adhesion reactions between the CTL and its target that are necessary to stabilize the binding of the CTL to its target cell. The leukocyte adhesion molecule LFA-1 found on CTL interacts with its ligand ICAM-1 (intracellular adhesion molecule) on the target cell surface. Antibodies to LFA-1 can block CTL-mediated killing, suggesting the importance of this molecule in conjugate formation between the CTL and the target cell. Other interactions include the association between CD3 and the T cell receptor on the CTL, the interaction of CD8 molecules on the CTL and class I MHC molecules on the target, and the interaction of CD2 on the CTL with its ligand LFA-3 on the target cell. Antibodies to CD2 or CD8 are also capable of blocking CTL-mediated killing, especially when the affinity between the T cell receptor and antigen-MHC is low. The role of these accessory molecules is to strengthen the adhesion between the CTL and its target, improving the efficiency of recognition and killing. The CD3 molecule is an essential part of the T cell-receptor complex, playing an important role in signal transduction of activation signals received through the T cell receptor.

Programming for lysis involves the delivery of intracellular signals to the T cell through the T cell receptor. During the first few minutes following interaction of the T cell receptor with antigen and MHC, a number of intracellular changes occur. There is a rapid influx of $Ca^{2+}$ and activation of protein kinase C and the phosphatidylinositol pathway. The phosphitidyinositol pathway generates $IP_3$, which releases $Ca^{2+}$ from intracellular stores. Transcription is increased within minutes, leading to a cascade of signaling molecules and, within a few hours, synthesis of such lymphokines as IL-2. There is also reorientation of cytoskeletal elements, and granules become polarized toward the target cell membrane.

There are two models for the mechanism of delivery of the lethal hit by the CTL. The granule exocytosis model proposes that CTL granules contain cytotoxic factors that are deposited in the space between the CTL and its target. One of the cytotoxic factors found in CTL granules is perforin. In the presence of $Ca^{2+}$, perforin assembles into a porelike structure on the target cell surface and can mediate killing by osmotic lysis. Perforin molecules can be seen on the target cell membrane following interaction with CTL. This model does not account for some killing observed in the absence of $Ca^{2+}$ and the observation of nuclear disintegration before lysis of the target (45). A second model for killing is that the T cell delivers signals to the target that induce the target cell to self-destruct, a process known as apoptosis. The mechanism of inducing target cell apoptosis is not understood. It has been proposed that elevated intracellular $Ca^{2+}$ levels within the target may activate $Ca^{2+}$-dependent DNAses and topoisomerases, leading to the rapid nuclear disintegration observed during CTL-mediated lysis events (86,87).

### Protective Role for CTL During Viral Infection

CTL are essential in the clearance of many viral infections. The CTL response to LCMV has been extensively investigated and has provided much insight into the role of CTL in the control of viral infection. LCMV is a member of the arenavirus family of viruses. It has a bisegmented ambisense RNA genome consisting of 7.2 and 3.4 kb RNA molecules. The major structural proteins are a nucleoprotein and two glycoproteins, GP-1 and GP-2, which are cleaved from a common precursor protein, GP-C. These structural proteins are all encoded on the 3.4 kb RNA segment. LCMV is a natural pathogen for mice. Infection of mice with LCMV can have three possible outcomes. Adult immunocompetent mice infected with LCMV develop an acute asymptomatic infection but generate a protective immune response that clears the viral infection. Immunocompromised or neonatal mice cannot clear virus and develop a lifelong, persistent infection with LCMV. Finally, mice infected intracerebrally with LCMV develop an acute fatal choriomeningitis. T cell depletion studies have revealed that $CD8^+$ T cells are required for clearance of LCMV. Adoptive transfer of spleen cells 7–8 days postinfection with LCMV clears virus from infected mice (73). Clearance by spleen cells is H-2 restricted and mediated by CTL. The specificity of the T cell response to LCMV varies in different inbred strains of mice. Cloning of CTL from C57B/6 (H-2b) mice revealed that 90% of the LCMV-reactive T cells were specific for a nine amino acid stretch (from amino acid 278 to 286) of the LCMV glycoprotein GP-2 presented by H-2$D^b$. Clones reactive with nucleoprotein and a different GP epitope (from amino acids 1 to 218) could also be identified, but these clones represented a small percentage of the total CTL response. Mice of different H-2 haplotypes have different immunodominant

CTL epitopes for LCMV. For example, in Balb/c mice the CTL response to LCMV is predominantly specific for a five amino acid epitope found in the LCMV nucleoprotein when presented by H-2L$^d$ (88). Vaccination of Balb/c mice with a recombinant vaccinia virus expressing the nucleoprotein epitope was capable of conferring complete protection from a lethal dose of LCMV (89). This vaccine could not protect H-2$^b$ mice from challenge, indicating the H-2 restriction of this epitope in conferring a protective CTL response (89). These studies have illustrated that CTL responses can be the major mechanism of viral clearance, that protective CTL responses can be directed primarily to a single immunodominant epitope, and that the nature of the epitope depends on the MHC background of the host.

### CTL-Mediated Tissue Damage

Although CTL are primarily involved in protection from viral disease, they have also been implicated in the pathology associated with some viral infections. Myocardial disease is commonly associated with the enterovirus, coxsackievirus B3. A model for coxsackievirus-induced myocarditis has been established in Balb/c mice with the Woodruff variant of coxsackievirus B3 (90). Mice infected with CVB3W develop acute myocarditis with lesions characterized by infiltration of mononuclear cells and necrosis of cardiac tissue. T cell-mediated immune responses play a role in the development of disease since T cell-depleted and thymectomized mice do not develop myocarditis in response to viral infection. During infection with CVB3W, mice develop CTL directed at both viral antigens and self antigens (91). The autoreactive CTL are capable of transferring disease to thymectomized infected mice. In vitro these CTL lyse both CVB3W-infected and uninfected myocytes, but not other cell types. It was recently reported that coxsackievirus has cross-reactive epitopes with the cardiac proteins adenosine translocator protein and cardiac myosin (92,93). Injection of these proteins into mice induces myocarditis resembling the disease induced by CVB3W (94). Therefore, molecular mimicry of cardiac proteins by coxsackieviruses B may be responsible for triggering a CTL response that is autoreactive.

## Vaccination Strategies

Viruses are the causative agents for some of the most devastating illnesses of humans and livestock. Strategies for treatment of viral illnesses have tremendous value to society. Because viruses are obligate intracellular parasites and often make use of host cellular machinery for replication assembly and release, eradication of viral infection without simultaneously interfering with the metabolic processes of normal uninfected cells is difficult to achieve. For this reason few chemotherapeutic strategies for the elimination of viral infection have been developed. The alternative strategy for combating viral infection is to boost the host immune system, which has evolved mechanisms to detect and eliminate virus and virally infected cells. Vaccination has been the most successful strategy for preventing and eradicating viral infections worldwide. The earliest strategy for vaccination was the use of live viral vaccines. With the advent of recombinant DNA technologies, vaccinations with purified viral antigen has become a feasible means of conferring protection for some viral diseases. Most recently, live recombinant viruses have proven to be a very effective means of inducing protective immunity. These three strategies are discussed here.

### Live Attenuated Virus

The first recorded incidence of vaccination using live viruses occurred during the tenth century in China and India to control smallpox infection, when pustular fluid from smallpox-infected individuals was inoculated into uninfected individuals (95,96). Disease resulted in the inoculated individuals, but it was often less severe and had a lower incidence of mortality than natural infection, and thus inoculation provided protection from severe smallpox infection. In 1796, Edward Jenner developed the first live attenuated vaccine by inoculating an 8-year-old boy with the pustular fluid from a milkmaid's cowpox lesion. When the boy was challenged 6 weeks later with smallpox virus, a lesion appeared at the inoculation site but no disease developed. This vaccination strategy gained rapid acceptance and eventually resulted in the eradication of smallpox (97). The use of live attenuated virus strains to develop protective immune responses, without causing disease, has been a successful means of protection from a wide variety of human and animal viruses. A few well-known examples of live attenuated vaccines include smallpox, yellow fever, measles, mumps, polio, rubella, and Marek's disease viruses. Live attenuated viruses have the advantages of establishing long-lasting protection, safety, and low-cost, thus allowing widespread vaccination. However, live viruses occasionally cause disease, and they also cannot be used in immunocompromised individuals.

### Recombinant Vaccines

The development of DNA cloning and gene expression technologies has led to the development of recombinant vaccines. Genes for immunodominant viral proteins are subcloned into a bacterial vector. Viral proteins can be produced in large quantities by the bacteria, purified, and injected into animals to stimulate protective immune responses. This type of vaccination is probably best for inducing humoral immune responses since antibody can efficiently recognize either native or denatured antigen. Recombinant vaccines have been developed and successfully induce a protective immune response to foot and mouth disease virus (98), a member of the picornavirus family and an important disease agent in livestock. Immunization with the VP3 capsid protein can induce a neutralizing antibody response that protects both cattle and swine from FMDV. A cDNA copy of the VP3 gene was subcloned into a plasmid, forming a fusion protein with the bacterial *trp* LE gene. Large quantities of the VP3-trp LE fusion protein were produced in *Escherichia coli*, purified and injected into cattle and swine. The fusion protein induced high titers of neutralizing antibody in cattle and swine that protected them from subsequent infection with FMDV (98).

Yeast can also be used to express recombinant viral proteins for the development of vaccines. A vaccine directed against hepatitis B virus surface glycoprotein has been developed in yeast (99).

Compared to live attenuated virus vaccine, recombinant vaccines have the disadvantage of being more complicated to produce. They are also not as effective at inducing cellular immune responses, because antigen is introduced into the animal extracellularly. Recombinant DNA vaccines have not gained widespread use.

### Viral Vectors

The use of vaccinia virus as a vector for the expression of heterologous viral sequences is gaining widespread experimental use in the study of the immune response to viruses (100). Vaccinia is the strain of smallpox virus used by the World Health Organization in the worldwide effort to eliminate smallpox virus. There are many advantages to its use in vaccination strategies. Because of its widespread use, much information is now available on the efficacy, immune response, and complications resulting from vaccinia virus inoculation. Vaccinia virus as a vaccine vector has the advantages of a wide host range, relative stability, and ease of production. Inoculation with vaccinia also induces long-lasting immunity with a single dose.

Creation of a recombinant vaccinia virus vaccine usually involves the subcloning of immunodominant viral gene sequences into a plasmid that also contains vaccinia virus gene sequences (101). The plasmid contains vaccinia virus promoter sequences upstream from a multiple cloning site, into which heterologous gene sequences are inserted. The promoter and multiple cloning sites are flanked on either side by a disrupted vaccinia virus thymidine kinase gene. The recombinant plasmid is transfected into cells infected with vaccinia virus. A genetic recombination event occurs inside infected cells between the TK genes found in the plasmid and the vaccinia virus TK genes, resulting in the insertion of the disrupted TK gene and the subcloned sequence into the vaccinia genome. Recombinant vaccinia viruses are selected on the basis of their lack of an active gene by growth of infected cells in the presence of 5-bromodeoxyuridine.

Recombinant vaccinia viruses have been used to develop protective immune responses to a wide variety of viruses, including rabies virus, dengue virus, hepatitis B virus, and many others. Vaccinia virus vaccines have been demonstrated to induce both protective neutralizing antibodies and protective CTL responses against many different viruses. Recombinant vaccinia viruses expressing rabies virus antigens have been used successfully in the wild to protect raccoons and foxes from infection (102). A recombinant vaccinia virus expressing HIV glycoprotein has been used in clinical trials on healthy individuals and has been demonstrated to induce serum antibody and T cell proliferative responses to HIV (103). No recombinant vaccinia virus vaccine has been approved for human or veterinary use so far, but with continued development and demonstration of safety, this method of vaccination may gain widespread acceptance and use.

Recombinant viral vaccines using Sindbis virus as the vector are also being developed (104,105). Sindbis virus is a member of the alpha virus family of viruses (106,107). Sindbis virus is transmitted through an insect vector, such as the mosquito, and it has been isolated in Europe, Africa, Asia, and Australia. It causes a mild disease in humans that can be asymptomatic or in some regions cause fever, a rash, and arthritis (107). Sindbis virus is a good candidate for the creation of recombinant vaccines for several reasons (107, 108). First, Sindbis virus has a very wide host range. It can infect mammalian, avian, reptilian, and some insect cell lines in vitro. Second, Sindbis virus replicates to a high titer in the cytoplasm of the host cell, producing large quantities of the protein of interest. The complete cDNA sequence of Sindbis virus is known and cloned, aiding in the construction of recombinant viruses. Finally, temperature-sensitive mutants of Sindbis are available that can be modulated to induce expression of cloned genes.

Sindbis virus has a positive-strand RNA genome of 11 kb (106,108). The 5′ two-thirds of the genome encode nonstructural genes for transcription and replication, and the 3′ one-third of the genome encodes genes for the viral structural proteins. The viral nonstructural proteins are translated directly from the infectious RNA genome. The structural proteins, however, are first transcribed from a negative-strand copy of the viral genome, as a "subgenomic RNA molecule" of 4.1 kb. The structural proteins are then translated from this subgenomic RNA. To create a recombinant Sindbis virus a viral gene of interest must first be subcloned into the structural gene region of a Sindbis virus cDNA. The gene of interest can either replace the structural genes or be incorporated into the structural genes to create a fusion protein. The recombinant cDNA is then subcloned into a plasmid containing

SP6 or T7 RNA polymerase promoter sequences, and RNA copies are transcribed in vitro. These RNA copies can then be transfected into cells to express the gene of interest. If the structural genes for Sindbis virus have been disrupted or replaced by the inserted genes, a helper virus may be necessary to package the RNA into infectious virions. The effectiveness of Sindbis virus as an expression vector was demonstrated by expression of the CAT gene (108). Chimeric viruses with Sindbis have been created using Ross River virus, equine arteritis virus, and Rift Valley fever viruses (104,105). An immunodominant epitope of Rift Valley fever virus was subcloned into the E2 structural protein of Sindbis virus by random insertion mutagenesis (105). Recombinant viruses expressing the epitope of Rift Valley fever virus were identified by western blot analysis with monoclonal antibodies to the Rift Valley fever virus epitope. These recombinant viruses were able to partially protect mice challenged with a lethal dose of Rift Valley fever virus (105). These preliminary studies suggest that Sindbis virus might provide a useful vector for the development of protective recombinant vaccines in the future.

## SUMMARY

The mammalian immune system has evolved multiple strategies for the defense against viral pathogens. Nonspecific mechanisms, such as complement and IFN, provide a first line of defense during viral infection. The main function of these systems is to limit the replication and spread of virus early after infection while specific immune responses are being generated. For some viruses, nonspecific defense mechanisms of the host provide a barrier to infection. However, other viruses have developed specific strategies to evade the host's immune system. For example, the vaccinia virus gp35 is homologous to C4 binding protein and can block the assembly of the classic pathway C3 convertases (8). HSV has proteins homologous to complement receptor type 1 (CR1) and decay accelerating factor, which can disassemble alternative pathway C3 convertases (8). Many viruses have evolved strategies to evade the antiviral actions of interferon as well (15). For example, adenovirus produces small transcripts that block the action of the IFN-induced P1/elf protein kinase (15). Therefore, host defense against many viruses requires a flexible antigen-specific immune response. Antiviral B and T cells provide such highly specific and efficient mechanism of viral elimination. Because of the tremendous potential for diversity in immunoglobulin and T cell receptor genes, the mammalian immune system can provide a response to literally billions of different viral antigen specificities (54). The specific immune system also provides the host with antiviral memory cells. After virus is cleared, antiviral T and B memory cells protect the host from reinfection. Thus, nonspecific and specific immune responses cooperate to protect us from a constant barrage of viruses in the environment.

## APPENDIX: ABBREVIATIONS

### Viruses

**CVB3W**, coxsackievirus B3, Woodruff variant
**EAV**, equine arteritis virus
**FMDV**, foot and mouth disease virus
**HIV**, human immunodeficiency virus
**HSV**, herpes simplex virus
**IBV**, infectious bronchitis virus
**LCMV**, lymphocytic choriomeningitis virus
**TMEV**, Theiler's murine encephalomyelitis virus
**VSV**, vesicular stomatitis virus

### Immunology

**ADCC**, antibody-dependent cellular cytotoxicity
**CSF**, colony-stimulating factor
**CTL**, cytotoxic T lymphocytes
**DAF**, decay accelerating factor
**DTH**, delayed-type hypersensitivity
**GM-CSF**, granulocyte-macrophage colony-stimulating factor
**IL**, interleukins
**INF**, interferons
**LT**, lymphotoxins
**MHC**, major histocompatibility complex
**NK**, natural killer
**NKCF**, natural killer cell cytotoxic factor
**TNF**, tumor necrosis factors

### Other

**AIDS**, acquired immunodeficiency syndrome
**ARC**, AIDS-related complex
**CAT**, chloramphenicol transacetylase
**CNS**, central nervous system
**ER**, endoplasmic reticulum
**IP**, inositol phosphate
**LAD**, leukocyte adhesion deficiency
**OVA**, ovalbumin
**RNA**, ribonucleic acid
**TK**, thymidine kinase

## REFERENCES


1. Hirsch RL. The complement system: its importance in the host response to viral infection. Microbiol Rev 1982; 46:71–85.
2. Bhakdi S, Tranun-Jensen J. Complement lysis: a hole is a hole. Immunol Today 1991; 12:318–20.
3. Hicks JT, Ennis FA, Kim E, Verbonitz M. The importance of an intact complement pathway in recovery from a primary viral infection: influenza in decomplemented and C5-deficient mice. J Immunol 1978; 121:1437–45.
4. Hirsch RL, Winkelstein JA, Griffin DE. The role of complement in viral infections. III. Activation of the classical and alternative pathways by Sindbis virus. J Immunol 1980; 124:2507–10.
5. Ljunggren HG, Karre K. Host resistance directed selectively against H-2 deficient lymphoma variants. J Exp Med 1985; 162:1745–59.
6. Aaby P, Bukh J, Hoff G, Lisse IM, Smits AJ. Humoral immunity in measles infection: a critical factor? Med Hypotheses 1987; 23:287–301.
7. Oldstone MBA, Sissons JGP, Fujinami RS. Action of antibody and complement in regulating virus infection. In: Fourgereau M, ed. Immunology 1980. 4th International Congress of Immunology. London: Academic Press, 1980; 599–621.
8. Radawan AI, Burger D. The role of sensitizing antibody in the neutralization of equine arteritis virus by complement or anti-IgG serum. Virology 1973; 53:366–71.
9. Berry DM, and Almeida JD. The morphological and biological effects of various antisera on avian infectious bronchitis virus. J Gen Virol 1968; 3:97–102.
10. Grewal AS, Rouse BT, Babiuk LA. Mechanism of recovery from viral infections: destruction of infected cells by neutrophils and complement. J Immunol 1980; 124:312–19.
11. West BC, Eschete ML, Cox ME, King JW. Neutrophil uptake of vaccinia virus in vitro. J Infect Dis 1987; 156:597–606.
12. Van Strijp JAG, Van Der Tol ME, Miltenburg LAM, Van Kessel KPM. Tumor necrosis factor triggers granulocytes to internalize complement-coated virus particles. Immunology 1991; 73:77–82.
13. Sissons PJG and Oldstone MBA. Antibody-mediated destruction of virus-infected cells. Adv Immunol 1980; 29:209–59.
14. Isaacs A, Lindemann J. Virus interference. I. The interferon. Proc R Soc Lond [Biol] 1957; 147:258–67.
15. Samuel CE. Antiviral actions of interferon: interferon-regulated cellular proteins and their surprisingly selective antiviral activities. Virology 1991; 183:1–11.
16. Stanton GJ, Weigent DA, Fleischmann WR, Dianzani F, Baron S. Interferon review. Invest Radiol 1987; 22:259–73.
17. Gastl G, Huber C. The biology of interferon actions. Blut 1988; 56:193–9.
18. Horisberger MA, Gunst MC. Interferon induced proteins: identification of Mx proteins in various mammalian species. Virology 1991; 180:185–90.
19. Speiser DE, Zurcher T, Ramseier H, et al. Nuclear myxovirus resistance protein Mx is a minor histocompatibility antigen. Proc Natl Acad Sci U S A 1990; 87:2021–5.

20. Chebath J, Benech P, Revel M, Vigneron M. Constitutive expression of (2′-5′) oligo A synthetase confers resistance to picornavirus infection. Nature 1987; 330:587–8.
21. Samuel CE. Mechanism of interferon action. Phosphorylation of protein synthesis initiation factor elF-2 in interferon-treated human cells by a ribosome-associated kinase possessing site specificity similar to hemin-regulated rabbit reticulocyte kinase. Proc Natl Acad Sci U S A 1979; 76:600–4.
22. Pestka S, Langer J, Zoon KC, Samuel CE. Interferons and their actions. Annu Rev Biochem 1987; 56:727–77.
23. Minato N, Reid L, Cantor H, Lengyel P, Bloom BR. Mode of regulation of natural killer activity by interferon. J Exp Med 1980; 152:124–37.
24. Adams DO, Hamilton TA. The cell biology of macrophage activation. Annu Rev Immunol 1984; 2:283–318.
25. Schreiber RD, Hicks LJ, Celada A, Buchmeier NA, Gray PW. Monoclonal antibodies to murine $\gamma$-interferon which differentially modulate macrophage activation and antiviral activity. J Immunol 1985; 134:1609–18.
26. Ellermann-Eriksen S, Sommerlund M, Morgensen SC. Differential sensitivity of macrophages from herpes simplex virus-resistant and -susceptible mice to respiratory burst priming by interferon $\alpha/\beta$. J Gen Virol 1989; 70:2139–47.
27. Maeda H, Akaike T. Oxygen free radicals as pathogenic molecules in viral diseases. FASEB J 1991; 5:721–7.
28. Van Kessel KPM, Verhoef J. A view to kill: cytotoxic mechanisms of human polymorphonuclear leukocytes compared with monocytes and natural killer cells. Pathobiology 1990; 58:249–64.
29. Goudsmit J, Ljunggren K, Smit L, Jonda M, Fenyo EM. Biological significance of the antibody response to HIV antigens expressed on the cell surface. Arch Virol 1988; 189–206.
30. Ljunggren K, Broliden PA, Morfeldt-Manson L, Jondal M, Wahren B. IgG subclass response to HIV in relation to antibody-dependent cellular cytotoxicity at different clinical stages. Clin Exp Immunol 1988; 73:343–7.
31. Wust CJ, Crombie R, Brown A. Passive protection across subgroups of alphaviruses by hyperimmune non-cross-neutralizing anti-Sindbis serum. Proc Soc Exp Biol Med 1987; 184:56–63.
32. Debrick JE, Campbell PA, Staerz UD. Macrophages as accessory cells for class I MHC-restricted immune responses. J Immunol 1991; 147:2846–51.
33. Townsend A, Ohlen C, Bastin J, Ljunggren HG, Foster L, Karre K. Association of class I major histocompatibility heavy and light chains induced by viral peptides. Nature 1989; 340:443–8.
34. Townsend ARM, Gotch FM, Davey J. Cytotoxic T cells recognize fragments of influenza nucleoprotein. Cell 1985; 42:457–67.
35. Durum SK, Schmidt JA, Oppenheim JJ. Interleukin 1: an immunological perspective. Annu Rev Immunol 1985; 3:263–87.
36. Heberman RB, Callewaert DM, eds. Mechanisms of cytotoxicity by NK cells. Orlando, FL: Academic Press, 1985.
37. Biron CA, Welsh RM. Blastogenesis of natural killer cells during viral infection in vivo. J Immunol 1982; 129:2788–95.

38. Trinchieri G. Biology of natural killer cells. Adv Immunol 1989; 47:187–376.
39. Ljunggren H, Karre K. In search of the "missing self": MHC molecules and NK cell recognition. Immunol Today 1990; 11:237–44.
40. Storkus WJ, Alexander J, Payne AJ, Dawson JR, Cresswell P. Reversal of natural killing susceptibility in target cells expressing transfected class I HLA genes. Proc Natl Acad Sci U S A 1989; 86:2361–4.
41. Sturmhofel K, Hammerling GJ. Reconstitution of H-2 class I expression by gene transfection decreases susceptibility to natural killer cells of an EL4 class I loss variant. Eur J Immunol 1990; 20:171–7.
42. Quillet A, Presse F, Marchiol-Fournigault C, et al. Increased resistance to non-MHC-restricted cytoxicity related to HLA A, B expression. J Immunol 1988; 141:17–20.
43. Fanger MW, Shen L, Graziano RF, Guyre PM. Cytotoxicity mediated by human Fc receptors for IgG. Immunol Today 1989; 10:92–9.
44. Suzuki T. Signal transduction mechanisms through FR$\gamma$ receptors on the mouse macrophage surface. FASEB J 1991; 5:187–93.
45. Henkart PA. Mechanisms of lymphocyte-mediated cytotoxicity. Annu Rev Immunol 1985; 3:31–58.
46. Wright SC, Bonavida B. Selective lysis of NK-sensitive target cells by a soluble mediator released from murine spleen cells and human peripheral blood lymphocytes. J Immunol 1981; 126:1516–21.
47. Paya CV, Kenmotsu N, Schoon RA, Leibson PJ. Tumor necrosis factor and lymphotoxin secretion by human natural killer cells leads to antiviral cytotoxicity. J Immunol 1988; 141:1989–95.
48. Biron CA, Byron KS, Sullivan JL. Severe herpes virus infections in an adolescent without natural killer cells. N Engl J Med 1989; 320:1731–5.
49. Piontek GE, Weltzin R, Tompkins WAF. Enhanced cytotoxicity of mouse natural killer cells for vaccinia and herpes virus-infected targets. J Reticuloendothel Soc 1980; 27:175–88.
50. Paya CV, Patick AK, Leibson PJ, Rodrigues M. Role of natural killer cells as immune effectors in encephalitis and demyelination induced by Theiler's virus. J Immunol 1989; 143:95–102.
51. Godeny EK, Gauntt CJ. Murine natural killer cells limit Coxsackie virus B3 replication. J Immunol 1987; 139:913–8.
52. Welsh RM. Natural cell-mediated immunity during viral infections. Curr Top Microbiol Immunol 1981; 92:83–106.
53. Kishimoto T, Hirano T. B lymphocyte activation, proliferation and immunoglobulin secretion. In: Paul WE, ed. Fundamental immunology, 2nd ed. New York: Raven Press, 1989; 385–411.
54. Abbas AK, Lichtman AH, Pober JS. T cell maturation in the thymus. In: Wonsiewicz MJ, ed. Cellular and molecular immunology. Philadelphia: W.B. Saunders, 1991; 169–85.
55. Melnick JL. Enteroviruses. In: Fields BN, Knipe DM, eds. Fields virology, 2nd ed. New York: Raven Press, 1990; 549–605.
56. Minor PD, Schild GC, Bootman J, et al. Location and primary structure of a major antigenic site for poliovirus neutralization. Nature 1983; 301:674–9.

57. Kohl S. Role of antibody-dependent cellular toxicity in defense against herpes simplex virus infections. Rev Infect Dis 1991; 13:108–14.
58. Kohl S. The neonatal human's immune response to herpes simplex virus infection: a critical review. Pediatr Infect Dis J 1989; 8:67–74.
59. Kohl S, Strynadka NCJ, Hodges RS, Pereira L. Analysis of the role of antibody dependent cellular cytotoxic antibody activity in murine neonatal herpes simplex virus infection with antibodies to synthetic peptides of glycoprotein D and monoclonal antibodies to glycoprotein B. J Clin Invest 1990; 86:273–8.
60. McKendall RR, Woo W. Antibody activity to herpes simplex virus in mouse Ig classes and IgG subclasses. Arch Virol 1988; 98:225–33.
61. Kipps TJ, Parham P, Punt J, Herzenberg LA. Importance of immunoglobulin isotype in human antibody-dependent cell-mediated cytoxicity directed by murine monoclonal antibodies. J Exp Med 1985; 161:1–17.
62. Casali P, Notkins AL. Probing the human B-cell repertoire with EBV. Annu Rev Immunol 1989; 7:513–35.
63. Hardin JA, Vos K, Kawano Y, Sherr DH. A function for ly1 + B cells. Immunol Today 1990; 11:172–82.
64. Kasaian MT, Ikematsu H, Casali P. CD5 + B lymphocytes. Immunol Today 1991; 12:226–41.
65. Peters PJ, Neefjes JJ, Oorschot V, Ploegh HL, Geuze HJ. Segregation of MHC class II molecules from MHC class I molecules in the Golgi complex for transport to lysosomal compartments. Nature 1991; 349:669–76.
66. Moore MW, Carbone FR, Bevan MJ. Introduction of soluble protein into the class I pathway of antigen processing and presentation. Cell 1988; 54:777–85.
67. Bjorkman PJ, Saper MA, Samraoui B, Bennett WS, Strominger J, Wiley DC. Structure of the human class I histocompatibility antigen, HLA-A2. Nature 1987; 329:506–12.
68. Robertson M. Proteasomes in the pathway. Nature 1991; 353:300–1.
69. Deverson EV, Gow IR, Coadwell WJ, Monaco JJ, Butcher GW, Howard JC. MHC class II region encoding proteins related to the multidrug resistance family of transmembrane transporters. Nature 1990; 348:738–41.
70. Trowsdale J, Hanson I, Mockridge I, Beck S, Townsend A, Kelly A. Sequences encoded in the class II region of the MHC related to the 'ABC' superfamily of transporters. Nature 1990; 348:741–4.
71. Spies T, Bresnaham M, Bahram S, et al. A gene in the human major histocompatibility complex class II region controlling the class I antigen presentation pathway. Nature 1990; 348:744–7.
72. Brown MG, Driscoll J, Monaco JJ. Structural and serological similarity of MHC-linked LMP and proteasome (multicatalytic proteinase) complexes. Nature 1991; 353:355–7.
73. Ahmed R, Butler LD, Bhatti L. $T4^+$ T helper function: differential requirements for induction of antiviral cytotoxic T-cell and antibody response. J Virol 1988; 62:2102–6.
74. Buller ML, Holmes KL, Hugin A, Frederickson TN, Morse HC. Induction of cytotoxic T-cell responses in vivo in the absence of $CD4^+$ helper cells. Nature 1987; 328:75–9.

75. Rahemtulla A, Fung-Leung WP, Schillham MW, et al. Normal development and function of CD8$^+$ cells but markedly decreased helper cell activity in mice lacking CD4. Nature 1991; 353:180–4.
76. Lipton HL. Theiler's virus infection in mice: an unusual biphasic disease process leading to demyelination. Infect Immun 1975; 11:1147–55.
77. Welsh CJR, Tonks P, Nash AA, Blakemore WF. The effect of L3T4 T cell depletion on the pathogenesis of Theiler's murine encephalomyelitis virus infection in CBA mice. J Gen Virol 1987; 68:1659–67.
78. Rodriguez M, Sriram S. Successful therapy of Theiler's virus-induced demyelination (DA strain) with mononuclear anti-Lyt-2 antibody. J Immunol 1988; 140:2950–5.
79. Sussman MA, Shubin RA, Kyuwa S, Stohlman SA. T-cell mediated clearance of mouse hepatitis virus strain JHM from the central nervous system. J Virol 1989; 63:3051–6.
80. Korner H, Schliephake A, Winter J, et al. Nucleocapsid or spike protein-specific CD4$^+$ T lymphocytes protect against coronavirus-induced encephalomyelitis in the absence of CD8$^+$ cells. J Immunol 1991; 147:2317–23.
81. Stohlman SA, Matsushima GK, Casteel N, Weiner LP. In vivo effects of coronavirus-specific T cell clones: DTH inducer cells prevent a lethal infection but do not inhibit virus replication. J Immunol 1986; 136:3052–6.
82. Townsend A, Bodmer H. Antigen recognition by class I restricted T lymphocytes. Annu Rev Immunol 1989; 7:601–24.
83. Byrne JA, Oldstone MBA. Biology of cloned cytotoxic T lymphocytes specific for lymphocytic choriomeningitis virus: clearance of virus in vivo. J Virol 1984; 51:682–6.
84. Oldstone MBA, Blount P, Southern PJ. Cytoimmunotherapy for persistent virus infection reveals a unique clearance pattern from the central nervous system. Nature 1986; 321:239–43.
85. Zinkernagel RM, Doherty PC. Immunological surveillance against altered self components by sensitized T lymphocytes in lymphocytic choriomeningitis. Nature 1974; 251:547–8.
86. Berke G. Functions and mechanisms of lysis induced by cytotoxic T lymphocytes and natural killer cells. In: Paul WE, ed. Fundamental immunology, 2nd ed. New York: Raven Press, 1989; 735–64.
87. Russel JH. Internal disintegration model of cytotoxic lymphocyte-induced target damage. Immunol Rev 1983; 72:97.
88. Whitton JL, Tishon A, Lewicki H, et al. Molecular analysis of a five-amino-acid cytotoxic T-lymphocyte (CTL) epitope: an immunodominant region which induced nonreciprocal CTL cross-reactivity. J Virol 1989; 63:4304–10.
89. Klavinskis LS, Whitton JL, Oldstone MBA. Molecularly engineered vaccine which expresses an immunodominant T-cell epitope induces cytotoxic T lymphocytes that confer protection from lethal virus infection. J Virol 1989; 63: 4311–6.
90. Woodruff JF, Woodruff JJ. Involvement of T lymphocytes in the pathogenesis of Coxsackie virus B3 heart disease. J Immunol 1974; 113:1726–34.
91. Wong CY, Woodruff JJ, Woodruff JF. Generation of cytotoxic T-lymphocytes during Coxsackie B-3 infection. J Immunol 1977; 118:1159–69.

92. Huber SA, Lodge PA. Coxsackie B-3 myocarditis in Balb/c mice. Evidence for autoimmunity to myocyte antigens. Am J Pathol 1984; 116:21–9.
93. Louon RP, Moraska AF, Huber SA, Schwimmbeck P, Schultheiss P. An attenuated variant of Coxsackie B3 preferentially induces immunoregulatory T cells in vivo. J Virol 1991; 65:5813–9.
94. Schultheiss HP, Shulze K, Kuhl U, Ulrich G, and Klingenbery M. The ADP/ATP carrier as a mitochondrial auto-antigen—facts and perspectives. Ann. NY. Acad. Sci. 1987; 448:44–68.
95. Allison AC, Gregoriadis G. Vaccines: recent trends and progress. Immunol Today 1990; 11:427–9.
96. Esposito JJ, Murphy FA. Infectious recombinant vectored virus vaccines. Adv Vet Sci Comp Med 1989; 33:195–247.
97. Fenner FDA, Henderson DA, Arita I, Jezek Z, Ladnyi ID. "Smallpox and its eradication." Geneva: World Health Organization, 1988; 69–168.
98. Kleid DG, Yansura D, Small B, et al. Cloned viral protein vaccine for foot and mouth disease: responses in cattle and swine. Science 1981; 214:1125–8.
99. Hadler SC. Vaccines to prevent hepatitis B and hepatitis A virus infections. Infect Dis Clin North Am 1990; 4:29–46.
100. Moss B. Vaccinia virus: a tool for research and vaccine development. Science 1991; 252:1662–7.
101. Witcor TJ, MacFarlan RI, Reagan KJ, et al. Protection from rabies by a vaccinia virus recombinant containing the rabies virus glycoprotein gene. Proc Natl Acad Sci U S A 1984; 81:7194–8.
102. Blancou J, Kieny MP, Lathe R, et al. Oral vaccination of the fox against rabies using a live recombinant vaccinia virus. Nature 1986; 322:373–5.
103. Cooney EL, Collier AC, Greenberg PD, et al. Safety of and immunological response to a recombinant vaccinia virus vaccine expressing HIV envelope glycoprotein. Lancet 1991; 337:567–72.
104. Kuhn RJ, Niesters HGM, Hong Z, Strauss JH. Infectious RNA transcripts from Ross River virus cDNA clones and the construction and characterization of defined chimeras with Sindbis virus. Virology 1991; 182:430–41.
105. London SD, Schmaljohn AL, Dalrymple JM, Rice CM. Infectious enveloped RNA virus antigenic chimeras. Proc Natl Acad Sci U S A 1992; 89:207–11.
106. Schlesinger S, Schlesinger MJ. Replication of Togaviridae and Flaviviridae. In: Fields BN, Knipe DM, etd. Fields virology, 2nd ed. New York: Raven Press, 1990; 697–711.
107. Peters CJ, Dalrymple JM. Alphaviruses. In: Fields BN, Knipe DM, eds. Fields Virology, 2nd ed. New York: Raven Press, 1990; 713–61.
108. Xiong C, Levis R, Shen P, Schlesinger S, Rice CM, Huang HV. Sindbis virus: an efficient, broad host range vector for gene expression in animal cells. Science 1989; 243:1188–91.

# Part II

## PARVOVIRUSES

# 3

# B19 Parvovirus

**Neal S. Young**

*National Heart, Lung and Blood Institute*
*Bethesda, Maryland*

## INTRODUCTION

Yvonne Cossart, a virologist working in London in the mid-1970s, discovered B19 parvovirus while investigating laboratory assays for hepatitis B (1). She used an immunoelectrophoretic technique in which sera from blood bank donors, serving as a source of antigen, were reacted with samples from patients with hepatitis, used as a source of antibody. In comparison with more specific assays, she noted a number of apparently false positive reactions. When she excised the precipitin lines from the agarose and examined them by electron microscopy, she noted particles typical in appearance of parvoviruses (Fig. 1). (One of the viremic blood bank donors serum was encoded "B19.") Using the same assay system, her British colleagues found antibodies in a high proportion of normal adults (2). Subsequently, evidence of acute infection, IgM or viral antigen, was seroepidemiologically linked to transient aplastic crisis of sickle cell anemia (3) and fifth disease in normal children (4). The genetic material of the particles present in acute-phase sera could be characterized as single-stranded DNA, allowing classification of the agent as a proper member of the Parvoviridae family (5,6), and in the mid-1980s the virus was cloned by Cotmore and Tattersall (7) and sequenced by Astell's laboratory in Vancouver (8). At about the same time, B19 parvovirus was first cultivated in vitro using human bone marrow cells by Ozawa and colleagues at the National Institutes of Health (9); human erythroid

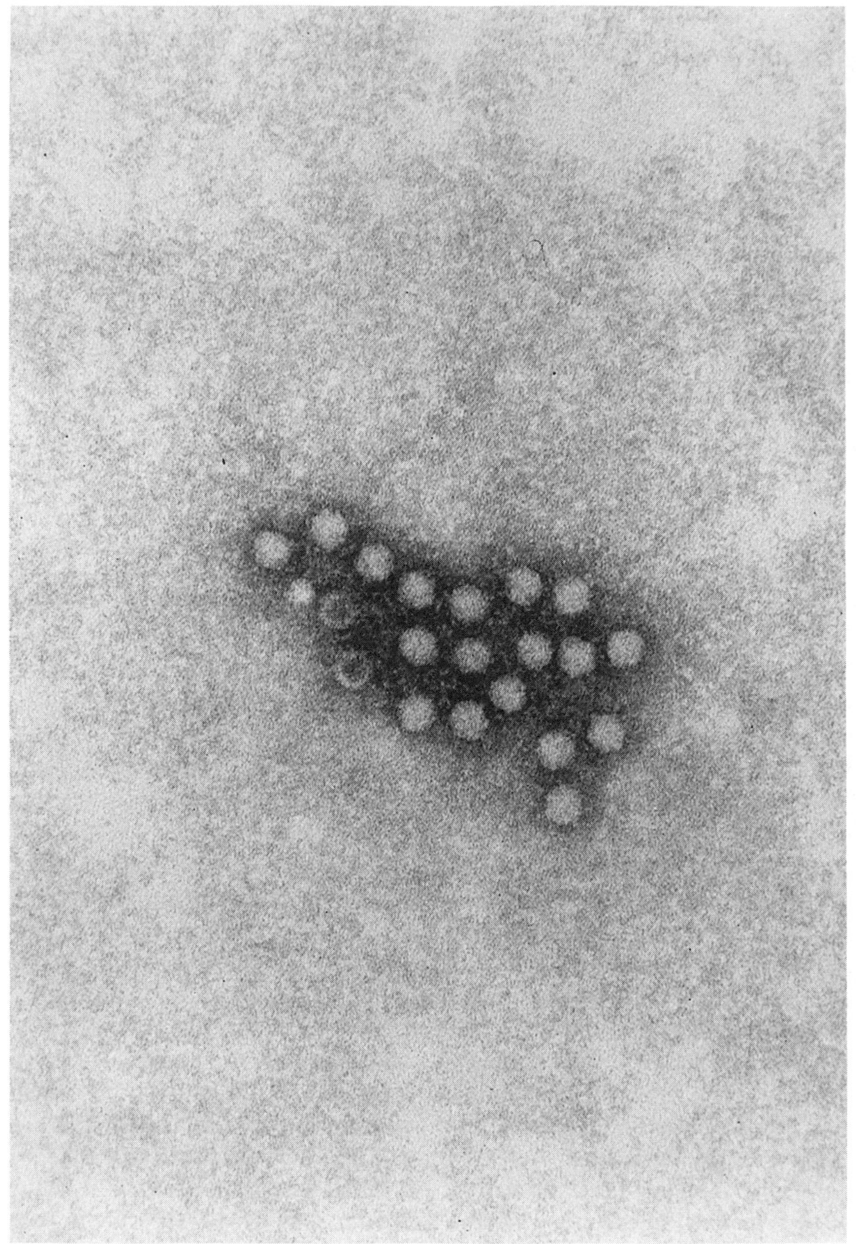

**Figure 1** Electron micrograph of B19 parvovirus particles showing icosahedral symmetry and empty capsids, both characteristic of members of the Parvoviridiae family. (Courtesy of Dr. Anne Field)

progenitors remain the most convenient productive tissue culture system, and inoculation of these cells has allowed a description of the molecular biology of the virus. Expression of B19 parvovirus capsid proteins using recombinant technology has been useful for the development of clinical assays for specific parvovirus antibodies, and engineered capsids should be suitable for a human vaccine (10).

## EPIDEMIOLOGY

B19 parvovirus is a common infection in humans. IgG antibody specific for the virus, which appears in the first 2 weeks after inoculation and persists for life (11–13), is the most convenient marker of past exposure. About 50% of adults have IgG antibody to B19 parvovirus; the proportion increases to more than 90% in the elderly (14); an annual seroconversion rate of 1.5% was estimated from studies of serial samples from women of childbearing age (15). Thus, most individuals acquire immunity during childhood, but susceptibility continues in others throughout adult life. Seroprevalence of IgG antibody is similarly high worldwide (16–18), except among some isolated Brazilian (19) and African (20) tribal populations.

Fifth disease is seasonal, with peak occurrence in spring and summer. Both fifth disease and transient aplastic crisis appeared to cycle in approximately 3 year periods, but more recent serologic surveys have suggested a more constant pattern of infection (21). Epidemics of fifth disease in normal children with clusters of transient aplastic crisis in patients with underlying hemolysis occur concurrently, but they are frequently recognized and treated by different physician specialists (22,23). Antibody to B19 parvovirus is common, but viral antigen is detected very rarely in normal persons: only 1 in 24,000 blood donors contained a high titer of virus in one purposeful screen (24).

B19 parvovirus is excreted from the nasopharynx, and the major route of transmission is probably through the upper airway (11). There is little evidence of virus excretion in feces or urine (11). In epidemics the attack rate is high: between 10 and 60% of susceptible school children develop fifth disease in school outbreaks (15,23,25), and for adult school and day-care personnel, parvovirus infections occurred in 20–30% (26). Sibling-to-sibling transfer is probably a major path of transmission (15). Although viremia is rare, B19 parvovirus can be transmitted in transfused blood products, especially pooled coagulation factor concentrates (27). Parvoviruses, including B19, are very heat resistant and can withstand the usual thermal treatment to destroy viral infectivity. Nonetheless, hemophiliacs who received factor VIII concentrates subjected to heating (80 °C for 72 h) had a lower rate of seroconversion than those who received unheated concentrate (28); nonetheless, parvovirus has been transmitted by dry- and steam-heated products

(29,30). Nosocomial transmission from infected patients to medical staff can occur (31) but is probably infrequent.

## THE PARVOVIRUSES

The Parvoviridae, small, single-stranded DNA viruses, are common animal pathogens (Table 1). Feline panleukopenia virus was one of the first viruses experimentally demonstrated to cause disease in animals; this virus infects cat hematopoietic and lymphocytic cells and causes often fatal neutropenia (see Chap. 4) (32). The canine, mink, and feline parvoviruses are similar enough to one another at the nucleotide and amino acid levels to be grouped as host-range variants (33). These parvoviruses are striking for the recent development of tropism for some species, like mink and dogs, and their host-dependent behavior. The global pandemic of canine parvovirus of the late 1970s was a new infection, no antiparvovirus antibody being present in pre-1978 stored sera (33). Even more recently, canine parvovirus has spread to

**Table 1** Autonomous Parvoviruses

| Virus | Host | Disease |
|---|---|---|
| Rat virus (RV) | Rat | Fetal death, stillbirth |
| H-1 virus (H-1) | Rat | Cerebellar ataxia |
| RT virus (RTV) | Rat | Congenital malformations |
| TVX (TVX) | | Murine |
| Minute virus of mice (MVM) | Mice | Enteritis, hepatitis |
| LuIII (LuIII) | Unknown | |
| Porcine parvovirus (PPV) | Domestic swine | Reproductive failure |
| Bovine parvovirus (BPV) | Cattle | Enteritis |
| Aleutian disease virus (ADV) | Mink | Hypergammaglobulinemia, arteritis |
| Feline parvovirus (FPV) | Cats | Enteritis, panleukopenia, ataxia |
| Mink enteritis virus (MEV)[a] | Mink | Enteritis |
| Canine parvovirus (CPV)[a] | Dogs | Enteritis, myocarditis |
| Racoon parvovirus (RPVP)[a] | Racoons | |
| Lapine parvovirus (LPV) | Rabbits | |
| Goose parvovirus (GPV) | Geese | Enteritis, myocarditis |
| B19 | Human | Red cell aplasia, erythema infectiosum, hydrops fetalis, congenital infection |

[a]Species host-range variant from FPV.

isolated wolf populations in Michigan's Upper Peninsula. There are interesting examples of the variety of clinical syndromes resulting from infection of these viruses in different hosts. Feline panleukopenia virus causes congenital ataxia in kittens as a result of a remarkably specific attack on cells of the developing fetal cerebellum (34). Canine parvovirus is notorious for myocarditis in puppies, which is rare in kittens, and feline panleukopenia virus often kills cats by marrow myeloid hypoplasia and neutropenia, which does not occur in dogs (33,35) [except puppies (36)].

Tropism for bone marrow hematopoietic progenitors may be a general feature of parvovirus biology. Hematopoietic suppression of murine progenitor and stem cells has been documented in vitro for minute virus of mice (37); this rodent parvovirus may infect a cell as primitive as the colony-forming unit–stem cell (CFU-S) (37). Aleutian disease virus causes an important disease of the immune system in minks (38) and replicates in vivo in their lymphocytes (39). A chicken marrow aplasia agent also has biochemical characteristics of a parvovirus (40).

Parvoviruses are defined by their size, symmetry, and genetic material. Parvum is Latin for small, and the parvoviruses are among the smallest viruses, usually 15–28 nm in diameter. In the electron microscope, they show icosahedral symmetry; the specific arrangement of viral proteins in the capsid has been determined by x-ray crystallography, described later. The absence of a lipid envelope contributes to the high heat stability of the parvoviruses, a major factor in their extremely contagious behavior in nature: B19 parvovirus has been transmitted in pasteurized blood products (27). For the same reason the virus resists solvent detergent treatment (41).

Contained within each parvovirus capsid is a single copy of the viral genome, composed of about 5000 bases of single-stranded DNA (Fig. 2). [For convenient reference, the entire genome is equated to 100 map units (mu).] Parvoviruses package either exclusively negative strands or an equal mixture of negative and positive strands depending on the virus species. For B19 parvovirus and the other vertebrate parvoviruses, only a single strand is used for coding genes. Parvoviruses have molecular weights ranging from $1.55$ to $1.97 \times 10^6$, about half of which represents DNA; their buoyant density in cesium chloride density gradients ranges from 1.36 to 1.43 g/ml, the less dense particles representing empty capsids.

## Genomic Organization

Most vertebrate parvoviruses share a similar genomic organization, with the capsid proteins encoded by genes on the right side of the genome and nonstructural proteins by genes of the left side. At both ends of the genome are

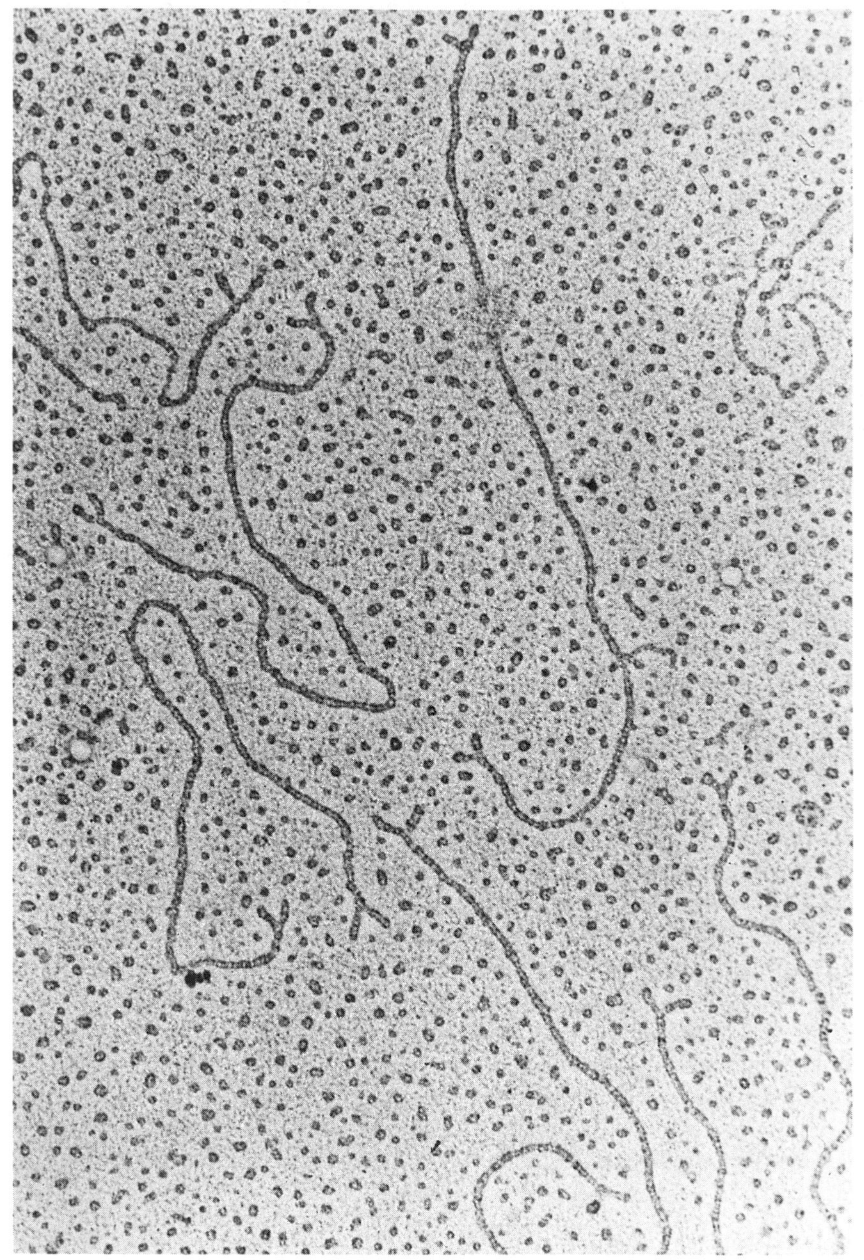

**Figure 2** Electron micrograph of B19 parvovirus DNA single strands were annealed in vitro. Note terminal hairpin structures. (Photograph courtesy of Dr. Bernard Cohen.)

terminal repeat sequences, palindromes of variable length and symmetry according to the species of virus. These inverted repeat elements serve as the double-stranded matix needed to initiate DNA synthesis, and they are therefore required for virus propagation (42,43). Somewhat surprisingly, the terminal repeats also appear to be necessary and sufficient for other virus functions, including not only replication but also packaging of DNA (44,45). B19 has the longest terminal repeats among the parvoviruses, 365 nucleotides, rivaled only by human adenoassociated virus and bovine parvovirus. In both B19 parvovirus and adenoassociated virus, the 5′ and 3′ ends of identical sequence (42). The length, the presence of several long direct repeat sequences, the high content of guanosine-cytosine pairs, and the resulting strong secondary structure of the B19 parvovirus terminal repeat sequences have made them resistant to molecular cloning in bacteria until the recent achievement of full-length cloning of a (presumably) infectious virus (46).

## Nonstructural Protein

The gene for nonstructural protein is fairly homologous among the parvoviruses, consistent with a required role in virus propagation. In particular, a 145 amino acid sequence in the middle of the gene is highly conserved among B19 parvovirus, adenoassociated virus, and minute virus of mice (8). Nonstructural protein is generally restricted to the nucleus and binds to DNA (47). Nickase, helicase, and endonuclease activities have been assigned to nonstructural protein of adenoassociated virus (48), but the nonstructural protein genes do not share homology with known cellular toxins or pore-forming proteins. Parvovirus nonstructural protein(s) are pleiotropic: they are required for parvovirus replication (49), including resolution of the terminal hairpin structures (50), and the gene also contains negative regulatory elements for replication (49). They are needed for RNA transcription (51, 52). Nonstructural proteins function as enhancer elements for the parvovirus structural gene promoter (53) and their own promoter (54), and they are required for excision of the parvovirus genome from transfecting plasmid (55). They may "lead" the DNA strand into the preformed capsid (56). The nonstructural proteins also cause host cell death (57,58): they can suppress heterologous promoter function (59), and they are the mediators of parvovirus "oncosuppressive" effects in a variety of cell culture systems (60,61). Some cells may be "resistant" to nonstructural protein toxic effects (58,62). Mutation and deletion analysis of the nonstructural protein gene have not allowed separation or assignment of the protein's functions to specific regions, and multiple activities can be abolished with an appropriate single amino acid substitution (51).

## Structural Proteins

The 2–3 capsid proteins are derived from overlapping reading frames and thus share substantial amino acid identity; for example, in B19 parvovirus, the minor capsid protein differs from the major capsid protein by an additional 227 amino acids at the amino terminus. By convention, the longest and least abundant minor capsid species is denoted VP1, and the shorter major capsid protein(s) is denoted VP2 (a VP3 is present in other parvoviruses). The virion is composed of 60 capsid proteins, 5–10% of which are VP1 and the remainder VP2. The structural proteins appear to have functions beyond simply providing the housing for viral DNA in a capsid. Tissue specificity for minute virus of mice (which has fibroblastotropic and lymphotropic strains) maps between mu 68 and 73 within the capsid protein genes (63–65), and for canine and feline parvoviruses, host range specificity has been mapped to a few nucleotide substitutions between mu 59 and 73 (66). The canine-feline differences are located on the virus surface in exposed loop regions and may affect binding (67). For murine parvovirus, tissue tropism is determined in the nucleus (68), suggesting multiple functional effects for the structural as well as nonstructural proteins.

With the recent solution at the atomic level of the structure of canine parvovirus, the three-dimensional organization of capsid proteins in the virion has been determined in detail (Fig. 3) (69). The central structural core motif of eight antiparallel $\beta$-pleated sheets is that of many other DNA and RNA viruses of the same size and symmetry. An unusual feature is the large protrusion on the threefold axes. The threefold axis forms a spike on the surface made up of VP2 loop regions that are important as antigen recognition sites for neutralizing antibodies. There are deep canyons about the fivefold axes that may represent, by analogy with other viruses, binding sites for receptors (70); alternatively, viral attachment protein may be a spike projection or even a disordered loop (see later) (71).

## Taxonomy

The classification of the family Parvoviridae is based on morphology and functional characteristics. The family is divided into three genuses. The insect parvoviruses occupy one genus, *Densovirus*. Most vertebrate disease-causing parvoviruses are autonomous parvoviruses (genus *Parvovirus*), meaning that they replicate in the absence of helper virus. Adenoassociated viruses occupy the third genus, *Dependovirus*, and require coinfection of target cells with adenovirus or herpesviruses for replication. The adenoassociated viruses infect human tissue culture cells and also human beings, but they appear to be entirely nonpathogenic (72). Adenoassociated viruses remain latent in the absence of helper virus, and in some cell lines they have the remarkable

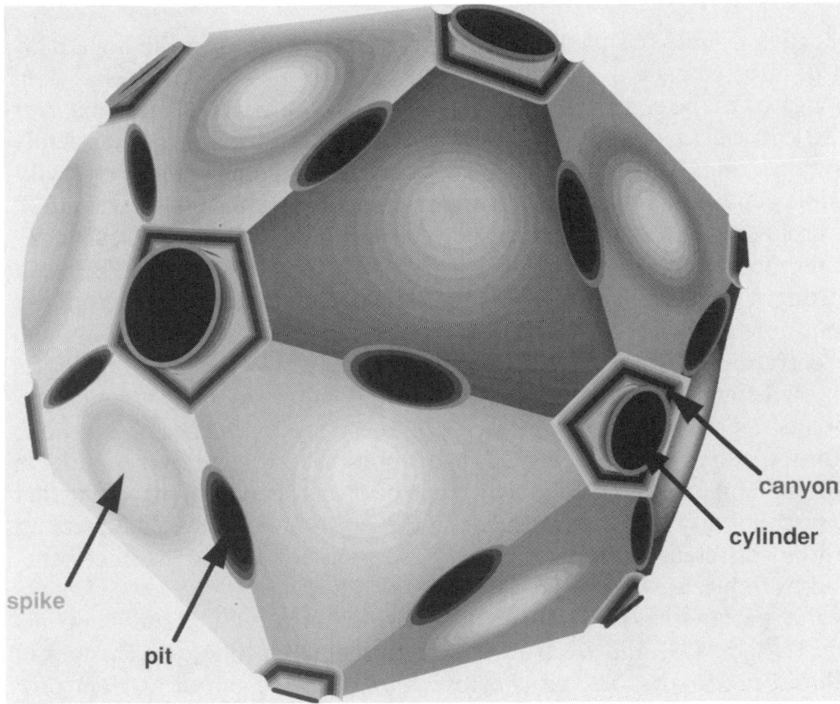


**Figure 3** Surface structure of canine parvovirus. (After Ref. 69.)

property of site-specific integration into chromosome 19 (73). One hypothesis is that the autonomous parvoviruses evolved from a defective parvovirus, originally a cellular transposon that functioned by interfering with viral infections (74). Perhaps consistent with this theory is the rather strange discovery that human herpesvirus 6 carried a portion of the nonstructural protein gene of adenoassociated virus (75). Sequence homology suggests that B19 parvovirus, minute virus of mice, and adenoassociated virus are equally different from each other and presumably separated at about the same evolutionary point in time (8). B19 parvovirus behaves like an autonomous parvovirus and is now classified in the genus *Parvovirus*, but its genomic organization and extremely limited tissue host range suggest a close relationship also to the adenoassociated viruses.

## B19 PARVOVIRUS

### B19 in Cell Culture

B19 parvovirus is extraordinarily tropic for human erythroid cells. Viral replication occurs at high levels only in erythroid progenitor cells (9), and replicative double-stranded DNA forms can be detected in the bone marrow of infected patients (76–78). In tissue culture, B19 parvovirus has been propagated in the erythroid cells of human bone marrow (79) and fetal liver (80,81), in cells from a patient with erythroleukemia that were transiently maintained in culture (82), and, most recently, in a human megakaryocytoblastoid cell line derived from a patient with leukemia and called UT-7 (62). Erythroid colony formation by the late erythroid progenitor cell, the CFU-E, and the more primitive erythroid progenitor, the burst-forming unit (BFU-E), is strongly inhibited by virus, but myelopoiesis, granulocyte-macrophage colony formation by the CFU-GM progenitor, is unaffected even by high concentrations of virus (83–85). The susceptibility of marrow cells increases with erythroid differentiation (86), and in all culture systems virus propagation is dependent on the presence of the erythroid cell-specific hormone erythropoietin. In the cell line UT-7, adaptation to growth over months in erythropoietin is required before virus can be propagated (62), suggesting that cell susceptibility to virus is related to the hormone's sustained effects on erythroid differentiation, not to the more transient alterations in cell metabolism induced by hormone exposure.

B19 parvovirus is directly cytotoxic to the host cell and induces characteristic light (79) and electron (87) microscopic morphologic changes in erythroid precursors. The virus cytopathic effect is manifest as giant pronormoblasts, first recognized by Owren in 1948 in the bone marrow of patients with transient aplastic crisis (88) and reproduced by tissue culture infection (79). Giant pronormoblasts are early erythroid cells with a diameter of about 25–32 $\mu$m, nuclear inclusions or multiple nucleoli, and cytoplasmic vacuolization; these cells are scattered throughout the aspirate smear of infected bone marrow and are striking in their disproportionate size (Fig. 4). The number of giant pronormoblasts in a specimen roughly corresponds to the virus content, but giant pronormoblasts themselves may not contain detectable B19 viral capsid proteins. Later, erythroid cells are absent from infected tissue culture or clinical specimens, and there may also be subtle dysplastic alterations in myeloid and megakaryocytic cells. Infected late erythroid progenitors from tissue culture inoculations show cytopathic ultrastructural changes on electron microscopy, including characteristic margination of chromatin, pseudopod formation, vacuolization, and capsid particles in lacunae within the nuclear chromatin (Fig. 5).

Virus toxicity is the result of expression of the single nonstructural protein of the virus. Cotransfection of the nonstructural protein gene and a selectable gene (antibiotic resistance) into certain nonpermissive cells abrogates colony formation of these cells in selective media (57). On the other hand, cell lines can express the parvovirus capsid proteins without any effect on cell proliferation (89). Limited expression of the nonstructural protein gene

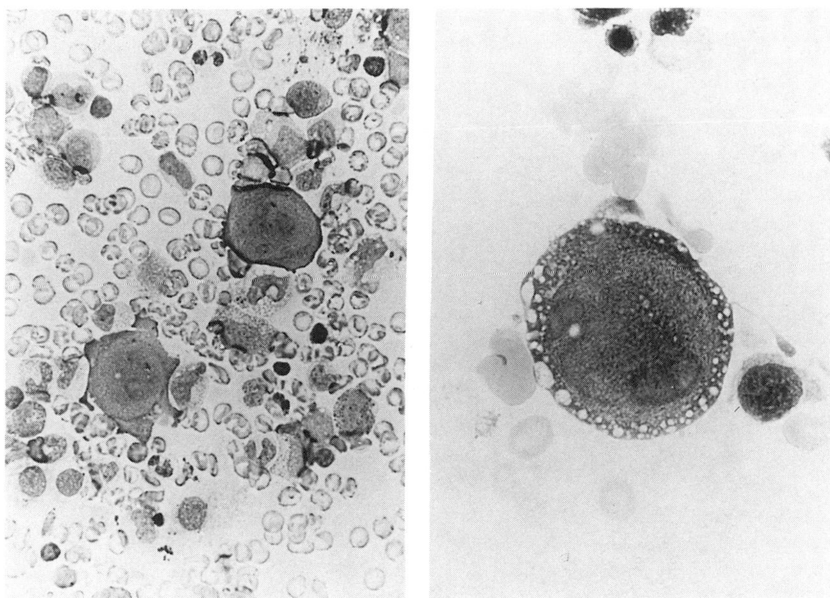

**Figure 4** Giant pronormoblasts in marrow aspirate smears from patients infected with B19 parvovirus.

may explain the inhibition of myelopoiesis and megakaryocytopoiesis in patients in the absence of virus replication in these cells. In vitro, B19 parvovirus depresses megakaryocytic colony formation; although replication of virus is not detectable by Southern analysis, there is low-level expression of RNA in these cells, and mutations within the nonstructural protein gene abrogate the inhibitory effect of virus on platelet progenitors (90).

## DNA Structure and Replication

Replication of parvovirus single-stranded DNA is initiated from brief, short double-stranded regions contained in self-annealing, terminal hairpin structures. For B19 parvovirus DNA, which is 5.6 kb in total length, DNA synthesis proceeds from the long palindromes to produce high-molecular-weight intermediates through a rolling hairpin model similar to that proposed for replication of eukaryotic chromosomal DNA (91). Parvovirus DNA replicative intermediates correspond to duplexes equivalent to two- or threefold the original single-stranded template; replicative intermediates can be distinguished from in vitro annealed duplexes because the covalent link between

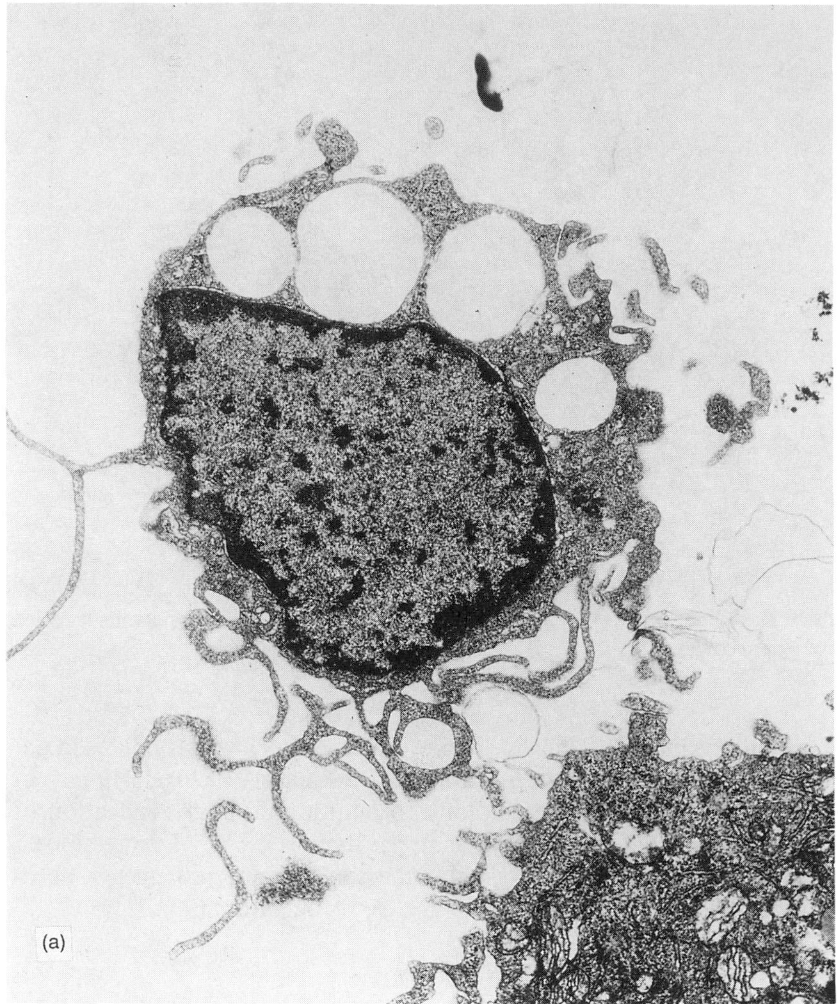


**Figure 5** Electron micrograph of an early erythroid precursor infected in vitro with B19 parvovirus showing margination of nuclear chromatin, vacuolization, and pseudopod formation in the cytoplasm. Virus particles are present in lancunae within the marginated chromatin.

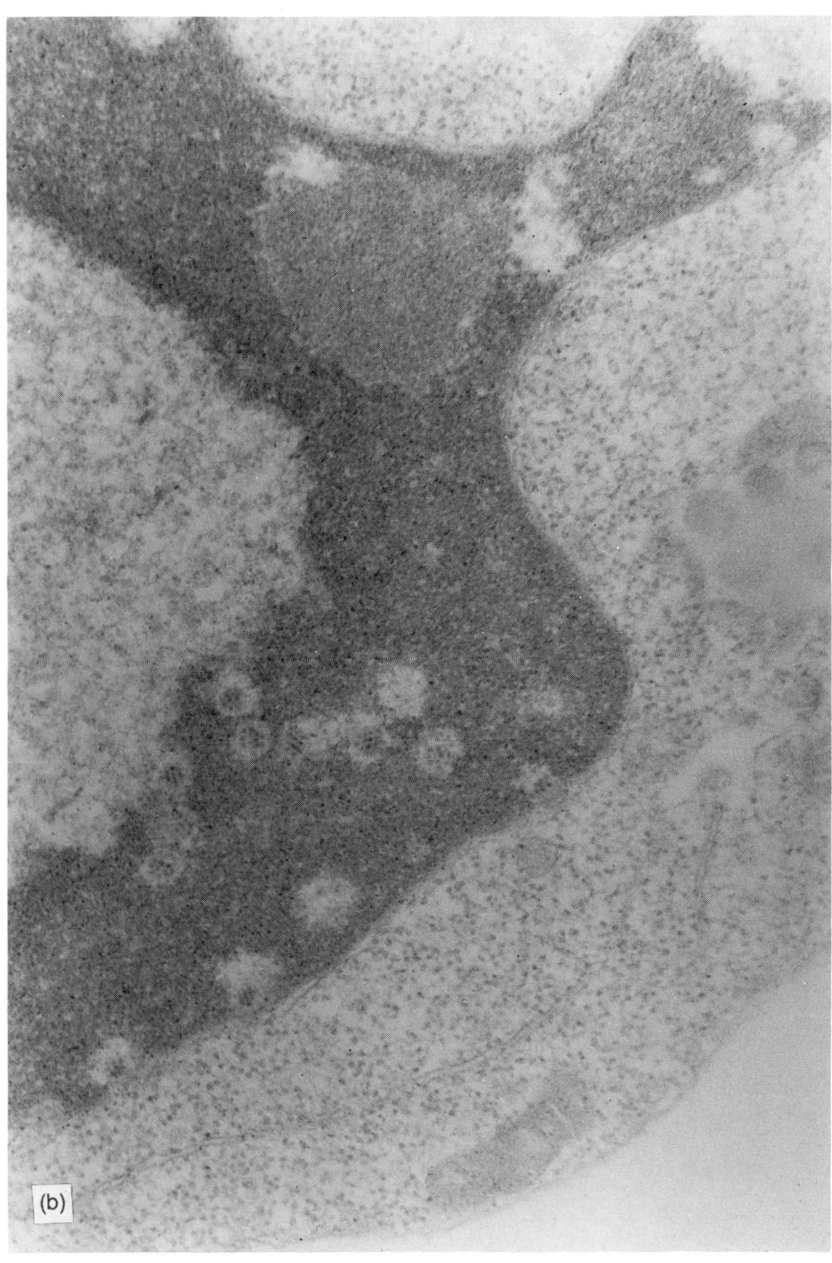
(b)

their strands allows "snapback" rather than simple separation of the double-stranded DNA structure after heating and quench cooling (9). High-molecular-weight parvovirus replicative intermediates can be detected directly by Southern analysis of DNA extracted under low salt conditions or after restriction enzyme digestion of DNA extracted with normal salt concentrations; asymmetric fragments are obtained after *Bam*HI digestion, resulting in characteristic doublets on electrophoresis and hybridization (Fig. 6). DNA analysis thus allows analysis for both the presence and propagation of parvovirus in tissue culture and clinical samples.

Late events in parvovirus DNA replication include exonuclease cleavage of the large DNAs, resolution of the hairpin structures, and packaging of the newly synthesized DNA single strands into capsids. Binding of cellular proteases and parvovirus nonstructural proteins to DNA are involved in these processes for animal parvoviruses and in adenoassociated virus, but the mechanics of these events have not been determined for B19 parvovirus in erythroid target cells.

## RNA Transcription

The scheme of DNA replication of B19 parvovirus is broadly similar to that of other autonomous parvoviruses, but the pattern of RNA transcription

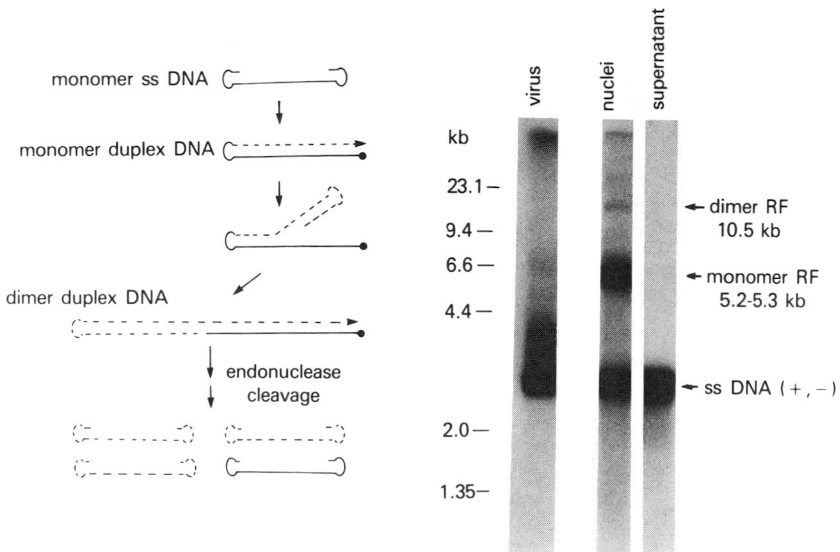


**Figure 6** Southern analysis of DNA from erythroid cells infected with B19 parvovirus. High-molecular-weight replicating monomers and dimers are present in the nuclei but not in the cytosol or supernatant of cultures, which contain only virions.

for B19 parvovirus sets it apart from most of the other Parvoviridae (Fig. 7). B19 parvovirus transcription is unusual in several important features (1) the large number of transcripts, (2) the extent of splicing and the large size of the introns removed, (3) the failure to coterminate all transcripts at the far right side of the genome, (4) the use of unusual polyadenylation signals for termination of transcripts in the middle of the genome, (5) the use of a single strong promoter at the far left side (at map unit 6, thus termed $P_6$), with an accompanying leader sequence to initiate transcription of all RNA species (Fig. 8). A TATA box exists in the middle of the genome, but these sequences do not represent a functional promoter either in bone marrow tar-

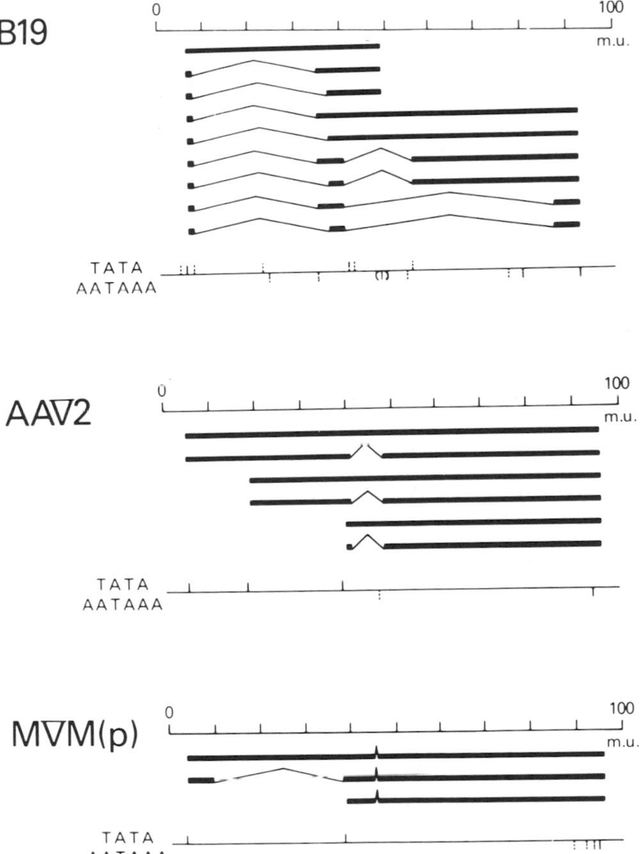


**Figure 7** Comparison of the transcription maps of representative parvovirus species. B19 is unusual in the large number of transcripts, abundant splicing, absence of a middle promoter, and failure of all transcripts to coterminate at the far right side of the genome.

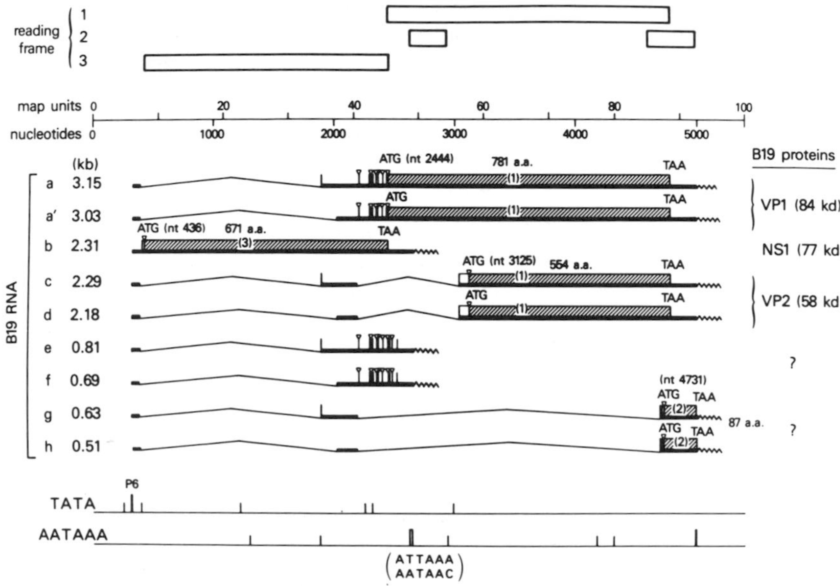


**Figure 8** Transcription map of B19 parvovirus. Nonstructural protein is encoded by the only unspliced RNA species from the left side of the genome. Unusual polyadenylation signals are utilized in the middle of the genome. Structural protein transcripts are located on the right side of the genome and encoded by overlapping RNAs in the same reading frame. Smaller peptides have been identified from the shortest RNA sequences, but their function, if any, is unknown (94).

gets or transfected cells (92,93). B19 parvovirus is thus denied the use of multiple promoters and enhancer elements in the regulation of transcript abundance. Although the parvovirus transcription map was considered unique on its discovery, bovine parvovirus and some Aleutian disease virus strains may also function by using a single promoter.

## Tissue Tropism of B19 Parvovirus

Permissivity, the ability of some cells to support B19 parvovirus propagation, may be tied to mRNA processing. In permissive erythroid progenitor cells, the major RNA species that accumulate not surprisingly encode the capsid proteins (92) [also abundant are short RNA species that encode small peptides of unknown function (94)]. The nonstructural protein gene transcript, the only unspliced RNA species, is relatively sparse in erythroid cells propagating parvovirus. In contrast, when the B19 parvovirus genome is tranfected into nonpermissive cell lines, the pattern of RNA transcription is altered so that the nonstructural protein transcript is overrepresented (95). A functional "block" in virus transcription in these nonpermissive cells can be demonstrated and localized to the middle of the parvovirus genome by RNAase protection experiments, and conversely, removal of about a kilobase of sequence from this region increases read-through transcription from the far right side of the genome (Fig. 9) (95). Attenuator sequences located downstream of parvovirus promoters have been demonstrated for rodent parvoviruses (96), and these results with B19 parvovirus suggest the possibility that, during evolution of the virus, a functional attenuator for the mid-

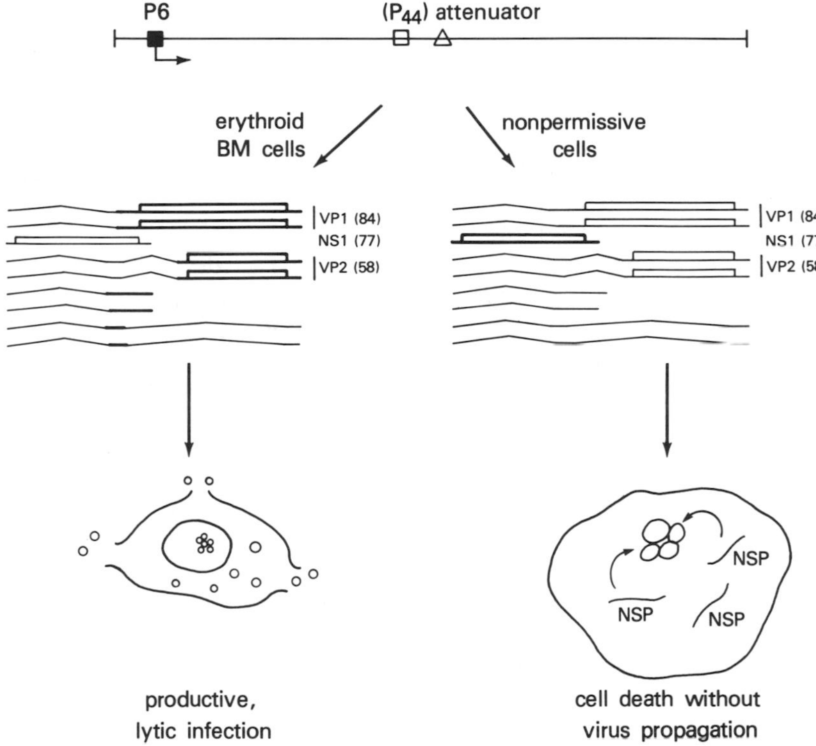


**Figure 9** Two routes to cell death after B19 parvovirus infection. Permissive cells allow full-length transcription of both the nonstructural and the capsid gene RNAs. Capsid RNAs are the predominant RNA species in erythroid cells. Nonpermissive cells have a functional RNA processing block in the middle of the genome that results in relative overexpression of nonstructural protein RNA and cell death without viral propagation.

dle promoter was retained while the promoter activity itself was lost. Qualitatively unique or quantitatively more abundant cellular transcription factors present in erythroid cells would explain the ability of the virus to propagate in these hematopoietic cells; predominant transcription of the nonstructural protein gene in nonpermissive cells would explain virus reduction of megakaryocytic progenitor number in vitro and platelets and white cell levels in infected persons in the absence of the ability of the virus to productively infect these cells.

Determination of B19 tissue trophism by RNA processing would be a unique mechanism among the parvoviruses. Tropism is regulated differently in other species of the family. The minute virus of mice has two strains of virus that exclusively infect either fibroblasts or lymphocytes. In the nonpermissive host cell, replication proceeds to dimers but no further (97), implicating an intranuclear factor required for completion of the processing of DNA to infectious monomers. For canine and feline parvoviruses, species specificity is apparently determined by binding to host cell surface receptors (67).

The presence of only one promoter and the extensive use of splicing suggest that much of the molecular regulation of B19 parvovirus occurs at the level of RNA. A further example concerns the control of the relative quantities of the minor and major capsid proteins, which are derived from overlapping sequences on the right side of the genome. Multiple upstream AUG codons are present before the authentic transcription initiation codon, and these spurious triplets reduce the efficiency of translation. The upstream AUG codons are removed by splicing of the VP2 RNA, greatly improving translation of the major capsid protein (98).

## CLINICAL SYNDROMES

### Fifth Disease

Acute infection with B19 parvovirus causes the childhood exanthem fifth disease (erythema infectiosum) (23,99,100). Children with fifth disease are usually not very ill. The characteristic rash—the "slapped cheek" facial erythema and a lacy, reticular, evanescent maculopapular eruption over the trunk and proximal extremities—combined with extreme contagion allow recognition of parvovirus infection in the individual patient and of the epidemic in the community (Fig. 10). Adults with fifth disease more commonly than children suffer joint paints or frank arthritis than a rash, and symptoms that mimic rheumatoid arthritis (101,102) or fibromyalgia (103) can occasionally persist for months, even years. Desquamation of the palms and soles in association with arthritis has been described (104). Acute parvovirus infec-

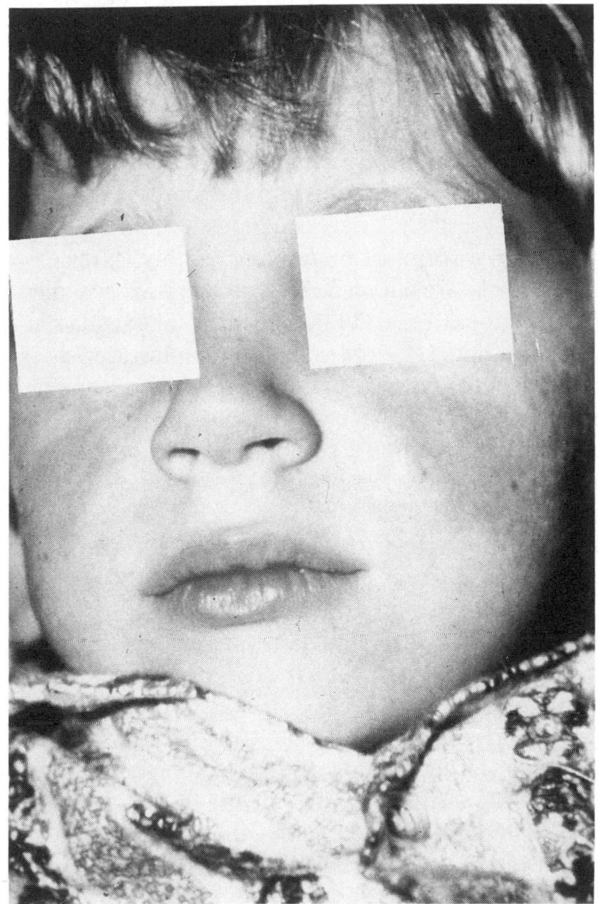

**Figure 10** "Slapped cheek" rash in a child with typical erythema infectiosum. (Photograph courtest of Dr. Mary Anderson.)

tion in adults is more frequently asymptomatic or results only in a nonspecific flulike illness (105).

## Transient Aplastic Crisis

This was the first B19 parvovirus illness identified, and the clear clinical relationship between acute virus infection and a specific form of marrow failure led to hematologists' interest in this pathogen. In persons with underlying hemolysis, acute parvovirus infection causes transient aplastic crisis, an abrupt cessation of erythropoiesis characterized by reticulocytopenia, absent erythroid precursors in the bone marrow, and precipitous worsening of anemia. The aregenerative quality of anemic crisis was recognized quite early from observations of hereditary spherocytosis in large Scandinavian kindreds (106), later appreciated also for other persons with underlying hemolysis (107). Owren introduced the term "aplastic crisis," and he stressed the relationship of anemic crisis to preceding infection and the temporary quality of red cell failure (88). Transient aplastic crisis occurs as a unique event in the life of patients with a variety of forms of underlying hemolysis (reviewed in Ref. 108), not only sickle cell disease but also congenital erythrocyte membrane defects (109,110), enzymopathies (111,112), and thalassemias and acquired hemolytic anemias in adults (113,114). Transient aplastic crisis can also occur under conditions of erythroid stress, such as hemorrhage and iron deficiency (115,116), and following bone marrow transplantation (117,118). In retrospect, parvovirus infection was almost certainly responsible for cases of transient erythropoietic failure that were blamed on kwashiorkor (119, 120), folic acid deficiency (121,122), some drugs (especially immunosuppressive agents), and bacterial infections (123,124). It is not accidental that many of the reported cases of aplastic crisis occurred in hospitalized patients, because the virus can be transmitted nosocomially (125,126). Parvovirus infection was likely responsible for cases of aplastic anemia (five of six of which occurred in sickle cell patients and were restricted to anemia only) that once were imputed to glue sniffing (127).

Although suffering from an ultimately self-limited illness, the patient with an aplastic crisis may be acutely and profoundly ill. Symptoms can include not only dyspnea and fatigue due to severe anemia but extreme lassitude, confusion, and congestive heart failure; death can occur. The anemia of transient aplastic crisis is readily treated by blood transfusion. Rarely, transient aplastic crisis may be complicated by bone marrow necrosis (128, 129). Transient pancytopenia (130–132) and a case of typical severe aplastic anemia (134) have been reported to follow acute parvovirus infection. Pancytopenia with hemophagocytosis, which can occur after many different viral infections, also has been reported following parvovirus infection (134). B19 parvovirus infection may worsen anemia in African children with malaria (135).

Transient aplastic crisis (77,136,137), as well as experimental parvovirus infection in humans (138), is often associated with variable degrees of neutropenia and thrombocytopenia; cases of idiopathic thrombocytopenic purpura and Henoch-Schönlein purpura (139,140) have apparently followed acute parvovirus infection. Thrombocytopenia may occasionally be the most prominent clinical feature of acute parvovirus infection (141), and serologic evidence of recent virus has been reported in some cases of idiopathic thrombocytopenic purpura of childhood (140,142–144) (but both this syndrome and IgM antibody to parvovirus are not uncommon in pediatric populations).

Community-acquired aplastic crisis is almost always due to parvovirus infection (145–148). B19 parvovirus should be the presumptive diagnosis in transient aplastic crisis and sought in any patient with anemia due to an abrupt cessation of erythropoiesis: aplastic crisis may be the first evidence of heriditary spherocytosis in a patient with compensated hemolysis (144,150). Patients with transient aplastic crisis are often viremic at presentation, with concentrations of viral genomes as high as $10^{14}$ $ml^{-1}$ as determined by DNA dot-blot hybridization of serum (151,152); IgM antibody appears during the first week of convalescence and is a specific indicator of recent infection (153). Testing for IgG antibody is not helpful, since IgG to parvovirus is present in about 50% of the adult population, and IgG may not be present in early serum specimens in transient aplastic crisis. Both IgG and IgM antibody to parvovirus can be measured in capture immunoassays (2).

Transient erythroblastopenia of childhood—temporary red cell failure production in very young children without underlying hemololysis—is almost certainly postviral in etiology but is not generally associated with serologic evidence of recent B19 parvovirus infection (154); the few cases assigned a B19 etiology (115,155) may be distinguished by associated mild thrombocytopenia and neutropenia (156,157).

## Hydrops Fetalis due to B19 Parvovirus

In utero infection is a cause of nonimmune hydrops fetalis, in which death occurs as a result of severe anemia (Fig. 11) (158,159). Hydropic infants, born of mothers infected with parvovirus, have similar pathologic features, including leukoerythroblastosis, iron deposition in the liver, and viral cytopathic alterations of erythroblasts in the liver; virus has been demonstrated by DNA hybridization and immunofluorecence for protein, mainly in the liver (160,161). The risk of a fatal outcome for the fetus is probably greatest if infection occurs during the first two trimesters, but although the probability of stillbirth has not been quantitated, it almost certainly is low: in one series of 170 reported cases of seroconversion during pregnancy, only a small minority have resulted in stillborn deliveries, including some cases in which the umbilical cord blood tested positive for IgM antibody to parvovirus (158). An increased risk of spontaneous abortion during the first trimester has been investigated in several large epidemiologic surveys; estimates of fetal death range from 5% (162)–9% (163) of infected women.

There have been a few congenital physical malformations associated with intrauterine parvovirus infection, either prospectively or in retrospective analysis of banked fetal tissue. One incomplete embryo at 9 weeks of

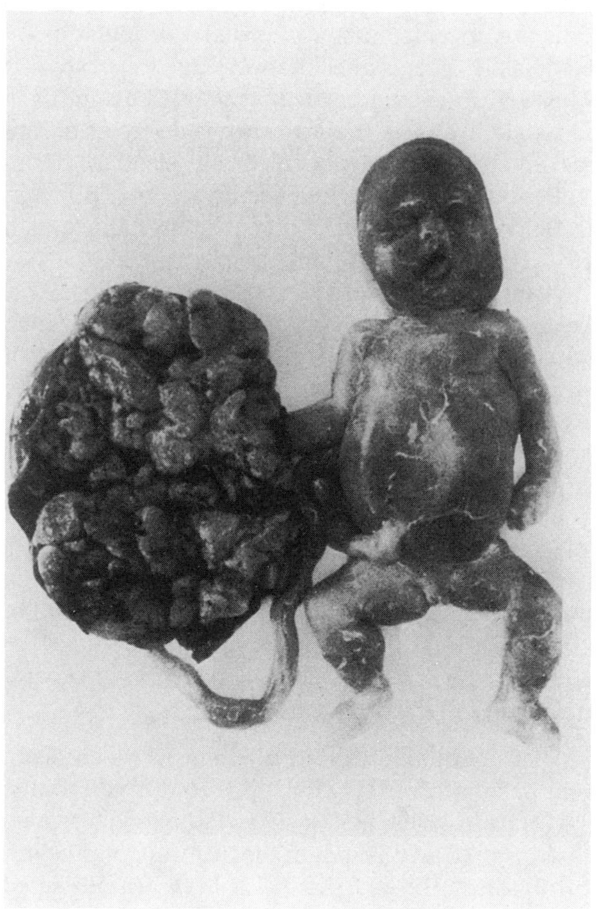

**Figure 11** Hydropic fetus and placenta after intrauterine B19 parvovirus infection. (From Ref. 205.)

development showed widespread vascular endothelial cell damage with associated T cell infiltrates, abnormal eye formation, and degenerative changes of skeletal and cardiac muscle; the mother had a viral arthralgia and elevated IgM antibody to B19 parvovirus earlier in pregnancy, and there were typical cytopathic changes in the fetus cells of parvovirus infection (164). Viral infection of myocardial cells was shown by in situ hybridization at autopsy of one hydropic infant (165) and advanced liver disease in another (166), and immune thrombocytopenia was observed in a third viremic newborn (167).

The overall risk of a poor outcome to pregnancy is probably low, but the concern of the potentially exposed pregnant mother is not. Parvovirus infection is extremely contagious. Pregnant women are commonly exposed to fifth disease through other children in the household, at schools and day-care centers, and, among nursing and medical personnel, by caring for persistently infected patients. About half of the pregnant population has acquired protective immunity, as determined by assay for IgG antibody to parvovirus. Evidence of seroconversion should be sought in IgG women. Hydrops can be detected by ultrasound, and treatment of a suspected hydropic infant with intrauterine red blood cell transfusion has been reported (168). The usefulness of this type of intervention, or of the administration of commercial immunoglobulins containing antiparvovirus antibodies as prophylaxis or treatment, needs to be determined.

## Congenital Infection

Parvovirus infection of the fetus need not be fatal but may persist after birth (167,169). We have studied an infant born with chronic anemia and susceptible to frequent infections; there was a history of maternal exposure to parvovirus during pregnancy and hydrops at birth. Congenital infection is distinctive among parvovirus syndromes by the low level of viral infection: virus can be detected in the bone marrow by gene amplification but does not circulate. Presumably, infection early in ontogeny allows more efficient suppression of red cell production than infection of a mature marrow. Our case terminated fatally, and virus was present in other tissues obtained at autopsy, including thymus, brain, heart, liver, and spleen, suggesting the possibility of congenital malformation of other organ systems as a result of B19 parvovirus infection in utero. Exposure of the fetal immune system to virus early in pregnancy is also predicted to result in tolerance to the capsid proteins and absence of an antibody response despite continued virus production.

## Persistent Infection

Patients with persistent B19 parvovirus infection have pure red cell aplasia. Persistently infected patients have failed to mount a neutralizing antibody response to the virus, and they lack the immune complex-mediated symptoms of fifth disease, fever, rash, and polyarthralgia and polyarthritis. Persistent parvovirus infection and pure red cell aplasia have been documented in four patient populations: congenital immunodeficiency (Nezelof's syndrome) (76,170), children with lymphoblastic leukemia and other similar malignancies in remission on chemotherapy (78,171–176), patients with the acquired immunodeficiency syndrome (177,178), and recipients of solid organ transplants (Antunez de Mayolo and Young, unpublished observations) (179). However, defective antibody production also occurs in other diseases associated with pure red cell aplasia, like chronic lymphocytic leukemia and malignancies treated with cytotoxic drugs, and some of these cases may also represent occult viral infection [since parvovirus infection has likely been unrecognized previously in the acquired immunodeficiency syndrome (AIDS) (180) and leukemia (181)].

Clinically, the anemia is severe and the patients are dependent on erythrocyte transfusions. There may be associated intermittent neutropenia (76), and in one case the major hematologic manifestation of persistent parvovirus infection was recurrent agranulocytosis (182). The bone marrow should contain some giant pronormoblasts, the cytopathic sign of parvovirus infection, although these are infrequent. The anemia may be intermittent, with periods of relapse associated with the viremia and remission with spontaneous disappearance of virus from the circulation, possibly due to depletion of the erythroid target cell population. The diagnosis is established by detection of B19 parvovirus genome in the serum, blood, or bone marrow cells by dot-blot hybridization; polymerase chain reaction amplification of viral DNA may be necessary in rare cases (183). Antibodies to parvovirus, as determined in immunoassays or enzyme-linked immunosorbent assay (ELISA), are not present in most patients, but a pattern of antibody response suggestive of early infection (IgM antibody and IgG antibody directed to the major capsid protein) may be found in patients with congenital immunodeficiency (184). A poor reaction on immunoblot testing is a consistent finding and correlates with poor neutralizing activity for the virus in erythroid colony assays (184). It should be stressed that persistent parvovirus infection may be the dominant manifestation of some inherited immunodeficient states.

Effective therapy consists of infusion of commercial immunoglobulin preparations, which are a good source of neutralizing antibodies because most of the adult population has been exposed to the virus. The best treatment regimen has not been established. One patient with congenital immunodeficiency was cured by a 10 day course followed by intermittent injections until virus disappeared from his serum (177). Patients with AIDS respond to a 5–10 day course but may relapse some months later; they can respond to a second course (177); in an occasional patient, virus may disappear from the circulation and yet anemia persist (185). Patients with AIDS have had very high virus serum concentrations, comparable to levels in acute infection of transient aplastic crisis and many orders of magnitude higher than in other patients with chronic parvovirus infection (177). Measurement of serum virus is helpful in predicting relapse and may assist in determining optimal treatment.

## IMMUNE RESPONSE

### Normal Humoral Response

Both virus-specific IgM and IgG antibodies are made following experimental (138) and natural (153) B19 parvovirus infection (Fig. 12). Following intranasal inoculation of volunteers, virus can first be detected at days 5–6 and levels peak at days 8–9. Virus is rarely detected in patients with clinical fifth disease, probably because the manifestations are secondary to immune complex formation and patients therefore present to medical attention after the period of viremia has passed. In patients with transient aplastic crisis, $10^8$–$10^{14}$ genome copies per ml of virus DNA may circulate (151,152). IgM antibody to virus appears about 10–12 days after experimental inoculation; IgM antibody may be present in patients with transient aplastic crisis at the time of reticulocyte nadir and during the subsequent 10 days. IgG antibody appears in normal volunteers about 2 weeks after inoculation; in patients with transient aplastic crisis, IgG is not present at the time of reticulocyte depression but appears rapidly with recovery. IgM antibody may be found in serum samples for several months after exposure (12). IgG presumably persists for life, and levels rise with reexposure (138). IgA antibodies to B19 parvovirus can also be detected and presumably play a role in protection against infection by the natural nasopharyngeal route (Anderson, personal communication).

A humoral immune response to B19 parvovirus is much more readily measured than a cellular response, but antibody appears to have a dominant role in containing parvovirus infection apart from these possibly technical considerations. Not only does normal recovery from infection correlate with the appearance of circulating specific antivirus antibody, but administration of commercial immunoglobulins can cure or ameliorate persistent parvovirus infection in immunodeficient patients (see later).

### Cellular Immune Response

Patients with persistent parvovirus infection suffer T cell as well as B cell immune deficits, and a cellular component to the normal immune response to parvovirus must exist. However, attempts to measure peripheral blood lymphocyte proliferation in response to free parvovirus antigen have been unsuccessful (184).

T cell responses have been examined for several other animal parvoviruses. Rat parvovirus persists in athymic neonatal animals (186). For canine parvovirus, delayed hypersensitivity responses can be positively transferred by lymphocytes exposed to virus in vitro, and T cells proliferate and secrete interleukin-2 in response to soluble viral antigen (187). Some T cell epitopes

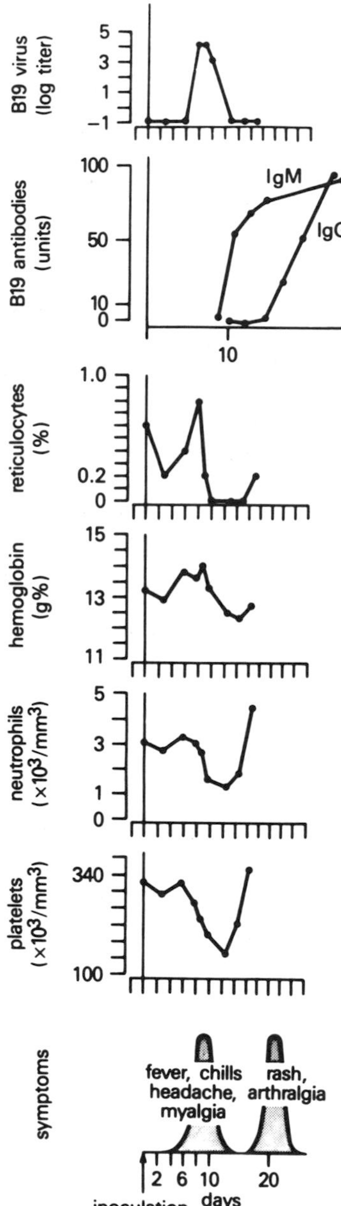


**Figure 12** Virologic, immunologic, and clinical course after B19 infection in a normal host. (Adapted from Ref. 138 with permission of Dr. Mary Anderson.)

of canine parvovirus have been mapped to the major capsid protein (187). For Aleutian disease virus, lymphocyte responses to virus have been measured only transiently or late in the course of the disease, and they may represent pathologic phenomena (188,189). For B19 parvovirus, more subtle experiments may be required to document a T cell response to virus, including measurement of lymphokine production in response to viral antigen or analysis of lymphocyte proliferation on presentation of cell-bound virus antigen in the appropriate histocompatibility protein context.

Many animal parvoviruses infect lymphocytes in vivo and replicate in immune system cells like lymphocytes and macrophages in vitro, including the lymphotrophic strain of minute virus of mice (190), porcine parvovirus (191), feline panleukopenia virus (192), and Aleutian disease virus (38). Lymphocyte infection by parvoviruses, as in retrovirus infection, may compromise immune function by direct cytotoxicity for the target cell or altered function of persistently infected viable cells (191). These considerations may be relevant to B19 parvovirus, in which persistent infection has been linked to subtle clinical syndromes of congenital immunodeficiency (see later).

## B Cell Neutralizing Epitopes

Several regions containing neutralizing epitopes have been localized to linear sequences of B19 parvovirus: one region at the amino terminus of VP2 at amino acids 38–87 (193) and six others distributed within the carboxyl terminal half of VP2 [amino acids 253–272, 309–330, 328–344, 359–382, 449–468, and 491–515 (194,195)]; neutralizing epitopes are also found in the unique region of VP1 (196). Some of the neutralizing epitopes of VP2, by analogy with the three-dimensional structure of canine parvovirus (69), would correspond to external loops of the protein present on the virus surface as major protrusions or spikes (Fig. 13) (196). Anti-VP2 antibodies directed against sequences in the $\beta$ barrel central structure are produced in animals immunized with VP2-only containing empty capsids, but these antibodies fail to neutralize virus activity (Rosenfeld, Young, and Saxinger, unpublished data). Addition of VP1 to the capsid has two effects: it allows presentation of the spike to the immune system and adds its own intrinsic neutralizing sequences. Antisera raised to the unique region of VP1, 227 amino acids at the amino terminus, precipitate empty capsids and virions, indicating that the unique region is expressed on the virus surface, and these antibodies also neutralize virus activity (196). Both anti-VP2 and anti-VP1 specificities are present in normal human covalescent antisera, and sera that predominate in either one or the other specificity both effectively neutralize virus; however, VP1 is the major antigen recognized on immunoblot by late convalescent phase antiserum or in commercial immunoglobulin preparations (184).

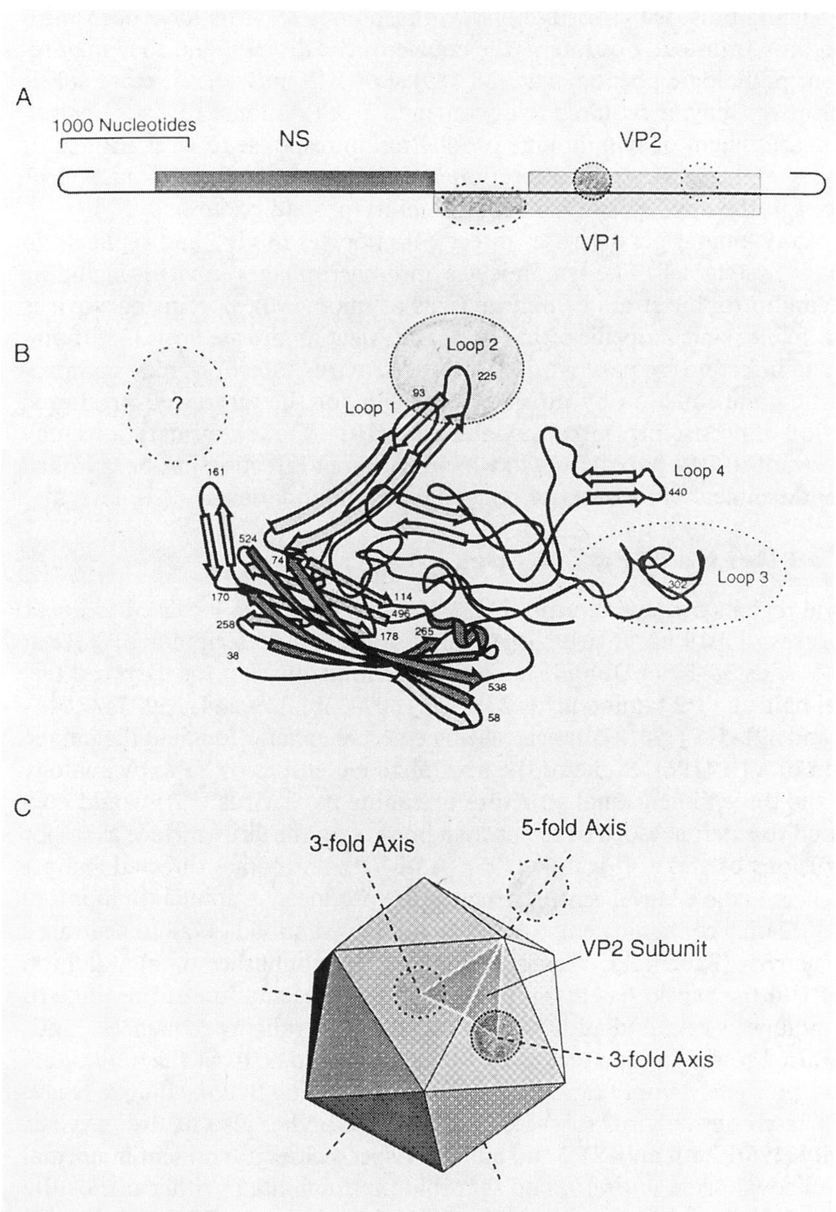


**Figure 13** Some neutralizing epitopes of B19 parvovirus, shown on the genome map of B19 and superimposed, after alignment by homology, on the "road map" of the major capsid protein and the surface structure determined by x-ray crystallography for canine parvovirus (From Ref. 51.)

Only a limited number of linear epitopes have been detected, but the majority of monoclonal antibodies that neutralize B19 parvovirus do not recognize peptide sequences within the capsid proteins and presumably bind to conformationally determined epitopes (193). The structure of B19 parvovirus may be more dynamic than suggested by the static picture presented in x-ray crystallography. Although VP2 contains neutralizing epitopes, as described, these are not presented to the immune system in VP2-only empty capsids (10), suggesting that the conformation of some VP2 determinants, particularly those on the prominent spike, is altered by insertion of one or two VP1 molecules per 60 protein subunit capsid. A further alteration likely occurs with insertion of DNA into empty capsids containing both proteins, because many monoclonal antibodies raised to virions and screened by ELISA fail to recognize VP1 plus VP2 empty capsids in the same test (Yoshimoto, Rosenfeld, Kennedy, and Young, unpublished data).

Persistent B19 parvovirus infection is the result of failure to produce effective neutralizing antibodies by the immunosuppressed host. Perhaps because of the limited epitopes presented to the immune system by B19 parvovirus, the congenital immunodeficiency states associated with persistent infection may be clinically mild, with susceptibility largely restricted to parvovirus, although multiple immune system defects are apparent once directed testing of T and B cell function is performed. Patients with persistent B19 parvovirus testing uniformly lack strong reactions on immunoblot analysis of their sera for antibodies to parvovirus, although congenitally immunodeficient patients may show normal reactivity on ELISA testing for IgG and IgM parvovirus-specific antibodies (184). These results suggest that the linear epitopes detected by immunoblotting are functionally very important, and the clinical findings in persistent infection are analogous to animal data showing the dependence of a neutralizing antibody response on presentation of specific epitopes, particularly the amino-terminal region of the minor capsid protein (discussed earlier).

## Passive Immunity and Vaccine Development

Antibodies play a dominant role in the normal immune response to parvovirus, and antibodies are protective in both passive and active immunizations. Convalescent antiserum can protect puppies against canine parvovirus infection (197), and commercial immunoglobulin from normal donors can cure or ameliorate persistent B19 parvovirus infection in immunosuppressed human patients (170,177). Human convalescent-phase antisera (184) and commercial immunoglobulin preparations (198) contain neutralizing antibodies to parvovirus as assessed in vitro using erythroid colony systems.

Effective vaccines have been produced for animals using attenuated or fixed virus preparations, including feline (33,199–201), canine (33), and porcine (202) parvoviruses. Antisera raised against peptide fragments of canine parvovirus, determined to contain neutralizing epitopes, have also been protective (203). Prospects for a B19 parvovirus vaccine are also good, although the immunogen almost certainly will be a recombinant capsid rather than attenuated or killed virus because of the difficulty of propagating B19 parvovirus in tissue culture and the potential danger of inadvertently modifying, for the worse, the host range of B19 parvovirus by selection in vitro. Recombinant B19 parvovirus capsids produced in baculovirus are suitable for inducing neutralizing antibodies in inoculated animals (10), even in the absence of adjuvant (204). The presence of VP1 protein in the capsid immunogen appears critical for the production of antibodies that neutralize virus activity in vitro: capsids with supernormal VP1 content are more efficient in inducing neutralizing activity in immunized animals, and neutralization correlates with anti-VP1 reactivity on immunoblot (204).

## CONCLUSIONS

The pattern of disease that follows parvovirus infection is the result of balance among virus, marrow target cell, and the immune response (Fig. 14). Bone marrow depression in parvovirus infection occurs during the early viremic phase and under normal conditions is terminated by a neutralizing antibody response. It is the immune response that produces the clinical manifestations of fifth disease, in children usually a rash illness and in adults often a rheumatic syndrome, which occur during the period of antibody formation and are immune complex mediated (fifth disease symptoms can be precipitated by treatment of persistent infection with immunoglobulin). In patients with hyperactive erythropoiesis, large amounts of virus are produced and the immune response may be weak, perhaps resulting in relatively greater quantities of antigen to antibody and little immune complex formation; rash and joint pains are rare in patients with transient aplastic crisis (136). In both persistent infection in children and adults and in utero infection, failure to mount a neutralizing antibody response allows parvovirus to persist and cause chronic anemia (183). In acute infection, the period of viremia is brief, usually 1–3 days, and virus titers are extremely high. In persistent infection, virus can be demonstrated in serum samples obtained months apart; the viral titer is often lower by orders of magnitude, although AIDS patients may have serum concentrations comparable to those seen in acute infection.

The basic biology of B19 parvovirus is well understood and directly relevant to human diseases caused by this agent. B19 parvovirus is cytotoxic to human erythroid target cells, but serious disease results only if the host's erythroid marrow is stressed or host immunity inadequate. The antibody response restricts virus propagation in the human host, and a very limited num-

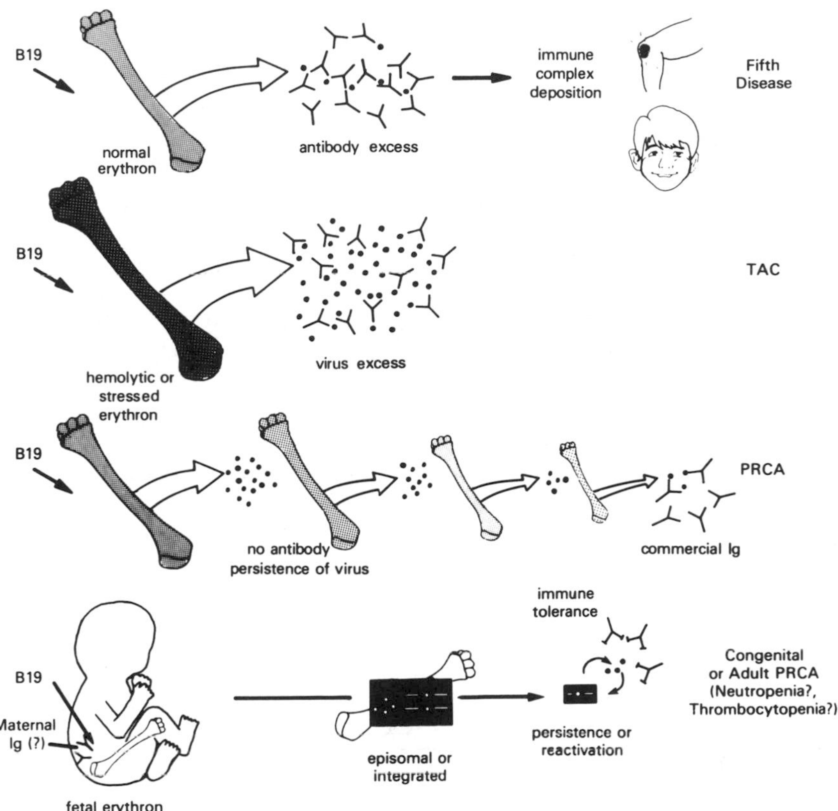


**Figure 14** Pathogenesis of human diseases caused by B19 parvovirus. TAC, transient aplastic crisis; PRCA, pure red cell aplasia.

ber of viral epitopes presented to the immune system may allow the virus to elude some genetically deficient immune systems. Development of recombinant empty capsids should provide a basis for vaccination and prevention of parvovirus disease.

Outstanding and interesting questions remain. What is the exact molecular basis of altered transcription in erythroid cells and its relation to tissue tropism? What is the mechanism of cell death induced by nonstructural protein? What is the cell surface receptor for parvovirus? Experimental approaches to these problems may yield gains in understanding the regulation of transcription, programmed cell death, and oncosuppression.

## REFERENCES

1. Cossart YE, Field AM, Cant B, et al. Parvovirus-like particles in human sera. Lancet 1975; 1:72–3.
2. Cohen BJ, Mortimer PP, Pereira MS. Diagnostic assays with monoclonal antibodies for the human serum parvovirus-like virus (SPLV). J Hyg 1983; 91:113–30.
3. Pattison JR, Jones SE, Hodgson J, et al. Parvovirus infections and hypoplastic crisis in sickle cell anemia. Lancet 1981; 1:664–5.
4. Anderson MJ, Jones SE, Fisher-Hoch SP, et al. Human parvovirus, the cause of erythema infectiosum (fifth disease)? Lancet 1983; 1:1378.
5. Summers J, Jones SE, Anderson MJ. Characterization of the genome of the agent of erythrocyte aplasia permits its classification as a human parvovirus. J Gen Virol 1983; 64:2527–32.
6. Clewley JP. Biochemical characterization of a human parvovirus. J Gen Virol 1984; 65:241–5.
7. Cotmore SF, Tattersall P. Characterization and molecular cloning of a human parvovirus genome. Science 1984; 226:1161–5.
8. Shade RO, Blundell MC, Cotmore SF, Tattersall P, Astell CR. Nucleotide sequence and genome organization of human parvovirus B19 isolated from the serum of a child during aplastic crisis. J Virol 1986; 58:921–36.
9. Ozawa K, Kurtzman G, Young NS. Replication of the B19 parvovirus in human bone marrow cultures. Science 1986; 233:883–6.
10. Kajigaya S, Fujii H, Field AM, et al. Self-assembled B19 parvovirus capsids, produced in a baculovirus system, are antigenically and immunogenically similar to native virions. Proc Natl Acad Sci U S A 1991; 88:4646–50.
11. Anderson MJ, Higgins PG, Davis LR, et al. Experimental parvoviral infection in humans. J Infect Dis 1985; 152:257–65.
12. Anderson LJ, Tsou C, Parker RA, et al. Detection of antibodies and antigens of human parvovirus B19 by enzyme-linked immunosorbent assay. J Clin Microbiol 1986; 24:522–6.
13. Yaegashi N, Shiraishi H, Tada K, Yajima A, Sugamura K. Enzyme-linked immunosorbent assay for IgG and IgM antibodies against human parvovirus B19: use of monoclonal antibodies and viral antigen propagated in vitro. J Virol Methods 1989; 26:171–82.
14. Cohen BJ, Buckley MM. The prevalence of antibody to human parvovirus B19 in England and Wales. J Med Microbiol 1988; 25:151–3.
15. Koch WC, Adler SP. Human parvovirus B19 infections in women of childbearing age and within families. Pediatr Infect Dis J 1989; 8:83–7.
16. Anderson LJ, Torok TJ. The clinical spectrum of human parvovirus B19 infections. Curr Clin Top Infect Dis 1991; 11:267–80.
17. Nascimento JP, Buckley MM, Brown KE, Cohen BJ. The prevalence of antibody to human parvovirus B19 in Rio de Janeiro, Brazil. Rev Inst Med Trop Sào Paulo 1990; 32:41–5.
18. Nunoue T, Okochi K, Mortimer PP, Cohen BJ. Human parvovirus (B19) and erythema infectiosum. J Pediatr 1985; 107:38–40.

19. de Freitas RB, Wong D, Boswell F, et al. Prevalence of human parvovirus (B19) and rubellavirus infections in urban and remote rural areas in northern Brazil. J Med Virol 1990; 32:203–8.
20. Schwarz L, Gurtler LG, Zoulek G, Deinhardt F, Roggendorf M. Seroprevalence of human parvovirus B19 infection. Int J Med Microbiol 1989; 271:231–6.
21. Anderson MJ, Cohen BJ. Human parvovirus B19 infections in United Kingdom 1984–86. Lancet 1987; 1:738–9.
22. Saarinen UM, Chorba TL, Tattersall P et al. Human parvovirus B19-induced epidemic acute red cell aplasia in patients with hereditary hemolytic anemia. Blood 1986; 67:1411–7.
23. Chorba TL, Coccia P, Holman RC, et al. Role of parvovirus B19 in aplastic crisis and erythema infectiosum (fifth disease). J Infect Dis 1986; 154:383–93.
24. Cohen BJ, Field AM, Gudnadottir S, Beard S, Barbara JA. Blood donor screening for parvovirus B19. J Virol Methods 1990; 30:223–38.
25. Plummer AF, Hammond WG, Forward K. An erythema infectiosum-like illness caused by human parvovirus infection. N Engl J Med 1985; 313:74–9.
26. Gillespie SM, Cartter ML, Asch S, et al. Occupational risk of human parvovirus B19 infection for school and day-care personnel during an outbreak of erythema infectiosum. JAMA 1990; 263:2061–5.
27. Mortimer PP, Luban NLC, Kelleher JF, Cohen BJ. Transmission of serum parvovirus-like virus by clotting-factor concentrates. Lancet 1983; 2:482–4.
28. Williams MD, Beddall AC, Pasi KJ, Mortimer PP, Hill FGH. Transmission of human parvovirus B19 by coagulation factor concentrates. Vox Sang 1990; 58: 177–81.
29. Bartolomei Corsi O, Azzi A, Morfini M, Fanci R, Rossi Ferrini P. Human parvovirus infection in hemophiliacs first infused with treated clotting factor concentrates. J Med Virol 1988; 25:165–70.
30. Lyon DJ, Chapman CS, Martin C, et al. Symptomatic parvovirus B19 infection and heat-treated factor IX concentrate. Lancet 1989; 1:1085.
31. Bell LM, Naides SJ, Stoffman P, Hodinka RL, Plotkin SA. Human parvovirus B19 infection among hospital staff members after contact with infected patients. N Engl J Med 1989; 321:485–91.
32. Kurtzman GJ, Platanias L, Lustig L, Frickhofen N, Young NS. Feline parvovirus propagates in cat bone marrow cultures and inhibits hematopoietic colony formation in vitro. Blood 1989; 74:71–81.
33. Parrish CR. Emergence, natural history, and variation of canine, mink, and feline parvoviruses. Adv Virus Res 1990; 38:403–50.
34. Kilham L, Margolis G. Viral etiology of spontaneous ataxia of cats. Am J Pathol 1966; 48:991–1011.
35. Macartney L, McCandlish IAP, Thompson H, Cornwell HJC. Canine parvovirus enteritis 1: clinical, haematological and pathological features of experimental infection. Vet Rec 1984; 115:201–10.
36. O'Sullivan G, Durham PJK, Smith JR, Campbell RSF. Experimentally induced severe canine parvoviral enteritis. Aust Vet J 1984; 61:1–4.
37. Segovia JC, Real A, Bueren JA, Almendral JM. In vitro myelosuppressive effects of the parvovirus minute virus of mice (MVMi) on hematopoietic stem and committed progenitor cells. Blood 1991; 77:980–8.

38. Porter DD, Larsen AE. Mink parvovirus infections. In: Tijssen P, ed. Handbook of parvoviruses, Boca Raton, FL: CRC Press, 1990; 87–101.
39. Mori S, Wolfinbarger JB, Miyazawa M, Bloom ME. Replication of Aleutian mink disease parvovirus in lymphoid tissues of adult mink: involvement of follicular dendritic cells and macrophages. J Virol 1991; 65:952–6.
40. Goryo M, Sugimura H, Matsumoto S, Umemura T, Itakura C. Isolation of an agent inducing chicken anaemia. Avian Pathol 1985; 14:483–96.
41. Rubinstein DB. Inability of solvent-detergent (S-D) treated factor VIII concentrate to inactivate parvoviruses and non-lipid enveloped non-A, non-B hepatitis virus in factor VIII concentrate: advantages to using sterilizing 100o C dry heat treatment (letter). Am J Hematol 1990; 35:142.
42. Tattersall P, Cotmore SF. Reproduction of autonomous parvovirus DNA. In: Tijssen P, ed. Handbook of parvoviruses, Boca Raton, FL: CRC Press, 1990; 123–40.
43. Berns KI. Parvovirus replication. Microbiol Rev 1990; 54:316–29.
44. McLaughlin SK, Collis P, Hermonat PL, Muzyczka N. Adeno-associated virus general transduction vectors: analysis of proviral structures. J Virol 1988; 62: 1963–73.
45. Srivastava CH, Samulski RJ, Lu L, Larsen SH, Srivastava A. Construction of a recombinant human parvovirus B19: adeno-associated virus 2 (AAV) DNA inverted terminal repeats are functional in an AAV-B19 hybrid virus. Proc Natl Acad Sci U S A 1989; 86:8078–82.
46. Deiss V, Tratschin J-D, Weitz M, Siegl G. Cloning of the human parvovirus B19 genome and structural analysis of its palindromic termini. Virology 1990; 175:247–54.
47. Cotmore SF, Tattersall P. The NS-1 polypeptide of minute virus of mice is covalently attached to the 5′ termini of duplex replicative-form DNA and progeny single strands. J Virol 1988; 62:851–60.
48. Im DS, Muzyczka N. The AAV origin binding protein Rep68 is an ATP-dependent site-specific endonuclease with DNA helicase activity. Cell 1990; 61:447- 57.
49. Tratschin J-D, Tal J, Carter BJ. Negative and positive regulation in trans of gene expression from adeno-associated virus vectors in mammalian cells by a viral rep gene product. Mol Cell Biol 1986; 6:2884–94.
50. Synder RO, Im DS, Muzyczka N. Evidence for covalent attachment of the adeno-associated virus (AAV) rep protein to the ends of the AAV genome. J Virol 1990; 64(12):6204–13.
51. Li X, Rhode SL III. Mutation of lysine 405 to serine in the parvovirus H-1 NS1 abolishes its functions for viral DNA replication, late promoter trans activation, and cytotoxicity. J Virol 1990; 64:4654–60.
52. Doerig C, Hirt B, Antonietti JP, Beard P. Nonstructural protein of parvoviruses B19 and minute virus of mice controls transcription. J Virol 1990; 64:387–96.
53. Rhode SL. Trans-activation of parvovirus P38 promoter by the 76k noncapsid protein. J Virol 1985; 55:886–9.
54. Hanson ND, Rhode SL III. Parvovirus NS1 stimulates P4-expression by interaction with the terminal repeats and through DNA amplification. J Virol 1991; 65:4325–33.

55. Rhode SL. Both excision and replication of cloned autonomous parvovirus DNA require the NS1 (rep) protein. Virology 1989; 63:4249–56.
56. Cotmore SF, Tattersall P. A genome-linked copy of the NS-1 polypeptide is located on the outside of infectious parvovirus particles. J Virol 1989; 63:3902–11.
57. Ozawa K, Ayub J, Kajigaya S, Shimada T, Young NS. The gene encoding the nonstructural protein of B19 (human) parvovirus may be lethal in transfected cells. J Virol 1988; 62:2884–9.
58. Caillet-Fauquet P, Perros M, Branderburger A, Spegelaere P, Rommelaere J. Programmed killing of human cells by means of an inducible clone of parvoviral genes encoding non-structural proteins. EMBO J 1990; 9:2989–95.
59. Labow MA, Graf LH Jr, Berns KI. Adeno-associated virus gene expression inhibits cellular transformation by heterologous genes. Mol Cell Biol 1987; 7: 1320–52.
60. Rommelaere J, Tattersall P. Oncosuppression by parvoviruses. In: Tijssen P, ed. Handbook of parvoviruses, Boca Raton, FL: CRC Press, 1990; 41–57.
61. Khleif SN, Myers T, Carter BJ, Trempe JP. Inhibition of cellular transformation by the adeno-associated virus rep gene. Virology 1991; 181:738–41.
62. Shimomura S, Komatsu N, Frickhofen N, Anderson S, Kajigaya S, Young NS. First continuous propagation of B19 parvovirus in a cell line. Blood 1992; 79: 18–24.
63. Antonietti JP, Sahli R, Beard P, Hirt B. Characterization of the cell type-specific determinant in the genome of minute virus of mice. J Virol 1988; 672:552–7.
64. Gardiner EM, Tattersall P. Mapping of the fibrotropic and lymphotropic host range determinants of the parvovirus minute virus of mice. J Virol 1988; 62: 2605–13.
65. Ball-Goodrich LJ, Moir RD, Tattersall P. Parvoviral target cell specificity: acquisition of fibrotropism by a mutant of the lymphotropic strain of minute virus of mice involves multiple amino acid substitutions within the capsid. Virology 1991; 184:175–86.
66. Parrish CR, Aquadro CF, Carmichael LE. Canine host range and a specific epitope map along with variant sequences in the capsid protein gene of canine parvovirus and related feline, mink and raccoon parvoviruses. Virology 1988; 166:293–307.
67. Parrish CR. Mapping specific functions in the capsid structure of canine parvovirus and feline panleukopenia virus using infectious plasmid clones. Virology 1991; 183:195–205.
68. Spalholz BA, Tattersall P. Interaction of minute virus of mice with differentiated cells: strain-dependent target cell specificity is mediated by intracellular factors. J Virol 1983; 46:937–43.
69. Tsao J, Chapman MS. Agbandje M, et al. The three-dimensional structure of canine parvovirus and its functional implications. Science 1991; 251:1456–64.
70. Rossmann MG. The canyon hypothesis. Viral Immunol 1989; 2(3):143–61.
71. Bass DM, Greenberg HB. Strategies for the identification icosahedral virus receptors. J Clin Invest 1992; 89:3–9.
72. Berns KI, Bohenzky RA. Adeno-associated viruses: an update. Adv Virus Res 1987; 32:243–306.

73. Kotin RM, Siniscalco M, Samulski RJ, et al. Site-specific integration by adeno-associated virus. Proc Natl Acad Sci U S A 1990; 87:2211–5.
74. Fisher RE, Mayor HD. The evolution of defective and autonomous parvoviruses. J Theor Biol 1991; 149:429–39.
75. Thomson BJ, Efstathiou S, Honess RW. Acquisition of the human adeno-associated virus type-2 rep gene by human herpesvirus type-6. Nature 1991; 351: 78–80.
76. Kurtzman G, Ozawa K, Hanson GR, Cohen B, Oseas R, Young N. Chronic bone marrow failure due to persistent B19 parvovirus infection. N Engl J Med 1987; 317:287–94.
77. Kurtzman G, Gascon P, Caras M, Cohen B, Young N. B19 parvovirus replicates in circulating cells of acutely infected patients. Blood 1988; 71:1448–54.
78. Kurtzman G, Cohen B, Myers P, Amanullah A, Young N. Persistent B19 parvovirus infection as a cause of severe anemia in children with acute lymphocytic leukemia in remission. Lancet 1988; 2:1159–62.
79. Ozawa K, Kurtzman G, Young N. Productive infection by B19 parvovirus of human erythroid bone marrow cells in vitro. Blood 1987; 70:384–91.
80. Yaegashi N, Shiraishi H, Takeshita T, Nakamura M, Yajima A, Sugamura K. Propagation of human parvovirus B19 in primary culture of erythroid lineage cells derived from fetal liver. J Virol 1989; 63:2422–6.
81. Westmoreland D, Cohen B. Human parvovirus B19 infected fetal liver as a source of antigen for a radioimmunoassay for B19 specific IgM in clinical samples. J Med Virol 1991; 33:1–5.
82. Takahashi T, Ozawa K, Mitani K, Miyazono K, Asano S, Takaku F. B19 parvovirus replicates in erythroid leukemic cells in vitro (letter). J Infect Dis 1989; 160:548–9.
83. Mortimer PP, Humphries RK, Moore JG, Purcell RH, Young NS. A human parvovirus-like virus inhibits hematopoietic colony formation in vitro. Nature 1983; 302:426–9.
84. Takahashi M, Koike T, Moriyama Y. Inhibition of erythropoiesis by human parvovirus-containing serum from a patient with hereditary spherocytosis in aplastic crisis. Scand J Haematol 1986; 37:118–24.
85. Srivastava A, Lu L. Replication of B19 parvovirus in highly enriched hematopoietic progenitor cells from normal human bone marrow. J Virol 1988; 62: 3059–63.
86. Takahashi T, Ozawa K, Takahashi K, Asano S, Takaku F. Susceptibility of human erythropoietic cells to B19 parvovirus in vitro increases with differentiation. Blood 1990; 75:603–10.
87. Young NS, Harrison M, Moore JG, Mortimer PP, Humphries RK. Direct demonstration of the human parvovirus in erythroid progenitor cells infected in vitro. J Clin Invest 1984; 74:2024–32.
88. Owren PA. Congenital hemolytic jaundice: the pathogenesis of the "hemolytic crisis." Blood 1948; 3:231–48.
89. Kajigaya S, Shimada T, Fujita S, Young NS. A genetically engineered cell line that produces empty capsids of B19 (human) parvovirus. Proc Natl Acad Sci U S A 1989; 86:7601–5.

90. Srivastava A, Bruno E, Briddell R, et al. Parvovirus B19-induced perturbation of human megakaryocytopoiesis in vitro. Blood 1990; 76:1997–2004.
91. Astell CR. Terminal hairpins of parvovirus genomes and their role in DNA replication. In: Tijssen P, ed. Handbook of parvoviruses, Boca Raton, FL: CRC Press, 1990; 59–79.
92. Ozawa K, Ayub J, Yu-Shu H, Kurtsman G, Shimada T, Young N. Novel transcription map for the B19 (human) pathogenic parvovirus. J Virol 1987; 61: 2395–406.
93. Liu JM, Fujii H, Green SW, Komatsu N, Young NS, Shimada T. Indiscriminate activity from the B19 parvovirus P6 promoter in nonpermissive cells. Virology 1991; 182:361–4.
94. St. Amand J, Beard C, Humphries K, Astell CR. Analaysis of splice junctions and in vitro and in vivo translation potential of the small, abundant B19 parvovirus RNAs. Virology 1991; 183:133–42.
95. Liu J, Green S, Shimada T, Young NS. A block in full-length transcript maturation in cells nonpermissive for B19 parvovirus. J Virol 1992; 66:4686–92.
96. Krauskopf A, Resnekov O, Aloni Y. A cis downstream element participates in regulation of in vitro transcription initiation from the P38 promoter of minute virus to mice. J Virol 1990; 64:354–60.
97. Spalholz BA, Tattersall P. Interaction of minute virus of mice with differentiated cells: strain-dependent target cell specificity is mediated by intracellular factors. J Virol 1983; 46:937–43.
98. Ozawa K, Ayub J, Young NS. Translational regulation of B19 parvovirus capsid protein production by multiple upstream AUG triplets. J Biol Chem 1988; 263:10922–6.
99. Ager EA, Chin TDY, Poland JD. Epidemic erythema infectiosum. N Engl J Med 1966; 275:1326–31.
100. Balfour HH Jr. Erythema infectiosum (fifth disease): clinical review and description of 91 cases seen in an epidemic. Clin Pediatr 1969; 8:721–7.
101. Reid DM, Reid TMS, Rennie JAN, Brown T, Eastmond CJ. Human parvovirus-associated arthritis: a clinical and laboratory description. Lancet 1985; 1:422–4.
102. White DG, Woolf AD, Mortimer PP, Cohen BJ, Blake DR, Bacon PA. Human parvovirus arthropathy. Lancet 1985; 1:419–22.
103. Leventhal LJ, Naides SJ, Freundlich B. Fibromyalgia and parvovirus infection. Arthritis Rheum 1991; 34:1319–24.
104. Dinerman JL, Corman LC. Human parvovirus B19 arthropathy associated with desquamation. Am J Med 1990; 89:826–8.
105. Woolf AD, Campion GV, Chishick A, et al. Clinical manifestation of human parvovirus B19 in adults. Arch Intern Med 1989; 149:1153–6.
106. Lyngar E. Samtidig optreden av anemisk kriser hos 3 barn i en familie med hemolytisk ikterus. Nord Med 1942; 14:1246.
107. Gasser C. Akute erythroblastopenie: 10 falle aplastischer erythroblastenkrisen mit riesenproerythroblasten bei allergisch-taxischen Zustandsbildern. Helv Paediatr Acta 1949; 4:107–43.
108. Young N. Hematologic and hematopoietic consequences of B19 parvovirus infection. Semin Hematol 1988; 25:159–72.

109. Mabin DC, Chowdhury V. Aplastic crisis caused by human parvovirus in two patients with hereditary stomatocytosis. Br J Haematol 1990; 76:153–4.
110. Cutlip AC, Gross KM, Lewis MJ. Occult hereditary spherocytosis and human parvovirus infection. J Am Board Fam Pract 1991; 4:461–4.
111. Rechavi G, Vonsover A, Manor Y, et al. Aplastic crisis due to human B19 parvovirus infection in red cell pyrimidine-5′-nucleotidase deficiency. Acta Haematol (Basel) 1989; 82:46–9.
112. Nibu K, Matsumoto I, Yanai F, Nunque T. Aplastic crisis due to human parvovirus B19 infection in glucose-6-phosphate dehydrogenase deficiency. Acta Haematol Jpn 1989; 52:1117–21.
113. Smith MA, Shah NS, Lobel JS. Parvovirus B19 infection associated with reticulocytopenia and chronic autoimmune hemolytic anemia. Am J Pediatr Hematol Oncol 1989; 11(2):167–9.
114. Chitnavis VN, Patou G, Makar YF, Kendra JR. B19 Parvovirus induced red cell aplasia complicating acute cold antibody mediated haemolytic anaemia. Br J Haematol 1990; 76:433–4.
115. Lefrère JJ, Bourgeois H. Human parvovirus associated with erythroblastopenia in iron deficiency anaemia. Can Nat Transf Sang 1992; 1277.
116. Kojima S, Matsuyama K, Ishii E. High serum iron in human parvovirus-induced aplastic crisis in iron deficiency anemia. Acta Haematol (Basel) 1988; 80:171–2.
117. Weiland HT, Salimans MMM, Fibbe WE, Kluin PM, Cohen BJ. Prolonged parvovirus B19 infection with severe anaemia in a bone marrow transplant recipient (letter). Br J Haematol 1989; 710:300.
118. Niitsu H, Takatsu H, Miura I, et al. Pure red cell aplasia induced by B19 parvovirus during allogeneic bone marrow transplantation. RinshoKetsueki 1990; 31:1566–71.
119. Kho L-K. Erythroblastopenia with giant pro-erythroblasts in kwashiorkor. Blood 1957; 12:171–82.
120. Zucker JM, Tchernia G, Vuylsteke P, Becart-Michael R, Giorgi R, Blot J. Acute and transitory erythroblastopenia in kwashiorkor under treatment. Nouv Rev Fr Hematol 1971; 11:131.
121. Pierce LE, Rath CE. Evidence for folic acid deficiency in the genesis of anemic sickle cell crisis. Blood 1962; 20:19.
122. Alperin JB. Folic acid deficiency complicating sickle cell anemia. Arch Intern Med 1967; 120:398.
123. Choremis CB, Megas HA, Liaromati AA, Michael SC. Aplastic crisis in the course of infectious diseases. Report of 10 cases. Helv Paediatr Acta 1961; 2:134–45.
124. Jootar S, Srichaikul R, Atichartakaran V. Pure red cell aplasia in Thailand: report of twenty four cases. Southeast Asian J Trop Med Public Health 1985; 16:291–5.
125. Evans JPM, Rossiter MA, Kumaran TO, Marsh GW, Mortimer PP. Human parvovirus aplasia: case due to cross infection in a ward (letter). Br Med J 1984; 288:681.
126. Shneerson JM, Mortimer PP, Vandervelde EM. Febrile illness due to a parvovirus. Br Med J 1980; 280:1580.

127. Powars D. Aplastic anemia secondary to glue sniffing. N Engl J Med 1965; 273:700–2.
128. Conrad ME, Studdard H, Anderson LJ. Case report. Aplastic crisis in sickle cell disorders: bone marrow necrosis and human parvovirus infection. Am J Med Sci 1988; 295:212–5.
129. Pardoll DM. Rodeheffer RJ, Smith RRL, Charache S. Aplastic crisis due to extensive bone marrow necrosis in sickle cell disease. Arch Intern Med 1982; 142:2223–5.
130. Frickhofen N, Raghavachar A, Heit W, Heimpel H, Cohen BJ. Human parvovirus infection (letter). N Engl J Med 1986; 314:646.
131. Saunders PWG, Reid MM, Cohen BJ. Human parvovirus induced cytopenias: a report of five cases (letter). Br J Haematol 1986; 63:407–10.
132. Hanada T, Koike K, Takeya T, Nagasawa T, Matsunaga Y, Takita H. Human parvovirus B19-induced transient pancytopenia in a child with hereditary spherocytosis. Br J Haematol 1988; 70:113–5.
133. Hamon MD, Newland AC, Anderson MJ. Severe aplastic anaemia after parvovirus infection in the absence of underlying hameolytic anaemia (letter). J Clin Pathol 1988; 41:1242.
134. Boruchoff ES, Woda AB, Pihan AG, Durbin AW, Burstein D, Blacklow RN. Parvovirus B19-associated hemophagocytic syndrome. Arch Intern Med 1990; 150:897–9.
135. Jones PH, Pickett LC, Anderson MJ, Pasvol G. Human parvovirus infection in children and severe anaemia seen in an area endemic for malaria. J Trop Med Hyg 1990; 93:67–70.
136. Nunoue T, Koike T, Koike R, et al. Infection with human parvovirus (B19), aplasia of the bone marrow and a rash in hereditary spherocytosis. J Infect 1987; 14:67–70.
137. Doran HM, Teall AJ. Neutropenia accompanying erythroid aplasia in human parvovirus infection (letter). Br J Haematol 1988; 69:287–8.
138. Anderson MJ. Higgins PG, Davis LR, et al. Experimental parvoviral infection in humans. J Infect Dis 1985; 152:257–65.
139. Lefrère JJ. Peripheral thrombocytopenia in human parvovirus infection (letter). J Clin Pathol 1987; 40:469.
140. Lefrère JJ, Courouсé AM, Kaplan C. Parvovirus and idiopathic thrombocytopenic purpura (letter). Lancet 1989; 1:279.
141. Nagai K, Morohoshi T, Kudoh T, Yoto Y, Suzuki N, Matsunaga Y. Transient erythroblastopenia of childhood with megakaryocytopenia associated with human parvovirus B19 infection (letter). Br J Haematol 1992; 80:131–2.
142. Lefrere JJ, Courouce AM, Muller JY, Clark M, Soulier JP. Human parvovirus and purpura (letter). Lancet 1985; 2:730–1.
143. Foreman NK, Oakhill A, Caul EO. Parvovirus-associated thrombocytopenic purpura (letter). Lancet 1988; 2:1426–7.
144. Lefrère JJ, Got D. Peripheral thrombocytopenia in human parvovirus infection (letter). J Clin Pathol 1987; 40:469.
145. Serjeant GR, Topley JM, Mason K, et al. Outbreak of aplastic crisis in sickle cell anaemia associated with parvovirus-like agent. Lancet 1981; 2:595–7.

146. Anderson MJ, Davis LR, Hodgson SE, et al. Occurrence of infection with a parvovirus-like agent in children with sickle cell anaemia during a two-year period. J Clin Pathol 1982; 35:744–9.
147. Rao KRP, Patel AR, Anderson MJ, Hodgson J, Jones SE, Pattison JR. Infection with parvovirus-like virus and aplastic crisis in chronic hemolytic anemia. Ann Intern Med 1983; 98:930–2.
148. Kelleher JF Jr, Luban NLC, Cohen BJ, Mortimer PP. Human serum parvovirus as the cause of aplastic crisis in sickle cell disease. Am J Dis Child 1984; 138:401–3.
149. Lefrère J-J, Couroucé A-M, Bertrand Y, Girot R, Soulier J-P. Human parvovirus and aplastic crisis in chronic hemolytic anemias: a study of 24 observations. Am J Hematol 1986; 23:271–5.
150. McLellan NJ, Rutter N. Hereditary spherocytosis in sisters unmasked by parvovirus infection. Postgrad Med J 1987; 63:49–50.
151. Anderson MJ, Jones SE, Minson AC. Diagnosis of human parvovirus infection by dot-blot hybridization using cloned viral DNA. J Med Virol 1985; 15: 163–72.
152. Clewley JP. Detection of human parvovirus using a molecularly cloned probe. J Med Virol 1985; 15:173–81.
153. Saarinen UM, Chorba TL, Tattersall P, et al. Human parvovirus B19-induced epidemic acute red cell aplasia in patients with hereditary hemolytic anemia. Blood 1986; 67:1411–7.
154. Young NS, Mortimer PP, Moore JG, Humphries RK. Characterization of a virus that causes transient aplastic crisis. J Clin Invest 1984; 73:224–30.
155. Guillot M, Lefrere JJ, Raventet N, Leveque E, Girot R. Acute anaemia and aplastic crisis without haemolysis in human parvovirus infection (letter). J Clin Pathol 1987; 40:1264–5.
156. Wodzinski MA, Lilleyman JS. Transient erythroblastopenia of childhood due to human parvovirus B19 infection. Br J Haematol 1989; 73:127.
157. Elian JC, Frappaz D, Possetto B, Taimi A, Jacquemard R, Freycon F. Erythroblastopenie et neutropenie transitoires revelatrices d'une infection a parvovirus humain B19. Pediatrie 1991; 46:673–5.
158. Anderson LJ, Hurwitz ES. Human parvovirus B19 and pregnancy. Clin Perinatol 1988; 15:273–86.
159. Leads from the MMWR: Risks associated with human parvovirus B19 infection. JAMA 1989; 261:1406–8; 1555–63.
160. Anand A, Gray ES, Brown T, Clewley JP, Cohen BJ. Human parvovirus infection in pregnancy and hydrops fetalis. N Engl J Med 1987; 316:183–6.
161. Cotmore SF, McKie VC, Anderson LJ, Astell CR, Tattersall P. Identification of the major structural and nonstructural proteins encoded by human parvovirus B19 and mapping of their genes by procaryotic expression of isolated genomic fragments. J Virol 1989; 60:548–57.
162. Rodis JF, Quinn DL, Gary GW Jr, Anderson LJ. Management and outcomes of pregnancies complicated by human B19 parvovirus infection: a prospective study. Am J Obstet Gynecol 1990; 163(4 pt 1):1168–71.

163. Public Health Laboratory Service Working Party on Fifth Disease. Prospective study of human parvovirus (B19) infection in pregnancy. Br Med J 1990; 300:1166–70.
164. Hartwig NG, Vermeij-Keers C, Van Elsacker-Niele AM, Fleuren GJ. Embryonic malformations in a case of intrauterine parvovirus B19 infection. Teratology 1989; 39:295–302.
165. Porter HJ, Quantrill AM, Fleming KA. B19 parvovirus infection of myocardial cells (letter). Lancet 1988; 1:535–6.
166. Metzman R, Anand A, DeGiulio A, Knisely AS. Hepatic disease associated with intrauterine parvovirus B19 infection in a newborn premature infant. J Pediatr Gastroenterol Nutr 1989; 9:112–4.
167. Wright IM, Williams ML, Cohen BJ. Congenital parvovirus infection. Arch Dis Child 1991; 66:253–4.
168. Schwarz TF, Roggendorf M, Hottentrager B, et al. Human parvovirus B19 infection in pregnancy (letter). Lancet 1988; 2:566–7.
169. Belloy M, Morinet F, Blondin G, Courouce AM, Peyrol Y, Vilmer E. Erythroid hypoplasia due to chronic infection with parvovirus B19. N Engl J Med 1990; 322:633–4.
170. Kurtzman G, Frickhofen N, Kimball J, Jenkins DW, Nienhuis AW, Young NS. Pure red-cell aplasia of 10 years' duration due to persistent parvovirus B19 infection and its cure with immunoglobulin therapy. N Engl J Med 1989; 321:519–23.
171. Smith MA, Shah NR, Lobel JS, Cera PJ, Gary GW, Anderson LJ. Severe anemia caused by human parvovirus in a leukemia patient on maintenance chemotherapy. Clin Pediatr 1988; 27:383–6.
172. Rao SP, Miller ST, Cohen BJ. Severe anemia due to B19 parvovirus infection in children with acute leukemia in remission. Am J Pediatr Hematol Oncol 1990; 12:194–7.
173. Carstensen H, Ornvold K, Cohen BJ. Human parvovirus B19 infection associated with prolonged erythroblastopenia in a leukemic child (letter). Pediatr Infect Dis J 1989; 8:56–7.
174. Azzi A, Macchia PA, Favre C, Nardi M, Zakrezewska K, Corsi OB. Aplastic crisis caused by B19 virus in a child during induction therapy for acute lymphoblastic leukemia. Haematologica 1989; 74:191–4.
175. Coulombel L, Morinet F, Mielot F, Tchernia G. Parvovirus infection, leukaemia, and immunodeficiency. Lancet 1989; 1:101–2.
176. Graeve JLA, de Alarcon PA, Naides SJ. Parvovirus B19 infection in patients receiving cancer chemotherapy: the expanding spectrum of disease. Am J Pediatr Hematol Oncol 1989; 11:441–4.
177. Frickhofen N, Abkowitz J, Safford M, et al. Persistent parvovirus infection in patients infected with human immunodeficiency virus-1: a treatable cause of anemia in AIDS. Ann Intern Med 1990; 113:926–33.
178. Mitchell SA, Welch JM, Weston-Smith S, Nicholson F, Bradbeer CS. Parvovirus infection and anaemia in a patient with AIDS: case report. Genitoruin Med 1990; 66:95–6.

179. Nield G, Anderson M, Hawes S, Colvin BT. Parvovirus infection after renal transplant (letter). Lancet 1986; 2:1226–7.
180. Berner YN, Green L, Handzel ZT. Erythroblastopenia in acquired immunodeficiency syndrome (AIDS) (letter). Acta Haematol (Basel) 1983; 70:273.
181. Sallan SE, Buchanan GR. Selective erythroid aplasia during therapy for acute lymphoblastic leukemia. Pediatrics 1977; 59:895–8.
182. Pont J, Puchhammer-Stöckl E, Chott A, et al. Recurrent granulocytic aplasia as clinical presentation of a persistent parvovirus B19 infection. Br J Haematol 1992; 80:160–5.
183. Frickhofen N, Young NS. Persistent parvovirus B19 infections in humans. Microbial Pathog 1989; 7:319–27.
184. Kurtzman G, Cohen R, Field AM, Oseas R, Blaese RM, Young N. The immune response to B19 parvovirus infection and an antibody defect in persistent viral infection. J Clin Invest 1989; 84:1114–23.
185. Bowman CA, Cohen BJ, Norfolk DR, Lacey CJN. Red cell aplasia associated with human parvovirus B19 and HIV infection: failure to respond clinically to intravenous immunoglobulin (letter). AIDS 1990; 4:1038–9.
186. Jacoby RO, Johnson EA, Paturzo FX, Gaertner DJ, Brandsma JL, Smith AL. Persistent rat parvovirus infection in individually housed rats. Arch Virol 1991; 117:193–205.
187. Rimmelzwaan GF, Van der Heijden RWJ, Tijhaar E, et al. Establishment and characterization of canine parvovirus-specific murine CD4+ T cell clones and their use for the delineation of T cell epitopes. J Gen Virol 1990; 71:1095–102.
188. An SH, Wilkie BN. Mitogen- and viral antigen-induced transformation of lymphocytes from normal mink and from mink with progressive or nonprogressive Aleutian disease. Infect Immun 1981; 34:111–4.
189. Alexandersen S, Bloom ME, Perryman S. Nucleotide sequence and genomic organization of aleutian mink disease parvovirus (ADV): sequence comparisons between a nonpathogenic and a pathogenic strain. Adv J Virol 1988; 62: 2903–15.
190. Tattersall P, Bratton J. Reciprocal productive and restrictive virus-cell interactions of immunosuppressive and prototype strains of minute virus of mice. J Virol 1983; 46:944–55.
191. Harding MJ, Molitor T. Porcine parvovirus: replication in and inhibition of selected cellular functions of swine alveolar macrophages and peripheral blood lymphocytes. Arch Virol 1988; 101:105–17.
192. Carlson JH, Scott FW, Duncan JR. Feline panleukopenia. III. Development of lesions in the lymphoid tissue. Vet. Pathol. 1978; 15:383–92.
193. Yoshimoto K, Rosenfeld S, Frickhofen N, Kennedy D, Kajigaya S, Young NS. A second neutralizing epitope of B19 parvovirus implicates the spike region in the immune response. J Virol 1991; 65:7056–60.
194. Sato H, Hirata J, Kuroda N, Shiraki H, Maeda Y, Okochi K. Identifrication and mapping of neutralizing epitopes of human parvovirus B19 by using human antibodies. J Virol 1991; 65:5845–490.

195. Sato H, Hirata J, Furukawa M, et al. Identification of the region including the epitope for a monoclonal antibody which can neutralize human parvovirus B19. J Virol 1991; 65:1667–72.
196. Rosenfeld SR, Yoshimoto K, Anderson S, et al. The unique region of the minor capsid protein of B19 parvovirus is exposed on the virion surface. J Clin Invest. 1992; 89:2023–9.
197. Meunier PC, Cooper BJ, Appel MJG, Lanieu ME, Slauson DO. Pathogenesis of canine parvovirus enteritis: sequential virus distribution and passive immunization studies. Vet Pathol 1985; 22:617–24.
198. Takahashi M, Koike T, Moriyama Y, Shibata A. Neutralizating activity of immunoglobulin preparation against erythropoietic suppression of human parvovirus (letter). Am J Hematol 1991; 37:68.
199. Davis EV, Gregory GG, Beckenhauer WH. Infectious feline panleukopenia. Developmental report of a tissue culture origin formalin-inactivated vaccine. Vet Med Sm Anim Clin 1970; 65:237–42.
200. Gorham JR, Hartsough GR, Burger D, Lust S, Sato N. The preliminary use of attenuated feline panleukopenia virus to protect cats against panleukopenia and mink against virus enteritis. Cornell Vet 1963; 559:566.
201. King DA, Gutekunst DE. A new mink enteritis vaccine for immunization against feline panleukopenia. Vet Med Sm Anim Clin 1970; 65:377–83.
202. Pye D, Bates J, Edwards SJ, Hollingworth J. Development of a vaccine preventing parvovirus-induced reproductive failure in pigs. Aust Vet J 1979; 67: 179.
203. Rimmelzwaan GF, Carlson J, UytdeHaag FG, Ostrhaus AD. A synthetic peptide derived from the amino acid sequence of canine parvovirus structural proteins which defines a B cell epitope and elicits antiviral antibody in BALB c mice. J Gen Virol 1990; 71:2741–5.
204. Bansal GP, Hatfield J, Dunn FE, et al. Immunogenicity studies of recombinant human parvovirus B19 proteins. Vaccines In press: 1991;
205. Caul OE, Usher JM, Burton AP. Intrauterine infection with human parvovirus B19: a light and electron microscopy study. J Med Virol 1988; 24:55–66.

# 4

# Feline Panleukopenia Virus

**Gary J. Kurtzman**

*Gilead Sciences, Inc.*
*Foster City, California*

## INTRODUCTION

An understanding of the causes and pathogenesis of infectious diseases in other animals has benefited humans in several ways. Most directly, the study of animal infectious diseases had led to the control of zoonoses, that is, diseases communicable between other animals and humans. In addition, since many species have value to the human, commercial and emotional, a large effort has been made to control diseases causing animals significant morbidity or mortality. Apart from these direct benefits, the diseases caused by agents that infect animals can serve as models for human illness. They provide the opportunity to study disease pathogenesis at a level not often possible in the human and have been valuable in the development of prophylaxis and treatment. As highlighted by research into infection by the human immunodeficiency virus (HIV), lack of an adequate animal model has significantly slowed progress toward understanding the disease pathogenesis and the development of effective therapies.

Viral infection may alter hematopoiesis either directly as a result of infection of bone marrow progenitor cells or indirectly by effects on accessory cell populations (1). Although animal models for studying viral effects on the bone marrow are few, two are fairly well characterized: disease in cats caused by infection by feline leukemia virus (FLV) and panleukopenia due to feline parvovirus (FPV) infection. Both are significant pathogens in their host species, and a great deal of effort has been made to devise vaccines to protect animals from these infections. Although there is no human disease directly analagous to FLV-induced disease in cats, study of this viral infection has suggested mechanisms by which as yet unidentified viruses, particularly retroviruses, may be involved in the etiology of human hematologic diseases, such as aplastic anemia or pure red cell aplasia (reviewed in Chap. 11).

Panleukopenia is one of the most important infectious diseases of cats, and before the advent of vaccines, it was the principal cause of feline infectious deaths (2–4). This clinical syndrome, in which bone marrow failure is a prominent feature, was first attributed to a virus over 60 years ago (5). Early investigators proposed feline panleukopenia as a model of agranulocytosis in humans (6). With the recent identification of the B19 parvovirus as a cause of bone marrow failure in humans (reviewed in Chap. 3), FPV infection provides a system in which to address questions about human parvovirus infection (e.g., tissue tropism, persistence, and immune response). This chapter describes the disease caused by FPV by reviewing over half a century of clinical and laboratory studies of the virus and considers the basis for the bone marrow failure that results from parvovirus infection.

## FELINE PARVOVIRUS

### FPV and Related Parvoviruses

Parvoviruses are among the smallest DNA-containing viruses (7). The family Parvoviridae includes the genus *Dependovirus*, whose members, the adeno-associated viruses (AAV), require coinfection with a helper virus to produce progeny. The AAV have not been associated with any disease. In contrast, the viruses of the genus *Parvovirus*, of which FPV is a member, can replicate autonomously in infected cells and are common agents of disease. Within the genus *Parvovirus*, there are four closely related viruses: FPV, mink enteritis virus (MEV), canine parvovirus (CPV), and racoon parvovirus (RPV). MEV, CPV, and RPV appear to have arisen as host-range variants of FPV (7,8–12), although whether CPV arose from FPV (or from MEV or RPV) directly or from an as yet undiscovered common ancestor is unclear (12). As pathogens, MEV and CPV have emerged fairly recently. MEV was first described in the late 1940s as the cause of outbreaks of severe enteritis in Canadian ranch mink (13). CPV clearly arose in the late 1970s and was first identified in 1978 as a cause of widespread outbreaks of myocarditis and enteritis in dogs; sera obtained from dogs before this time reveal no evidence of infection (i.e., antibodies to CPV capsid proteins) (14).

## Virion Structure

Parvoviruses are nonenveloped, icosahedral viruses with a diameter of approximately 20–25 nm and a molecular mass of between $5.5 \times 10^3$ and $6.2 \times 10^3$ kD (15). The capsid of FPV and its related viruses consist of one major and two minor polypeptides. Two are primary translation products with the entire sequence of the major capsid protein, VP2 (64–66 kD), contained within the sequence of the minor species, VP1 (83–86 kD), which contains additional amino acids at the amino terminus. A third protein, VP3 (60–62 kD), is produced by proteolytic cleavage of 15–20 amino acids from the amino terminus of VP2 (15). Recently, the three-dimensional structure of CPV was determined (16); infectious subunits contain approximately 60 protein subunits that are predominantly VP2.

## Antigenic Structure

Antigenically, FPV, CPV, MEV, and RPV are similar, although differences are clearly apparent on the basis of their patterns of reactivity to panels of monoclonal antibodies (8,10). Based on their restriction maps and DNA sequences, FPV, RPV, and MEV appear to be more closely related to each other than to CPV, but all are 95–98% identical at the nucleotide level and 98–99% identical at the amino acid level (9,17–19). Differences appear to be clustered in a few areas within the capsid protein. As expected, the three-dimensional structure of CPV revealed that amino acids accounting for the antigenic properties of this virus are located in peptide loops on exteriorly exposed regions of the capsid (16).

## Virus Entry

Although little is known about how parvoviruses enter cells, entry is probably initiated by binding to specific cell surface receptors (15,20). The exact nature of these receptors is unknown and have been best characterized for the minute virus of mice (MVM). MVM appears to bind to a cell surface glycoprotein(s) because treatment of the cell with neuraminidase or trypsin abolishes binding (15). The number of binding sites per cell is large (between 1 and $5 \times 10^5$) , but the receptor is not ubiquitously expressed: some cell types appear to lack the receptor and are resistant to infection. Analysis of binding of CPV to polarized MDCK cells reveals a large number ($10^5$ per cell) of high-affinity binding sites ($K_d$ 29 pM). Interestingly, specific binding and virus entry in MDCK cells is polarized; that is, it occurs only on the basolateral surface of these cells (20). The three-dimensional structure of CPV reveals a depression on its surface. This "canyon" is reminiscent of similar depressions on the surface of rhino- and picornaviruses (16), which are implicated as the sites of cell receptor attachment.

## Viral Genome

The FPV genome consists of approximately 5000 bases of single-stranded DNA. The negative DNA strand is "infectious," and FPV, as do most of the autonomous parvoviruses, primarily packages the negative strand (7). The genomes of a number of parvoviruses have been cloned and sequenced (17,18,21–24), and for a few, detailed transcription maps have been determined (25–27). The major common feature of parvovirus transcription are two large open reading frames, each encompassing roughly half the viral genome. A number of proteins with overlapping amino acid sequence are translated from RNA transcripts initiated from several sites within the genome [this, however, does not appear to be the case for B19 parvovirus, for which only a single 5′ promoter has been defined (27)] and which is subject to alternative splicing patterns. The left-side ORF codes for the nonstructural or rep proteins. The rep proteins have pleomorphic functions involved in DNA replication, transcriptional regulation, and excision of multimeric DNA strands to produce monomer single-stranded viral DNA (28–35). In addition, there is evidence that at least one of the proteins encoded for by the left-side ORF has cytotoxicity activity (36–38). The right-hand ORF generally encodes the single major and one or more minor structural or capsid proteins (39). The FPV (17,19) and CPV genomes (18) have been sequenced, and both these viruses conform to this overall pattern.

## DNA Replication

The mechanism of parvovirus DNA replication is well understood (15,40). The parvovirus genome is characterized by 5′ and 3′ terminal inverted repeat sequences that form hairpin structures. The 5′ hairpin serves as a double-stranded primer, which is extended, presumably by the action of cellular DNA polymerases, to form the double-stranded monomer replicative form. This process is repeated at the newly synthesized 3′ terminus, and then, by an iterative process of self priming and DNA synthesis, multimeric replicative intermediates are produced. DNA strand cleavage follows replication, resulting in the formation of single-stranded monomer viral DNA. (This scheme is termed the rolling hairpin model of parvovirus DNA replication.) That FPV follows this scheme of DNA replication has been inferred from the results of experiments in which viral DNA is harvested at intervals after infection of cells in culture and subjected to Southern blot analysis (41).

## Virus-Host Interactions

Parvoviruses have limited genomic coding capacity and are dependent upon factors provided by the host cell to successfully replicate (42). At least some of these host factors appear to be produced during the *S* phase of the cell cycle; cells that are blocked in *S* phase by agents that inhibit cellular DNA synthesis (hydroxyurea and thymidine at high concentration) (43,44) can still support viral propagation. The diseases caused by parvovirus infection reflect the viral dependence on actively proliferating tissue, and the ability of a tissue to proliferate is to a large degree determined by the age of the animal at the time of infection (42). Infection of the fetus often results in abortion and congenital malformations; the pattern of fetal disease is determined by both the tissue tropism of the virus and the state of organogenesis at the time of infection. Indeed, parvoviruses are an important cause of reproductive failure in domestic animals (42), and B19 parvovirus infection in utero causes spontaneous abortion or hydrops fetalis (45–47). Pre- and postnatal infections result in a variety of syndromes (myocarditis, enteritis, hepatitis, cerebellar ataxia, and panleukopenia), whereas disease in susceptible adults is mainly a reflection of the remaining actively proliferating tissues (gastrointestinal epithelium and hematolymphoid tissues) (42).

## Host-Range Specificity

The small differences in the amino acid sequences between FPV, CPV, MEV, and RPV give rise to *in vivo* and *in vitro* differences in susceptibility to infection. FPV has broad infectivity in that it can cause disease in all members of the cat family in addition to the racoon and the mink (3). FPV replicates poorly in dogs, and likewise, CPV replicates poorly in cats, racoons, and mink (12). All four viruses productively infect feline cells in culture, but only CPV can infect canine cells in addition, indicating a wider *in vitro* host range for this virus (12). Upon continued passage of CPV in feline cells, CPV loses the ability to grow in canine cells, a property that can be mapped to a mutation in the VP2 gene (48). Analysis of chimeric viruses produced by interchanging regions of the capsid proteins between CPV and FPV likewise reveals a correlation between the small differences in amino acid sequence of the capsid proteins and host-range specificity (12,48). The mechanism by which these small differences influence this specificity is unknown but may reflect an interaction between the virus capsid and some cellular factor. Two strains of the MVM, the prototype p and immunosuppressive i strain, are serologically identical, but each is restricted for growth in the other's productive host cell. Similar to FPV and CPV, chimeras between these two strains map the determinant of host-range specificity to a 235 nucleotide region within the capsid region. Both strains bind to and compete for binding to the other's productive cell type, and some viral replication takes place. However, no detectable levels of capsid, virion, or single-stranded DNA are produced in restrictive infection, suggesting that some viral determinant is interacting with a cellular factor(s) to regulate viral gene expression (15,49)

## FELINE PANLEUKOPENIA

### Historical Perspectives

Feline gastroenteritis was one of the first animal diseases attributed to a viral infection. The first reports of an extremely contagious feline gastroenteritis with an exceptionally high mortality ("distemper") date to the early part of this century (50). In 1928, Verge and Christofroni passaged gastroenteritis between cats via cell free filtrates made from organs of animals that had previously died from the disease (5). This observation was confirmed by Hindle and Findlay, who in 1932 excluded the bacterial species that superinfect the gut of sick cats as the primary cause of infectious gastroenteritis; the disease could not be reproduced upon inoculation of cats with the same organisms (51). In 1934, Leasure et al. reported that cats could be immunized successfully with formalinized tissue preparations from infected animals and that protection was passively transferred by hyperimmune homologous and heterologous serum (50).

That infection with the same virus resulted in bone marrow suppression was first suggested in 1938, when Lawrence and Syverton reported transmission of a syndrome that they termed spontaneous agranulocytosis (6). During the course of routine blood count determination in cats, they found one animal with only 350 white blood cells per $mm^3$ of peripheral blood and the complete absence of neutrophils. When they injected a suspension of ground liver from that animal into five additional cats, two of the five developed the same clinical picture. This process was continued, and serial transmission of the agranulocytosis was confirmed. A year later, as the result of an investigation into the etiology of a disease that broke out among their laboratory stock of kittens, Hammon and Enders published the first complete clinical and pathologic study of "a virus disease of cats characterized by aleukocytosis, enteric lesions and the presence of intranuclear inclusion bodies" in which "fulminating" leukopenia was the outstanding clinical finding (52). Although both groups reported pathologic changes in the gut, clinically, gastroenteritis was not prominent. Rather, the hematologic manifestations were the most striking feature of the syndrome with bone marrow involvement ranging from suppression of myeloid elements to complete marrow aplasia.

Because of the differences in disease manifestations (predominant gastroenteritis versus agranulocytosis or panleukopenia), it took several decades before it could be concluded that infection with the same virus, later identified as FPV, was responsible for the variety of clinical manifestations observed. Over a quarter of century after the first reports appeared in the literature, the spectrum of disease caused by FPV was broadened with the finding that the transmissible agent causing feline ataxia was identical to that causing feline panleukopenia (53). As described in subsequent sections, the differences in clinical signs observed by these early investigators may have arisen from differences in viral strains studied or host factors, such as the age of the cat or endogenous bacterial flora (3,52).

## Panleukopenia

The early studies of Lawrence and colleagues and Hammon and Enders remain the best clinical description of the disease. Lawrence et al. first described "spontaneous agranulocytosis in the cat" in 1938, and their first detailed study of the hematologic findings of what they termed infectious feline agranulocytosis was published 2 years later as a report of their observations on 113 animals with this syndrome (55). The clinical course was variable, and the symptoms—listlessness, vomiting, diarrhea, and nasal and occular discharge—if they occurred, appeared from the 6–9 days after inoculation. Mortality was high. Hematologically, the animals fell into two groups based on a gradual or precipitous pattern of decline in leukocyte counts (Fig. 1). Mortality was greater in those animals whose leukocyte count fell rapidly. The average nadir of the white blood cell count (WBC) was 1350 per $mm^3$ (normal 15,000 per $mm^3$), with a range of 0–6400. The effects of virus infection on the differential counts were more striking. Over 70% of the animals had absolute neutrophil counts (ANC) of less than 200 per $mm^3$ during the course of the disease. Although a relative lymphocytosis was noted, the number of peripheral blood lymphocytes was also decreased. There was no consistent change in eosinophil, basophil, or monocyte numbers and only slight decrements in the hemoglobin and red cell count. Recovery was heralded by the appearance of band forms in the peripheral blood, with a marked left shift persisting for several days. Nucleated red cells were also occasionally noted during the recovery period. The findings of Hammon and Enders generally agreed with those reported by Lawrence et al., but they noted more prominent involvement of the lymphoid tissue (52,56), leading to their characterization of the hematologic manifestations as "aleukocytosis" rather than agranulocytosis. Leukopenia was the constant feature, with the majority of animals having white blood cell counts below 1000 per $mm^3$ of blood at the height of disease. They did not observe a relative lymphocytosis rather, both neutrophils and lymphocytes were severely depleted from the blood. Although a decrease in red blood cell count was occasionally noted, anemia was rarely seen.

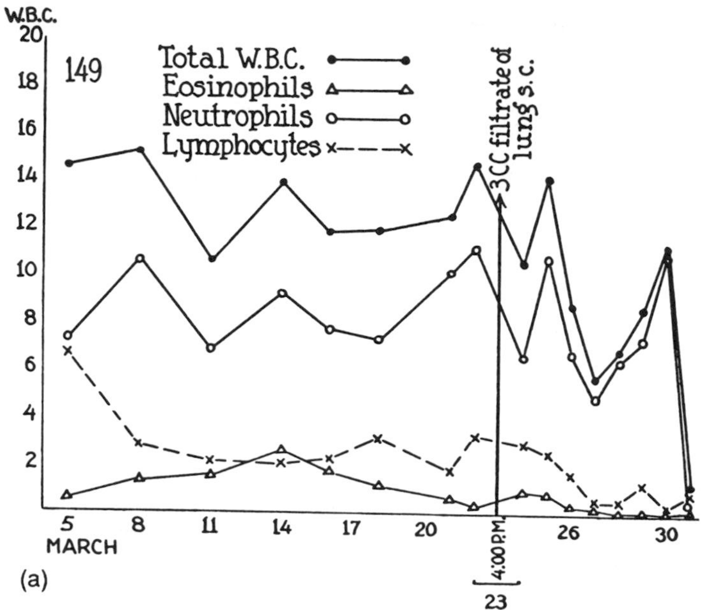


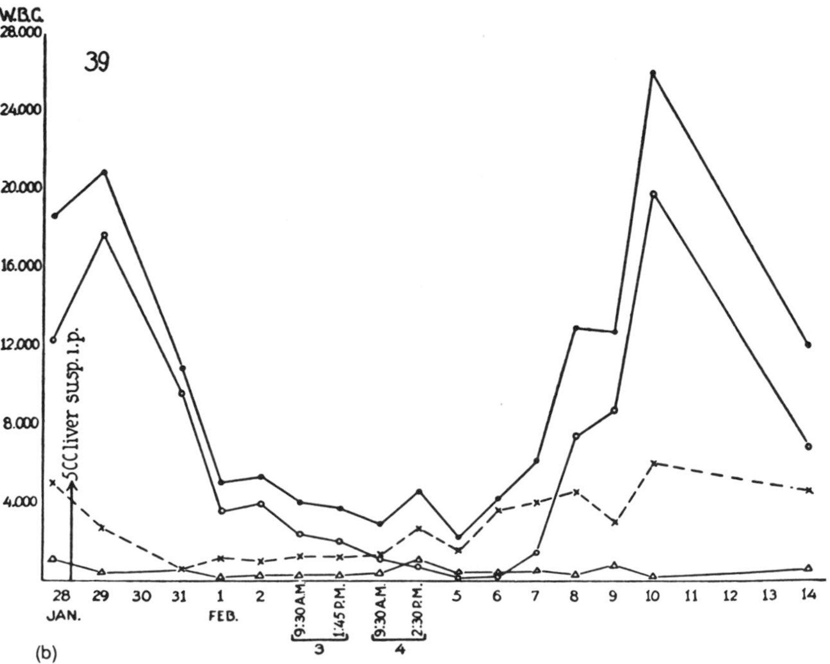


**Figure 1** Response of the peripheral blood leukocyte count in two representative animals infected with FPV. The course of the animal depicted in (b) was characterized by a gradual decline in both total count and neutrophil number and that in (a) by a more precipitous decline. [From Lawrence et al. (55).]

Subsequent clinical and pathologic descriptions of feline panleukopenia showed that although many of the signs and symptoms of panleukopenia may vary, a decrease in the white blood cell count and, more specifically, in the number of neutrophils, is a constant finding in natural infection with FPV (4). Symptomatic infection is more common in younger animals (57), and in the most severely affected, an incubation time of 3–7 days is followed by anorexia, apathy, abdominal pain, emesis, diarrhea, and pyrexia. Disease duration is short, with death ensuing within a few days; recovery, if it occurs, is rapid and complete. The disease may be subclinical because many adult, unvaccinated animals have antibodies to FPV (2). Pathologically, the bone marrow, gastrointestinal tract, and lymph nodes are invariably involved (2–4,50,54,56).

## Pathology

### Bone Marrow

The bone marrow findings described by Lawrence et al. were striking (Fig. 2). On gross examination the marrow appearance ranged from normally cellular to fatty and aplastic. At the height of disease, there was a marked diminution of myeloid elements; the remaining myeloid cells consisted primarily of myeloblasts. Erythroid cells were less affected, although there was some shift toward immature forms. Megakaryocytes were unaffected in number or state of differentiation. Upon recovery, there was a rapid increase in total cellularity and the progressive reappearance of mature myeloid cells. All the bone marrow samples described by Hammon and Enders were severely hypoplastic. They noted depletion of both erythroid and myeloid cells in some animals at the height of disease, and in a few, the red cell elements appeared to be more severely depleted than the myeloid cells. Erythrophagocytosis was also present. In general, the marrow picture reflected the peripheral blood with the most severe peripheral cytopenias associated with the more hypoplastic or aplastic marrows, although normal peripheral red cell counts were occasionally seen even in the presence of severely affected marrows. Most conspicuous among cells that persisted were the megakaryoctyes. Of note in the marrow were "larger mononuclear cells, sometimes binucleated" that contained "eosinophilic intranuclear inclusions."

### Lymphoid Tissue

Lawrence et al. (55) described moderate involvement of the lymph nodes, which showed hyperplasia of the reticuloendothelial cells. There was some decrease in lymphocytes in the germinal centers, but cortical lymphocyte numbers were normal. Hammon and Enders noted marked depletion of mature lymphocytes from the germinal centers in the lymph nodes, and some

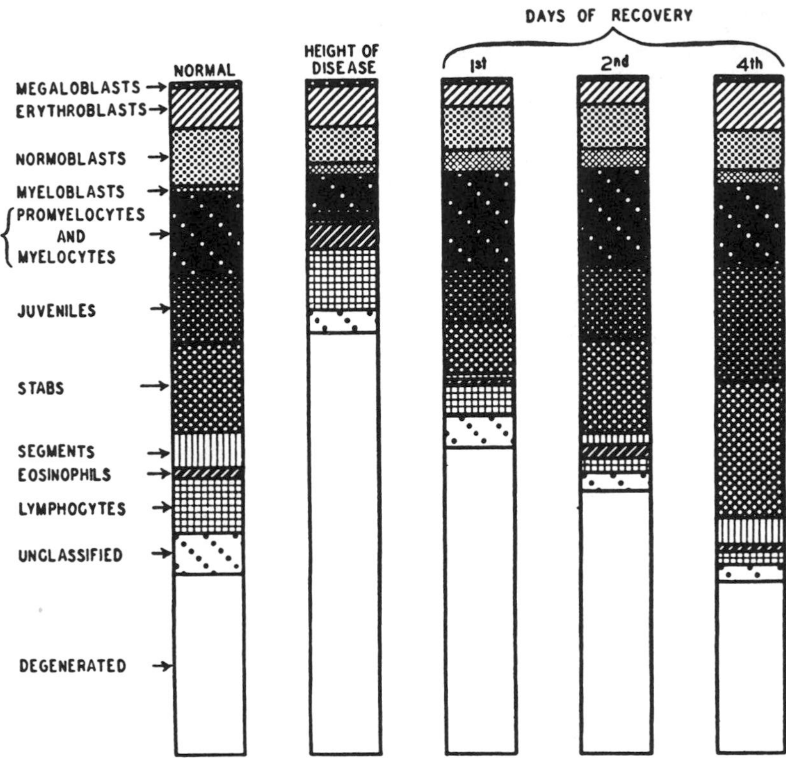


**Figure 2** Differential bone marrow counts in normal cats and during the course of infection with FPV. At the height of disease there is a marked decrease in the proportion of myeloid cells in the marrow, which returns very rapidly upon recovery. [From Lawrence et al. (55).]

cells contained intranuclear inclusion bodies. Increased phagocytic cells, some containing ingested red cells, were also seen. The spleen was also involved, but the most marked abnormalities were generally confined to the lymphoid elements.

## Gastrointestinal Tract

Evidence of infection of the gut is a constant finding with FPV infection, although the degree of symptomatic gastrointestinal infection is quite variable (4,52,55,58–60). A broad range of lesions can be seen; in some animals, there is only microscopic evidence of involvement; in others, there is gross disease, including sloughing of the villi, effacement of the mucosal architecture, and necrosis. The jejunum and ileum are most frequently involved, with the duodenum and colon generally less affected. Microscopically, marginated chromatin and eosinophilic nuclear inclusions are the most frequent finding, and although the incidence of these findings is variable, they can be seen in cells from both slightly affected and severely involved mucosa. Lesions begin in the crypts, particularly flattening, probably resulting from the lack of replacement of new cells, not direct infection of nondividing, undifferentiated cells farther up the villi. In natural infection, the submucosal infiltrate consists mostly of histiocytes and plasma cells; neutrophils and lymphocytes are remarkably absent (52). Invasion of damaged mucosa by bacteria and fungi can complicate the intestinal manifestations of infection with FPV (4).

#### Cerebellum

Although not part of the panleukopenia syndrome, cerebellar involvement is another striking feature of infection with FPV. Cerebellar ataxia arises at 2–3 weeks of age as kittens become ambulatory and is the result of intrauterine or neonatal infection with FPV. Pathologically, the cerebellum may be grossly hypoplastic, and on microscopic examination, there is loss of germinal and Purkinje's cells (2,3,60). Basophilic intranuclear inclusions can also be seen in infected cells (61).

### CPV and MEV

The major clinical manifestations of infection of dogs with CPV and mink with MEV is usually fatal enteritis. Myocarditis can also occur as the result of *in utero* or neonatal infection of canine pups with CPV (14,42,61,62). Leukopenia can be a prominent feature of infection with either virus, and both neutrophils and lymphocytes are decreased (63–66). The marrow findings in dogs infected either naturally or experimentally are similar to those described with FPV infection, including marked diminution of the marrow myeloid content; involvement of the erythoid precursors and megakaryocytes is variable (62,67). Similarly to FPV infection, residual myeloid progenitors are quite abnormal, with cytoplasmic basophilia, vacuolization, nuclear swelling, and hyalinization. Depletion of lymphoid tissues also occurs. With CPV infection, the gut can often be so severely involved that intranuclear inclusions cannot be distinguished, but in milder disease, infected mucosal cells with inclusion bodies are clearly evident.

## PATHOGENESIS

### In Vivo

FPV is cytotoxic to rapidly dividing cells. Irradiation, which is known to be lethal to rapidly proliferating crypt cells of the gut, produces intestinal lesions identical to those seen in pankeukopenia (59,68). Variability in disease manifestations seen clinically results, at least in part, from differences in proliferative rates of susceptible tissues. Cell proliferation, in turn, is determined by the stage of development of the animal and its exposure to environmental agents.

To determine the factors that influence the pathogenicity of the feline parvovirus, several investigators have experimentally infected well-defined populations of cats and followed the disease both clinically and pathologically. Infection of newborn cats obtained from females without previous exposure to FPV is characterized by marked and prolonged diminution of the leukocyte count (69). However, when animals were sacrificed at various times postinfection, the principal gross lesions include thymic atrophy and cerebellar hypoplasia (70). Microscopically, viral inclusions can be seen in cells from almost all tissues, and virus can be detected by immunofluorescence. The thymus, lymph nodes, and cerebellum are the most severely depleted tissues. The cerebellum may be a target because it develops late in gestation and the early neonatal period. The degree of ensuing clinical neurologic disease evidently results from the stage of differentiation of the cerebellum at the time of infection (61). In older cats (12–27 weeks) cerebellar lesions are notably absent (58).

Infection of germ-free cats has been employed to determine the contribution of the microbial flora in the gut to disease pathogenesis. Preinfection, germ-free cats generally have lower total white blood cell counts (59) and higher lymphocyte counts (71) than specific pathogen-free (SPF) cats (i.e., cats without previous exposure to a number of defined infectious agents including FPV) or conventional cats; in the marrow, a higher proportion of immature myeloid and erythroid cells has been seen in germ-free animals. Upon infection with FPV, few germ-free animals develop symptomatic disease, and histologic evidence for intestinal involvement, if any, is mild (59,71–73). In the peripheral blood, germ-free animals show a decrease in the total leukocyte count in response to infection (59,71), but the largest component of this drop results from a marked decrease in the number of lymphocytes (71). The most consistent pathologic lesion in these animals is depletion of cells in the thymus and lymph nodes (57,71–73). A seeming paradox with infection of germ-free cats is the lack of the pronounced bone marrow disease that is seen with natural infection. In the one study in which it was adequately documented, marrow cellularity in infected germ-free cats was not significantly different from that in uninfected controls, and the number of myeloid cells actually increased with infection (71). If the ability of a tissue to support viral propagation, and hence to be susceptible to the cytopathic effects of infection, is dependent on its proliferative rate, one might expect less overall disease in a germ-free animal. Intestinal epithelium has a decreased turnover rate in germ-free animals (74), and one predicts that the proliferation of myeloid precursor cells is also decreased in the absence of exposure to microbial agents. In addition, the less pronounced neutropenia seen in germ-free cats may result from lack of the additional stress to respond to other microbial insults or to an increased baseline reserve in the postmitotic myeloid pool in germ-free animals. The bone marrow picture, however, indicates that the postmitotic pool is not increased in germ-free cats (71). That infection continues to markedly deplete the lymphoid tissues in germ-free cats, particularly in the thymus and germinal centers of lymph nodes, suggests a comparably high turnover of lymphoid cells in both germ-free and conventional cats (58). However, a consistent problem with these studies is the lack of controls for variables that may influence the outcome of infection, especially viral strain and the dose of viral inoculum.

Factors other than the ability of a cell to divide likely also influence susceptibility to infection. This is highlighted by one study that addressed the effect of canine parvovirus on erythroid progenitor cells in phenylhydrazine-induced regenerative hemolytic anemia in dogs (75). In animals treated with sufficient doses of phenylhydrazine, the severe hemolysis that resulted stimulated the proliferation of erythroid cells in the marrow. Under these conditions, dogs infected with CPV failed to show reduction in hematocrit, reticulocyte count, or erythroid content in the marrow. An increase in the number of committed erythroid progenitor cells, the colony-forming units–erythroids (CFU-E), that resulted from treatment with phenylhydrazine was not significantly altered by infection. The inability to produce an aplastic crisis in this model was intepreted as a lack of susceptibility of rapidly proliferating erythroid progenitor cells to inhibition by CPV.

## In Vitro

The first cell culture system to support the growth of FPV was reported in 1965 by Johnson, who successfully isolated virus from primary kitten cells inoculated with an extract of infected tissue (76,77). The ability to propagate the virus *in vitro* made it possible to study the cellular effects of viral infection. The cytopathic effect (CPE) of FPV can be demonstrated in vitro by infecting either primary or immortalized feline cells (78,79) and following the cultures morphologically. Intranuclear inclusions arise within 8–12 h, defined by the appearance of prominently staining material that surrounds a distinct nucleolus (by hemotoxylin and eosin stain this material initially can be eosinophilic but becomes more basophilic as the lesion progresses). A clear zone surrounds the inclusion, creating a halo appearance. The larger inclusions displace the normal chromatin, which becomes marginated at the nuclear membrane; they darken and obliterate the nucleolar architecture and eventually the entire nucleus. By 24 h there is rounding of the cytoplasm around the nucleus. Electron microscopy reveals that in the advanced stages of infection, the nucleus is packed with structures of approximately 20 nanomers, the size of viral particles. The majority of these particles appear to contain DNA, but some are empty. The chromatin marginates to the periphery of the nucleus, and recognizable nucleolar material disappears. The cytoplasm becomes disrupted and pale, and there is gross swelling of organelles. Identical changes can be seen in canine cells infected with CPV (80). These *in vitro* findings correlate well with what is described histologically *in vivo* following infection with either virus (4,52,54,81).

This cytopathic effect is dependent, at least in part, on cell division (78, 82). Johnson first noted that only a small percentage (less than 5%) of cells in infected confluent monolayers demonstrated a cytopathic effect and that this effect was transient within the culture; within a number of days, the cytopathic effect generally disappeared from the monolayer altogether (78). Older monolayers were less susceptible than younger, and monolayers that had lost the CPE regained it when the cells were repassaged. Consistent with the requirement of the *S* phase, the cytopathic effect of virus can be extended to the majority of cells in culture by synchronizing the cells so that they all traverse the *S* phase within a short time after infection. Under certain conditions, feline cells that are stalled in *S* phase can still support viral replication (44,83). The cellular factor(s) necessary for viral replication are still unknown, but clearly replication of viral DNA can occur in cells in which cellular DNA synthesis is blocked (44). The proliferative rate of tissues may in part be genetically determined, or alternatively, other host cell factors may influence the ability of a cell to support productive infection. The extent of cytopathicity varies depending on the animal from which the primary cells are derived; it is similar on monolayers of cells derived from littermates but shows a high degree of variability among those obtained from animals from different litters (82).

FPV propagates in cultures of cat bone marrow, and we used this system to investigate the mechanism underlying the hematopoietic depression caused by this virus (41). Bone marrow mononuclear cells were obtained from the marrow of specific pathogen-free cats and placed in suspension culture under conditions that support the proliferation of committed myeloid and erythroid progenitor cells (the colony-forming units–granuloctye-macrophage, CFU-GM, and the burst-forming units–erythroids, BFU-E, respectively). In these hematopoietic cultures, FPV propagated with kinetics similar to those seen with primary or immortalized feline fibroblasts. By 24 h after infection, viral DNA was detected in cells as determined by hybridization to a $^{32}$P-labeled cloned fragment from CPV (greater than 95% homologous to the same region of FPV). DNA content peaked at 48 h and decreased thereafter; within a day of the appearance of DNA in the cells, there was the release of new virus into the supernatant. At high virus innocula, the number of targets cells was the limit to virus production, as expected from the self-limited nature of these primary cultures of bone marrow. Monomer and dimer replicating forms were clearly demonstrated by Southern blot analysis of viral DNA obtained from the infected marrow cultures. Viral nucleic acid was also detected in individual marrow cells by in situ hybridization and capsid antigen by immunofluorescence.

Direct infection and inhibition of bone marrow progenitor cells accounts for the pathogenesis of feline panleukopenia. In addition, myeloid progenitor cells were relatively more susceptible to inhibition than erythroid progenitors. In suspension culture, virus production was specific for hematopoietic cells and could not be accounted for by propagation in T lymphocytes. Virus production in the marrow cultures was enhanced by the addition of a source of hematopoietic growth factors (PHA-LCM, phytohemagglutinin-stimulated lymphocyte-conditioned media) and was not increased under conditions in which T lymphocytes were stimulated (protein A). In contrast, virus propagated in the peripheral blood upon protein A stimulation. After inoculation of suspension cultures of cat marrow with FPV, reduced numbers of cells of the myeloid lineage were seen compared to control, uninfected cultures. Granulocytes were absent, and the cultures consisted predominantly of macrophages, lymphocytes, and occasional erythroblasts a week after infection.

FPV inhibited clonal hematopoietic colony formation. To demonstrate this, mononuclear cells were isolated from cat marrow and cultured in methylcellulose in the presence of hematopoietic growth factors. Under these conditions, the progenitors CFU-GM, BFU-E, and CFU-E are detected by the morphology of colonies that result from their proliferation and differentiation of progeny. When marrow cells were infected at a high virus-to-cell ratio, there was nearly complete inhibition of colony formation by all three progenitor cell types (Fig. 3). This effect was abrogated by neutralizing antibody or under physical conditions known to inactivate the virus. CFU-GM were about six times more susceptible than BFU-E, as demonstrated by the dose-dependent inhibition of colony formation, but there was no statistically different susceptibility between CFU-GM and CFU-E. The relative specificity of FPV for myeloid progenitors was clearly demonstrated by its effects on the formation of colonies stimulated by the addition of specific hematopoietic growth factors. For these experiments, bone marrow mononuclear cells were depleted of monocytes by adherence to plastic and of T lymphocytes by rosetting with heterologous lymphocytes and then plated in low concentrations of serum. Recombinant human granulocyte colony-stimulating factor (G-CSF) specifically supported the growth of feline CFU-G (colony-form-

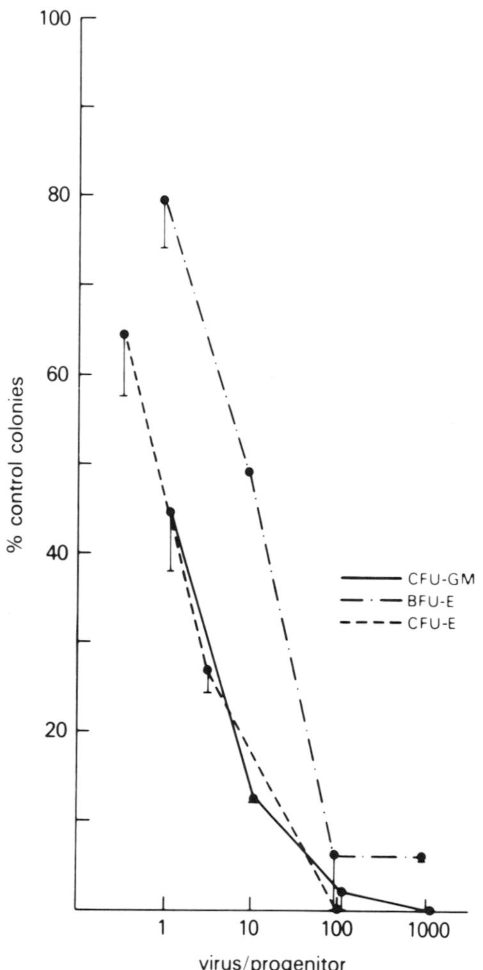


**Figure 3** Inhibition of clonal feline hematopoietic colonies by FPV. The percentage of control numbers of myeloid (CFU-GM) and erythroid (BFU-E and CFU-E) colonies infected at varying ratios of virus to progenitor cells is plotted. Represented here are the results of a typical experiment; the values plotted represent the mean number of colonies from duplicate cultures and the error bars the standard error of the mean. At low virus-progenitor cell ratios, CFU-GM and CFU-E are clearly more susceptible to inhibition by FPV than BFU-E. [From Kurtzman et al. (41).]

ing units–granulocytes), and recombinant human granulocyte-macrophate colony-stimulating factor (GM-CSF) supported the formation of CFU-GM. Growth of cat BFU-E was specifically stimulated by conditioned media from a feline leukemia-infected feline embryo fibroblast cell line (FLV-A-FEF) that contains burst-promoting activity. In this assay, the formation of CFU-G and CFU-GM was completely inhibited by FPV but the formation of BFU-E was only modestly affected. These results could not be explained on the basis of differences in cycling rates between the progenitor cells because the cycling rates of CFU-G, CFU-GM, and BFU-E were similar. By contrast, a greater than twofold difference in cycling rate for CFU-E relative to the other progenitors may at least partially contribute to their susceptibility to FPV.

## SUMMARY

Hammon and Enders were perplexed that no anemia could be found in animals infected with FPV even though at autopsy the marrow samples often appeared quite aplastic. They speculated that the longer life span of mature red cells in the blood compared to that of leukocytes protected against anemia. Since viral damage appeared to be confined to primitive blood-forming elements, anemia would not be expected during the course of an illness that lasted only 3–4 days (56). In contrast, the half-life of normal circulating neutrophils is of the order of 1–2 days and even shorter as a result of polymicrobial insult. The loss of myeloid precursors in the marrow is expected to result in a dramatic drop in neutrophil number under these conditions. An analogous situation occurs in humans upon infection with the B19 parvovirus, which shows relative or absolute specificity for erythroid progenitor cells (84). In otherwise normal individuals, the erythrocyte count may drop modestly postinfection, but because of the long half-life of circulating red blood cells (approximately 120 days), demonstrable anemia does not occur (85). In contrast, marked anemia occurs upon infection of individuals with underlying hemolysis, in which the half-life of circulating red cells is markedly decreased, or in individuals in whom infection is prolonged, as in persistent infection in immunosuppressed individuals (86,87). FPV infection carries a higher mortality than transient erythroid aplastic crisis in humans because of the relative tolerance of animals to short periods of anemia versus neutropenia.

The disease course of panleukopenia is most analogous to that of B19 infection in individuals with underlying hemolysis (transient aplastic crisis). Both tend to be monophasic diseases whose major manifestations occur with and result from the direct cytotoxic effect of the virus (86). In contrast, infection of normal individuals with B19 results in erythema infectiosum or fifth disease, a biphasic disease in which asymptomatic marrow suppression can be temporally separated from the major symptoms (fever, rash, and arthralgias) that occur as the result of immune complex formation (85). These symptoms are generally lacking in transient aplastic crisis. Individuals with an increased erythroid mass produce more virus than an infected, otherwise normal individual, and it has been postulated that a higher ratio of antigen to antibody results in less immune complex formation. The same may be true with FPV infection, for, as in an individual with underlying hemolysis, the number of targets for FPV in the conventional cat is likely to be high. Morphologically, the most consistent marrow finding in FPV infection is the loss of myeloid cells; with B19 infection, erythroid hypoplasia is most evident. The large mononuclear cells containing eosinophilic intranuclear inclusions described in infected marrow samples by Hammon and Enders are analogous to the giant pronormoblasts seen in marrow infected with B19 (86).

Although cats can continue to shed virus for a long time even in the presence of high titers of specific antibodies, no clinical syndrome attributible to persistent FPV infection has been described (88). By contrast, B19 persists and causes chronic bone marrow failure in individuals with underlying congenital or acquired immunodeficiency (87). A number of features of the recently described feline immunodeficiency virus (89–91), particularly neutropenia and gastrointestinal disease, are suggestive of concomitant infection with FPV, but it remains to be seen whether FPV can cause persistent infection during this or other immunodeficiency states in the cat.

Although not precisely characterized, B19, like FPV and the other parvoviruses, probably also requires active cell proliferation to successfully replicate. Both have similar kinetics in marrow culture (41,92), and both show dependence on the addition of specific hematopoietic growth factors. In cultures of bone marrow, B19 shows rather strict tropism for erythroid progenitors (84,92) and FPV shows relative specificity for myeloid cells. In general, FPV is a more promiscuous virus than B19. FPV infects a number of tissues and can be passaged in culture; B19 has been most successfully propagated in self-limited cultures of human erythroid bone marrow (84, 88). At high viral inocula, some in vitro inhibition of erythroid progenitor cells can be demonstrated for FPV, but there is no in vitro inhibition of neutrophil or platelet progenitor cells by B19 even though clinically the neutrophil and platelet counts are often decreased with infection (93). Cell cycling rate alone cannot completely account for the infectivity of FPV, and other host cell factors must in part influence a cell's susceptibility to productive infection. The host cell factor(s) that permit successful propagation of B19 are likely much more specific and restrictive than those for FPV.

Viruses can result in bone marrow failure by at least three mechanisms: (1) they can direct inhibit or be cytotoxic to hematopoietic progenitor cells;

(2) they can directly inhibit or be cytotoxic to accessory cells necessary to support hematopoiesis; or (3) they can stimulate the production of inhibitory lymphokines or cytotoxic lymphocytes that inhibit or destroy hematopoietic cells (1). The bone marrow suppression that results from FPV infection most likely results from direct cytotoxicity to bone marrow progenitor cells. That recovery from infection is complete reflects both the large reserve of bone marrow progenitor cells and the lack of susceptibility of nonproliferating stem cells to infection. It remains to be defined whether infections with common viruses, such as FPV or B19, have much more protracted effects on hematopoiesis under conditions in which the stem cell reserve is limited, for instance following chemotherapy or bone marrow transplantation. In these situations, unexplained and prolonged cytopenias are common. The cat system offers a convenient model with which to address these types of questions.

## REFERENCES

1. Kurtzman G, Young N. Viruses and bone marrow failure. Balliere's Clin Hematol, 1989; 2:51-67.
2. Greene CE. Feline panleukopenia. In: Clinical microbiology and infectious diseases of cats. CE, Greene ed. Philadelphia: W. B. Saunders, 1984; 479–89.
3. Bruner DW, Gilespie JH. Hagan's infectious diseases of domestic animals. Ithaca, NY: Cornell University Press, 1973; 1086–96.
4. Langheinrich KA, Nielsen SW. Histopathology of feline panleukopenia: a report of 65 cases. J Am Vet Med Assoc 1971; 158:863–72.
5. Verge J, Christoforoni N. La gastro-enterite infectieuse des chats est-elle duc a un virus filtrable? C R Soc Biol (Paris) 1928; 99:312–4.
6. Lawrence JS, Syverton JT. Spontaneous agranulocytosis in the cat. Proc Soc Exp Biol Med 1938; 38:914–8.
7. Siegl G, Bates RC, Berns KI, et al. Characteristics and taxonomy of Parvoviridae. Intervirology 1985; 23:71-3.
8. Parrish CR, Carmichael LE. Antigenic structure and variation of canine parvovirus type-2, feline panleukopenia virus, and mink enteritis virus. Virology 1983; 129:401-14.
9. Tratschin JD, McMaster GK, Kronauer G, Siegl G. Canine parvovirus: relationship to wild-type and vaccine strains of feline panleukopenia virus and mink enteritis virus. J Gen Virol 1982; 61:33-41.
10. Parrish CR, Carmichael LE, Antczak DF. Antigenic relationships between canine parvovirus type 2, feline panleukopenia virus and mink enteritis virus using conventional antisera and monoclonal antibodies. Arch Virol 1982; 72:267–78.
11. Mengeling WL, Paul PS, Bunn TO, Ridpath JF. Antigenic relationships among autonomous parvoviruses. J Gen Virol 1986; 67:2389–844.
12. Parrish CR, Aquadro CF, Carmichael LE. Canine host range and a specific epitope map along with variant sequences in the capsid protein gene of canine par-

vovirus and related feline, mink, and racoon parvoviruses. Virology 1988; 155: 293–307.
13. Shoenfield FW. Virus enteritis in mink. North Am Vet 1949; 30:651.
14. Siegl G. Canine parvovirus: origin and significance of a "new" pathogen. In: Berns KI, ed. The parvoviruses. New York: Plenum Press, 1984; 363–88.
15. Tatersall P, Cotmore SF. The nature of parvoviruses. In: Pattison JR, ed. Parvoviruses and human disease. Boca Raton, FL: CRC Press, 1988; 5–42.
16. Tsao J, Chapman MD, Agbandje M, et al. The three-dimensional structure of canine parvovirus and its functional implications. Science 1991; 251:1456–64.
17. Carlson J, Rushlow K, Maxwell I, Winston S, Hahn W. Cloning and sequence of DNA encoding structural proteins of the autonomous farvovirus feline panleukopenia virus. J Virol, 1985; 55:574–82.
18. Reed AP, Jones EV, Miller TJ. Nucleotide sequence and genome organization of canine parvovirus. J Virol 1988; 62:266–76.
19. Martyn JC, Davidson BE, Studdert MJ. Nucleotide sequence of feline panleukopenia virus: comparison with canine parvovirus identifies host-specific differences. J Gen Virol 1990; 71:2747–53.
20. Basak S, Compans RW. Polarized entry of canine parvovirus in an epithelial cell line. J Virol 1989; 63:3164–7.
21. Astell CR, Thomson M, Merchlinsky M, Ward DC. The complete DNA sequence of minute virus of mice, an autonomous parvovirus. Nucleic Acids Res 1983; 11: 999–1018.
22. Rhode SL, Paradiso PR. Parvovirus genome: nucleotide sequence of H-1 and mapping of its genes by hybrid arrest translation. J Virol 1983; 45: 173–84.
23. Shade RO, Blundell MC, Cotmore SF, Tattersall P, Astell CR. Nucleotide sequence and genome organization of human parvovirus B19 isolated from the serum of a child during aplastic crisis. J Virol 1986; 58:921–36.
24. Chen KC, Shull BC, Moses EA, Lederman M, Stout ER, Bates RC. Complete nucleotide sequence and genome organization of bovine parvovirus. J Virol 1986; 60:1085–97.
25. Carter BJ, Laughlin CA, Marcus-Sekura CJ. Parvovirus transcription. In: Berns KI, ed. The parvoviruses. New York: Plenum Press, 1984; 153–208.
26. Lebovitz RM, Roeder RG. Parvovirus H-1 expression: mapping of the abundant cytoplasmic transcripts and identification of promoter sites and overlapping transcription units. J Virol 1986; 58:271–80.
27. Ozawa K, Ayub J, Yu-Shu H, Kurtzman G, Shimada T, Young N. Novel transcription map for the B19 (human) pathogenic parvovirus. J Virol 1987; 61:2395–406.
28. Senapathy P, Teatschin JD, Carter BJ. Replication of adeno-associated virus DNA: complementation of naturally occurring *rep*-mutants by a wild-type genome or an *ori-* mutant and correction of terminal palindrome deletions. J Mol Biol 1984; 179:1–20.
29. Tratschin JD, Miller IL, Carter BJ. Genetic analysis of adeno-associated virus: properties of deletion mutants constructed in vitro and evidence for an adeno-associated virus replication function. J Virol 1984; 51:611–9.
30. Labow MA, Hermonat PL, Berns KI. Positive and negative autoregulation of the adeno-associated virus type 2 genome. J Virol 1986; 60:251–8.

31. Rhode SL. Trans-activation of parvovirus $P_{38}$ promoter by the 76K noncapsid protein. J Virol 1985; 55:886–9.
32. Rhode SL. Characterization of the trans-activation-responsive element of the parvovirus H-1 P38 promoter. J Virol 1987; 61:2806–15.
33. Tratschin JD, Tal J, Carter BJ. Negative and positive regulation in trans of gene expression from adeno-associated virus vectors in mammalian cells by a viral rep gene. Mol Cell Biol 1986; 6:2883–94.
34. Doerig C, Hirt B, Antonietti J, Beard P. Nonstructural protein of parvoviruses B19 and minute virus of mixe controls transcription. J Virol 1990; 64:387–96.
35. Rhode SL. Both excision and replication of clone autonomous parvovrs DNA require the NS1 (*rep*) protein. J Virol 1989; 63:4249–56.
36. Labow MA, Graf LH, Berns KI. Adeno-associated virus gene expression inhibits cellular transformation by heterologous genes. Mol Cell Biol 1987; 7:1320–5.
37. Rhode SL. Construction of a genetic switch for inducible trans-activation of gene expression in eucaryotic cells. J Virol 1987; 61:1448–56.
38. Ozawa K, Ayub J, Kajigaya S, Shimada T, Young N. The gene encoding the non-structural protein of B19 (human) parvovirus may be lethal in transfected cells. J Virol 1988; 62:2884–9.
39. Johnson FB. Parvovirus proteins. In: Berns KI, ed. The parvoviruses. New York: Plenum Press, 1984; 259–96.
40. Hauswirth WW. Autonomous parvovirus DNA structure and replication. In: Berns KI, ed. The parvoviruses. New York: Plenum Press, 1984; 129–52.
41. Kurtzman GJ, Platanias L, Lustig L, Frickhofen N, Young NS. Feline parvovirus propagates in cat bone marrow cultures and inhibits hematopoietic colony formation in vitro. Blood 1989; 74:71–81.
42. Siegl G. Biology and pathogeneicity of autonomous parvoviruses. In: Berns KI, ed. The parvoviruses. New York: Plenum Press, 1984; 297–362.
43. Yakobson B, Koch T, Winocour E. Replication of adeno-associated virus in synchronized cells without the addition of a helper virus. J Virol 1987; 61:972–81.
44. Lenghaus C, Mun TK, Studdert MJ. Feline panleukopenia virus replicates in cells in which cellular DNA synthesis is blocked. J Virol 1985; 53:345–9.
45. Brown T, Anand A, Ritchie LD, Clewley JP, Reid TMS. Intrauterine parvovirus infection associated with hydrops fetalis. Lancet 1984; 2:1033–4.
46. Knot PD, Welply GAC, Anderson MJ. Serologically proved intrauterine infection with parvovirus. Br Med J 1984; 289:1660.
47. Anand A, Gray ES, Brown T, Clewley JP, Cohen BJ. Human parvovirus in pregnancy and hydrops fetalis. N Engl J Med 1984; 316: 183–6.
48. Parrish CR, Carmichael LE. Characterization and recombination mapping of an antigenic and host range mutation of canine parvovirus. Virology 1986; 148: 121–32.
49. Spaholz BA, Tattersall P. Interaction of minute virus of mice with differentiated cells: strain-dependent target cell specificity is mediated by intracellular factors. J Virol 1983; 46:937.
50. Leasure EE, Leinhardt HF, Taberner FR. Feline infectious enteritis. North Am Vet 1934; 15:30–44.

51. Hindle E, Findlay GM. Studies on feline distemper. J Comp Pathol Ther 1932; 45:11–26.
52. Hammon WD, Enders JF. A virus disease of cats, principally characterized by aleucocytosis, enteric lesions and the presence of intranuclear inclusion bodies. J Exp Med 1939; 69:327–51.
53. Johnson RH, Margolis G, Kilham L. Identigy of feline ataxia virus with feline panleukopenia virus. Nature 1967; 214:175–7.
54. Lawrence JS, Syverton JT, Ackart RJ, et al. The virus of infectious feline agranulocytosis. II. Immunological relation to other viruses. J Exp Med 1943; 77:57–64.
55. Lawrence JS, Syverton JT, Shaw JS, Smith FP. Infectious feline agranulocytosis. Am J Pathol 1940; 16:333–54.
56. Hammon WD, Enders JF. Further studies on the blood and hematopoietic tissues in malignant panleucopenia of cats. J Exp Med 1939; 70:557–64.
57. Carpenter JL. Feline panleukopenia: clinical signs and differential diagnosis. J Am Vet Med Assoc 1971; 158:857–9.
58. Larsen S, Flagstad A, Aalbaek B. Experimental feline panleucopenia in the conventional cat. Vet Pathol 1976; 13:216–40.
59. Carlson JH, Scott FW, Duncan JR. Feline panleukopenia. I. Pathogenesis in germfree and specific pathogen-free cats. Vet Pathol 1977; 14:79–88.
60. Johnson GR, Koestner A, Rohovsky MW. Experimental feline infectious enteritis in the germfree cat: an electron lmicroscopic study. Pathol Vet 1967; 4:275–88.
61. Siegl G. Patterns of parvovirus disease in animals. In: Pattison JR, ed. Parvoviruses and human disease. Boca Raton, FL: CRC Press, 1988; 43–68.
62. Robinson WF, Wilcox GE, Flower RLP. Canine parvoviral disease: experimental reproduction of the enteric form with a parvovirus isolated from a case of myocarditis. Vet Pathol 1980; 17:589–99.
63. Reynolds HA. Some clinical and hematological features of virus enteritis of mink. Can J Comp Med 1969; 33:155–9.
64. Woods CB, Pollock RVH, Carmichael LE. Canine parvoviral enteritis. J Am Anim Hosp Assoc 1980; 16:170–9.
65. Jacobs RM, Weiser MG, Hall RL, Kowalski JJ. Clinicopathologic features of canine parvoviral enteritis. J Am Anim Hosp Assoc 1980; 16:809–14.
66. Carman PS, Pover RC. Pathogenesis of canine parvovirus-2 in dogs: hematology, serology and virus recovery. Res Vet Sci 1985; 38:134–40.
67. Boosinger TR, Rebar AH, DeNicola DB, Boon GD. Bone marrow alterations associated with canine parvovirual enteritis. Vet Pathol. 1982; 19:558–61.
68. Thomassen RW. Acute intestinal radiation injury in the cat (abstract). Vet Pathol 1972; 9:78.
69. Csiza CK, Scott FW, De Lahunta A, Gillespie JH. Pathogenesis of feline panleukopenia virus in susceptible newborn kittens. I. Clinical signs, hematology, serology, and virology. Infect Immun 1971; 3:833–7.
70. Csiza CK, Del Lahunat A, Scott FW, Gillespie JH. Pathogenesis of feline panleukopenia virus in susceptible newborn kittens. II. Pathology and immunofluorescence. Infect Immun 1971; 3:838–46.

71. Rohovsky MW, Griesemer RA. Experimental feline infectious enteritis in the germfree cat. Pathol Vet 1967; 4:391–410.
72. Rohovsky MH, Fowler EH. Lesions of experimental feline panleukopenia. J Am Vet Med Assoc 1971; 158:872–5.
73. Johnson GR, Koestner A, Rohovsky MW. Experimental feline infectious enteritis in the germfree cat: an electron microscopic study. Pathol Vet 1967; 4: 275–88.
74. Carlson JH, Scott FW. Feline panleukopenia. II. The relationship of intestinal mucosal cell proliferation rates to viral infection and the development of lesions. Vet Pathol 1977; 14:173–81.
75. Brock CV, Jones JB, Schull RM, Potgieter LND. Effect of canine parvovirus on erythroid progenitors in phenylhudrazine-induced regenerative hemolytic aniemia in dogs. Am J Vet Res 1989; 50:965–9.
76. Johnson RH. Isolation of a virus from a condition simulating feline panleucopenia in a leopard. Vet Rec 1964; 76:1008–13.
77. Johnson RH. Feline panleucopenia. I. Identification of a virus associated with the syndrome. Res Vet Sci 1965; 6:466–71.
78. Johnson RH. Feline panleucopenia virus. II. Some features of the cytopathic effects in feline kidney monolayers. Res Vet Sci 1965; 6:472–81.
79. O'Shea JD, Studdert MJ. Growth of an autonomously replicating parvovirus (feline panleucopenia): kinetics and morphogenesis. Arch Virol 1978; 57:107–22.
80. Paradiso PR, Rhode SL, Singer IW. Canine parovirus: a biochemical and ultrastructural characterization. J Gen Virol 1982; 62:113–24.
81. Yasoshima A, Doi K, Kojima A, Okaniwa A. Electron microscopic findings on epithelial cells of Lieberkühn's crypts in canine parvovirus infection. Jpn J Vet Sci 1982; 44:81–8.
82. Johnson RH. Feline panleucopenia virus. IV. Methods for obtaining reproducible in vitro results. Res Vet Sci 1967; 8:256–64.
83. Endo M, Shinagawa M, Goto H, Shimizu K. Growth characteristics of feline panleukopenia virus in synchronized kitten kidney cells. Jpn J Vet Sci 1981; 43:63–70.
84. Ozawa K, Kurtzman G, Young N. Replication of the B19 parvovirus in human bone marrow cell cultures. Science 1986; 233:883–6.
85. Anderson MJ, Higgins PG, Davis LR, et al. Experimental parvoviral infection in humans. J Infect Dis 1985; 152:257–75.
86. Young NS. Hematologic and hematopoietic consequences of B19 parvovirus infection. Semin Hematol 1988; 25:158–72.
87. Frickhofen N, Young NS. Persistent parvovirus B19 infection in humans. Microb Pathog 1989; 7:319–27.
88. Csiza CK, Scott FW, DeLahunta A, Gillespie JH. Immune carrier state of feline panleukopenia virus-infected cats. Am J Vet Res 1971; 32:419–26.
89. Pedersen NC, Ho E, Brown ML, Yamamoto JK. Isolation of a T-lymphotropic virus from domestic cats with an immunodeficiency-like syndrome. Science 1987; 235:790–3.
90. Yamamoto JK, Sparger E, Ho EW, et al. Pathogenesis of experimentally induced feline immunodeficiency virus infection in cats. Am J Vet Res 1988; 49: 1246–58.

91. Shelton GH, Linenberger ML, Grant CK, Abkowitz JL. Hematologic manifestations of feline immunodeficiency virus infection. Blood 1990; 76:1104–9.
92. Ozawa K, Kurtzman G, Young N. Productive infection by B19 parvovirus of human erythroid bone marrow cells in vitro. Blood 1987; 70:384–91.
93. Mortimer PP, Humphires RK, Moore JG, Purcell RH, Young NS. A human parvovirus-like virus inhibits hematopoietic colony formation in vitro. Nature 1983; 302:426.

# III

# HERPESVIRUSES

# 5

# Epstein-Barr Virus

**Bruce G. Baranski**

*University of Wisconsin—Madison*
*Madison, Wisconsin*

**Ian T. Magrath**

*National Cancer Institute*
*Bethesda, Maryland*

## INTRODUCTION

Hematologic abnormalities occurring during an acute infection with Epstein-Barr virus (EBV) are so common that they are considered part of the normal spectrum of the disease. Whether these hematologic changes are due to the virus itself or to the host immune response against the virus is not always clear. In individuals with abnormal immunity to EBV, however, particularly severe, even fatal, hematologic manifestations of an acute EBV infection are often encountered. Similar consequences can occur as a result of impairment of the host's immune response many years after primary infection, because virus-infected cells persist for life. The hematologic changes induced by infection with EBV vary widely, from transient cytopenias or self-limited lymphoproliferations to bone marrow failure. EBV may also induce fatal lymphoproliferation and is associated with some forms of monoclonal lymphoma.

In this chapter, we review the biology of EBV, the normal host immune response to the virus, the variety of hematologic changes seen in normal and abnormal hosts, and the malignant manifestations of EBV infection. The emphasis of this chapter is to review the hematologic manifestations of EBV infection in a comprehensive fashion; for details, the reader is guided to the appropriate reviews.

## HISTORICAL BACKGROUND

The clinical manifestations of primary infection with EBV—"glandular fever" or infectious mononucleosis—were noted long before the actual discovery of the virus, but Burkitt's lymphoma, a tumor frequently associated with EBV, was firmly established as a clinicopathologic entity only 6 years before EBV was discovered (1,2). In fact, it was a hypothesis that Burkitt's lymphoma is caused by a vectored virus that led to the discovery of EBV. The term "infectious mononucleosis" (IM) was first used in 1920, and in the same year, the atypical lymphocytes associated with IM were described. The first diagnostic test for EBV-induced infectious mononucleosis, the pathologic basis of which is still poorly understood, was described by Paul and Bunnel in 1932 when they noted the presence of the heterophil antibody in a medical student with infectious mononucleosis. A modified version of this test remains the predominant laboratory tool used in the diagnosis of this disease.

EBV was discovered in 1964 when Epstein, Achong, and Barr described the presence of herpeslike viral particles in a continuous cell line derived from tumor cells sent to them by Burkitt from patients with the "African lymphoma." Henle and Henle subsequently described an immunofluorescent assay for the detection of EBV antibodies in 1968 when a technician was seen to seroconvert after an episode of infectious mononucleosis. Since these early findings established the link between EBV, infectious mononucleosis, the Burkitt's lymphoma, the virus has been completely sequenced and our understanding of EBV biology and the host response to the virus has expanded at a rapid pace.

## EPSTEIN-BARR VIRUS BIOLOGY

### The Virus and Its Genome

EBV is a member of the human herpesvirus family. The viral particle is 150–180 nm in diameter and shares the four main characteristics of other human herpesviruses: (1) a core containing double-stranded DNA, (2) an icosahedral capsid with capsomere subunits, (3) a tegument surrounding the viral capsid, and (4) an envelope containing glycolipids and glycoproteins (3–5). An electron micrograph of EBV is shown in Figure 1. The EBV genome is approximately 170,000–190,000 base pairs in length and codes for 50–100 proteins. The entire genome has been sequenced for the B958 strain, and portions of the genome have been studied in other virus isolates.

The general organization of the EBV genome is similar to that of other herpesviruses (Fig. 2). There are multiple terminal repeats (TR) of approximately 500 base pairs each at both ends of the EBV genome. The number of

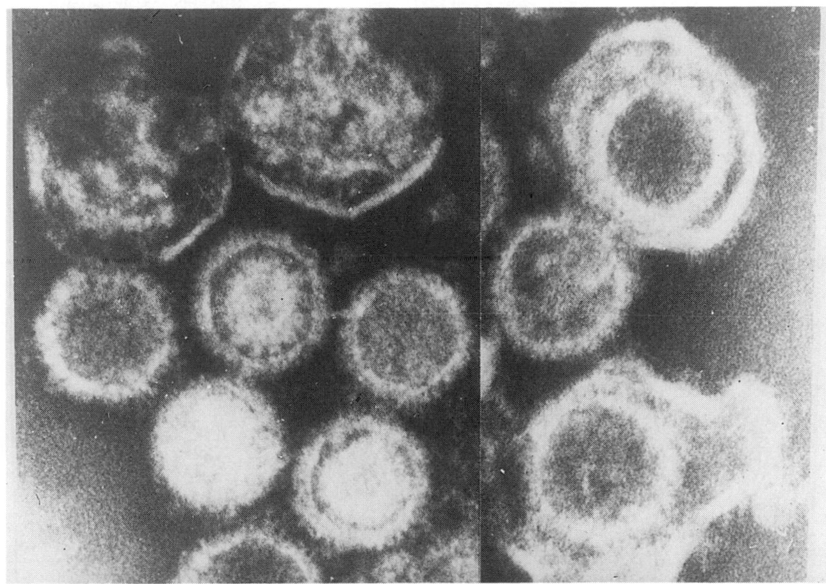

**Figure 1** EBV structure by electron micrography. The viral icosohedral capsid and the core are best seen on the left. On the right, the viral envelope is demonstrated in more detail (as seen in the particles at the top and bottom of the right panel).

terminal repeats varies considerably between EBV isolates, a phenomenon that has been exploited to differentiate between EBV clones in or between individuals. Latently infected cells contain episomal genomes fused at these terminal repeats. There are an additional four tandem internal repeat regions within the EBV genome. These internal repeats serve to divide the genome into five unique regions (U1–5) which are the primary coding regions of EBV. The U2 portion of the genome, which contains the EBNA-2 gene, varies considerably between EBV isolates and is almost entirely deleted in the nontransforming strain of EBV, P3HR–1, and in the virus present in the cell line, Daudi. Other regions of the EBV genome also vary among EBV isolates, the most widely recognized being sequence differences in the EBNA-2, 3a, 3b, and 3c (also known as 3, 4, and 6) genes, which are sufficiently reproducible to lead to the designation of two major EBV types 1 or 2, or A or B. To date, however, no other differences between genomes have been found to alter the known biologic activity of EBV in a significant manner. Some strains contain separate small pieces of DNA known as het (heterogeneous) fragments, some of which may contain sequences important in the switch from a latent infection to a productive infection.

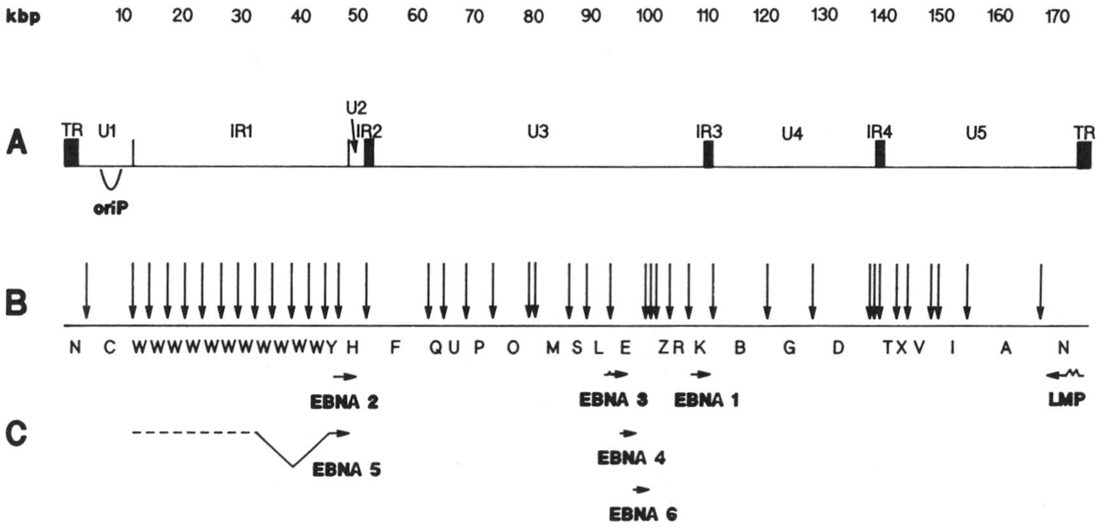


**Figure 2** General structure of the EBV genome. The size of the genome is shown in kbp (kilobase pairs). The scale is located over the map of the genome. (A) General structure of the virus showing the unique coding regions (U), the internal repeats (IR), the terminal repeats (TR), and the origin of replication (oriP). (B) A restriction map of the genome showing the fragments generated by digestion of EBV DNA with the restriction enzyme *Bam*HI. The restriction sites are designated by arrows. A letter is assigned to each restriction fragment generated; the coding regions of the genome are named by the DNA fragment in which they reside. (C) RNA transcripts coding for the EBNA genes. Each transcript is located directly below the area of the genome (B) from which it is transcribed.

The EBV DNA fragments generated by digestion with *Bam*HI provide a convenient means of mapping the genome. Each *Bam*HI fragment is assigned a letter, according to size (beginning with A, the largest fragment). Most coding and regulatory regions of EBV are designated by the *Bam*HI fragment in which they reside (see Fib. 2B).

## Route of Infection

Upon entering the host through saliva, the main target of the EBV appears to be the epithelial cells lining the oropharynx (2,5,6). The EBV genome and virus-encoded antigens are present within these cells during acute infectious mononucleosis. The C3d receptor (CD21), known to mediate virus entry into B cells, is also expressed on epithelial cells and presumably provides the portal of entry into such cells. Other cells, such as T lymphocytes, may contain low quantities of the C3d receptor capable of binding EBV (7). However, it is likely that there are other viral receptors because cell lines capable of binding EBV that do not bear the C3d receptor have been described.

Cervical epithelial cells also contain EBV in vivo and can be infected in vitro with EBV, suggesting that epithelial cells at other sites may also be targets of EBV infection. Only wild-type EBV is capable of infecting cervical epithelial cells, however, suggesting that laboratory strains of EBV may be selected for their ability to infect B cells (8).

Infection of B lymphocytes primarily takes place in pharyngeal lymphoid tissue. The virus appears to spread to other parts of the body via B cells infected while circulating through the pharynx. EBV genome and antigens have been detected, using in situ hybridization, within the cervical lymph nodes of patients with acute mononucleosis. Surprisingly, most cells containing EBV genome were found within the paracortex and pulp cords, areas known to contain predominantly T lymphocytes.

EBV binds to the C3d receptor via glycoprotein gp350/220, present in the viral envelope. Once the virus binds to the cell surface receptor, the receptor is phosphorylated and the virus enters the cell. The cell is then activated, enters the *G*1 phase, and expresses cell surface antigens, such as Blast-2 (CD23) (9). The surface CD23 molecule is cleaved and shed into the cellular space as a smaller fragment, where it may act as an autocrine or paracrine growth factor for B cells. These early internalization and activation steps can be induced with ultraviolet (UV)-inactivated EBV or antibodies to the C3d receptor. However, the transition to the *S* phase of the cell cycle and immortalization of B cells is dependent on the presence of an intact virus genome, since expression of viral genes, including EBNA-2, EBNA-5 (leader protein), and latent membrane protein (LMP) is necessary. These genes probably act on cellular genes involved in proliferation, including, perhaps, those encoding growth factors and growth factor receptors that may result in the establishment of an autocrine loop. Not all cells infected with EBV are induced to proliferate, and only 50% of the latter are transformed into permanent cell lines (10). Lymphocytes induced to proliferate by EBV infection are capable of producing polyclonal immunoglobulins.

The true host cell range of EBV is currently under investigation. The EBV genome and antigens have been found in many other cell types (see Tables 1 and 2). This list of cells that are infected by EBV can be expected to expand as newer and more sensitive detection techniques for EBV become available.

Infection of cells resistant to EBV in vitro and expression of EBV antigens within these cells is possible when the C3d receptor is transfected and expressed in cells not readily infectable with EBV. Multiple cell types transfected or microinjected with EBV DNA express EBV antigens and may be transformed, implying that the EBV host range may be limited more by cell surface receptor expression than by host cell metabolic differences.

## Productive Infection and Viral Replication

Upon entering the host cell, the viral particles are stripped of their envelope, tegument, and capsid (29,30). The viral DNA enters the nucleus, and expres-

**Table 1** Known In Vivo Tissue Distribution of EBV[a]

| Tissue | Cell type infected | Method of detection (Ref.) |
|---|---|---|
| Oral cavity | Epithelial cell | ISH, IF, CX (11,12) |
| Tongue (HL) | Epithelial cell | SH, ISH, IF (13) |
| Cervix | Epithelial cell | ISH, IF (14) |
| Lymph node | Unknown | SH, ISH, IF (15) |
| Lung | Epithelial cell | SH, ISH, IF (16) |
| Non-Hodgkin's lymphoma | Unknown | SH, IF, ISH (17) |
| Hodgkin's | Reed-Sternberg cell | SH, IF, ISH (18) |
| NPC | Unknown | SH, IF (19) |
| Parotid | Unknown | SH, IF (20) |
| Leukemia | B cells | SH, IF (21) |
| | T cells | SH, IF (22) |
| | Hairy cells | IF, ISH (23) |
| | Myeloid cells | SH, IF (24) |
| Thymus | Unknown | IF (25) |

[a]ISH, in situ hybridization; IF, immunofluorescence; SH, Southern hybridization; NH, northern hybridization; CX, culture.

**Table 2** Cells That Can Be Infected with EBV In Vitro[a]

| Cell type | Detection method(s) | References |
|---|---|---|
| B cell | IF, SH, ISH, CX | 4, 5, 10 |
| Erythroid progenitor | IF, ISH | 26 |
| Monocyte | IF, SH | 27 |
| Megakaryocyte | IF | 28 |
| Cervical epithelium | IF, ISH | 29 |
| Oral epithelium | IF, ISH | 11 |

[a]ISH, in situ hybridization; IF, immunofluorescence; SH, Southern hybridization; NH, northern hybridization; CX, culture.

sion of viral genes begins. EBV DNA integration into the host cell genome is uncommon, but cell lines containing only integrated EBV genomes exist. During productive infection ("lytic" phase), many early RNA transcripts are produced that lead to the production of viral DNA polymerase, thymidine kinase, alkaline exonucleases, early antigens [EA-R (restricted) and EA-D (diffuse)], viral capsid antigen (VCA), and membrane antigens (MA). The EBNA genes are primarily expressed during latent infection and may be down-regulated during lytic infection (see Fig. 2C for EBNA and LMP coding regions). Other proteins are produced during the replicative cycle but are not yet characterized. The EBV genome is packaged in a linear form. In vivo, epithelial cells are known to produce virus, but there is no information regarding other cell types. In vitro only a small percentage of infected lymphoid cells produce virus, regardless of whether they are of malignant or nonmalignant origin. Even in cell lines like P3HR-1, produce nontransforming virus at higher levels, treatment with exogenous agents is required to raise the proportion of virus-producing cells to greater than the usual 1–5%.

Data from bone marrow transplant patients suggest that EBV can be eradicated from the host by the pretransplant conditioning regimen and that patients reinfected posttransplant may be infected with a different virus (as determined by EBNA types) (31). In one case, the virus isolated from a transplanted patient matched the virus isolated from the patient's spouse. These data suggest that lymphocytes are the permanent reservoir for EBV, since epithelial cells are not readily destroyed by pretransplant conditioning and therefore presumably are repeatedly reinfected from the B cell pool or by exogenous virus under normal circumstances.

## Latent Infection and Immortalization

Latent infection is an important part of the EBV life cycle and has considerable clinical relevance (30–33).

Latently infected, immortalized lymphocytes consistently express at least eight genes. Of these, the functional properties of three of the gene products have been studied in vitro (33): EBNA-1, EBNA-2, and BNLF-1 (LMP). EBNA-1 is a trans-activating factor required for the replication of EBV episomes in replicating cells, and it also activates an enhancer that increases the transcription of other latent genes. EBNA-2 is believed to be required for EBV-induced transformation, since this gene is deleted in nontransforming strains of EBV. EBNA-2 also induces the expression of CD23. The BNLF-1 gene encodes a latent membrane protein that increases the expression of several cell adhesion molecules and also acts as an oncogene in rodent cells. The other EBV gene products made in latently infected cells include EBNA-3, EBNA-5, and EBER small RNAs. The function of these is less well understood, although EBNA-3 is also believed to play a role in transformation.

The possible role of EBV-encoded proteins in the etiology of Burkitt's lymphoma (which consistently contains an 8;14 chromosomal translocation involving the c-*myc* gene) remains to be elucidated. In fact, many of these molecules (EBNA-2, EBNA-5, and LMP) present in lymphoblastoid cell lines are not consistently expressed in Burkitt's lymphoma cells (34). EBNA-1, however, appears to be uniformly expressed in all latently infected cells.

## HOST IMMUNE RESPONSE TO EBV

A number of clinical observations have suggested a major role of the cellular immune system in the regulation of EBV-infected cells (6,35). These observations include the following: (1) renal allograft recipients receiving immunosuppressive therapy shed more virus from their throats than normal individuals, (2) some aspects of cellular immunity, including T cell responses to EBV-infected cells, in patients in regions endemic for Burkitt's lymphoma are consistently impaired; and (3) individuals with the X-linked lymphoproliferative disease (discussed in detail later in this chapter) cannot control EBV infections despite a strong humoral response to the virus.

The immune response to EBV infection invokes many arms of the immune system. Initially, the host response is nonspecific and consists of activation of natural killer (NK) cells, nonspecific cytotoxic T lymphocytes, suppressor T lymphocytes that inhibit the abnormal polyclonal production of antibodies, and the release of soluble factors, such as interferons and interleukin-1 (IL-1), which help control the expansion of EBV-infected cells. Following this initial nonspecific phase of the immune response, EBV-specific HLA class I-restricted cytotoxic T lymphocytes and EBV neutralizing antibodies appear.

Svermyr et al. (36) described a case of a young man whose immune function was followed prospectively after his girlfriend developed IM. The first abnormalities noted were the presence of transformed B lymphocytes and detectable (50 U/ml) interferon levels in the peripheral blood. Once the subject developed symptoms of IM, EBNA-positive B cells, anti-EBV antibodies, activated suppressor lymphocytes (as determined by surface phenotype analysis), nonspecific lymphocyte-mediated cytoxic activity, and functional B cell suppressor activity appeared. During the convalescent phase of the illness, the lymphocytc phenotype returned to normal and only EBV-specific cytoxic T cells and anti-EBV antibodies persisted. The peripheral blood lymphocyte response was studied in greater detail by other investigators, who confirmed the presence of activated suppressor lymphocytes, high levels of soluble IL-2 receptors, and an inversion in the helper-suppressor ratio of subjects with acute IM. The acute nonspecific immune response may serve to clear EBV-infected B lymphocytes rapidly and prevent the exuberant polyclonal antibody production, further spread of the infection to other cells, and uncontrolled proliferation of EBV-transformed B lymphocytes.

In vitro, lymphokines (interferon $\alpha$ and $\gamma$ and tumor necrosis factor, TNF) are capable of preventing EBV-induced B cell transformation and may be the factor(s) produced by nonspecific cytotoxic lymphocytes, which both prevent the spread of EBV and attenuate the intense nonspecific antibody production. These molecules can all inhibit hematopoiesis and may be partially responsible for the transient cytopenias noted during IM.

Although the initial response to an acute EBV infection is nonspecific, a more specific immune response that prevents the outgrowth of EBV-transformed lymphocytes persists throughout the lifetime of the host. As mentioned earlier, any perturbation of this arm of the immune system can lead to reactivation of EBV production (as measured by oral virus shedding) and outgrowth of EBV-transformed lymphocytes (B cell proliferative disorders and lymphomas).

EBV-neutralizing antibody levels persist for life in infected individuals, but they appear to play only a minor role in the control of EBV immortalized cells in vivo. Individuals who are treated with immunosuppressive drugs can develop EBV-associated lymphomas despite the presence of normal antibody levels. In an animal model, cottontop tamarins that have been immunized with purified gp350 produce strong neutralizing antibodies but still develop tumors on inoculation with EBV within 2–3 weeks (37). Conversely, animals vaccinated with vaccinia containing the EBV gp350 membrane protein are protected against tumorigenic doses of EBV without developing neutralizing antibodies, suggesting that the T cell response evoked by presentation of antigen in the context of MHC antigens prevents EBV-induced lymphomas.

T lymphocytes are essential for the long-term control of EBV outgrowth. This control is EBV specific and restricted by class I HLA antigens. The frequency of EBV-specific T cells appears to be approximately 1 in 1000–10,000 in individuals seropositive for EBV, and these cells are found in virtually all seropositive individuals. Progress has been made recently in identifying the surface antigens against which the T cell response is directed, antigens that, before their identification, were referred to as LYMDA (lymphocyte-detected antigen). Attempts to further define LYMDA have led to the isolation of T cell clones specific for LMP, GP350, EBNA-2, and EBNA-3; T cell clones specific for different variants of EBNA-2 (Fig. 2A versus 2B) have been isolated from individuals infected with the respective virus. The role of EBNA is entirely consistent with studies demonstrating that influenza nuclear antigens may be processed and presented to T cells as small polypeptides within the cleft of class I HLA antigens. Attempts to define the antigenic epitopes of EBV latent genes are ongoing.

The humoral response to EBV in normal individuals is well characterized (38). Antibodies directed toward viral capsid antigens and early antigens (both produced during the productive cycle) are first detected in the peripheral blood early in the symptomatic phase of IM. Only later are antibodies found that react with EBNA and surface molecules (membrane antigens). Low-level IgG antibodies to EBNA and VCA are then detectable for the remainder of the host's life span. Reactivation of EBV or the proliferation of large numbers of EBV-containing cells (a small fraction of which produce virus), as occurs in EBV-associated neoplasia, is accompanied by a rise in antibody levels to EA. Nasopharyngeal carcinoma is associated with a high-level IgA response to EBV antigens.

Measurement of antibody levels for diagnostic purposes is performed in most clinical laboratories using indirect immunofluorescence techniques (anti-VCA and anti-EA) or anticomplement immunofluorescence (anti-EBNA). Recently, enzyme-linked immunosorbent assay (ELISA) techniques for measurement of a broad range of anti-EBV antibodies have been introduced.

Reliance only upon serology in the diagnosis of EBV-related hematologic disorders may be misleading. Immunosuppressed patients may not respond to EBV antigens in a normal fashion, and some patients with massive EBV-associated lymphoproliferation, for example, may not have detectable antibody to EBV. The host immune responses to EBV infection have been reviewed in detail elsewhere (6,35).

## DETECTION OF EBV IN TISSUES

The use of serologic techniques alone to document the presence of EBV is neither sensitive nor specific. Linking EBV with a specific disease or organ involvement requires the demonstration of viral antigens or nucleic acids within the affected tissue (39). Even this approach has limitations, since negative results may be seen if tissue damage is mediated by immunologic mechanisms independent of the presence of viral antigens. A list of diagnostic techniques is presented in Table 3.

Initially, the presence of EBV within samples was defined by the spontaneous outgrowth of EBV immortalized lymphocytes, the transformation of B lymphocytes (cord blood or cells from seronegative individuals) in vitro, and the demonstration of viral antigens in the resultant cell lines or tissue samples using immunofluorescent techniques. Although these techniques are sensitive (one genome copy per cell may be detected in a latently infected cell using EBNA immunofluorescence) fresh tissue must be obtained and inadequate processing of samples may lead to rapid loss of sensitivity (particularly with EBNA detection). Transformation of B lymphocytes may not always be an accurate assay for the presence of EBV because some clinical isolates are not capable of transforming B cells (40,41) and the efficiency of transformation is not 100% (10).

The cloning of the EBV genome and the subsequent use of cloned portions of the EBV genome as molecular probes have improved EBV detection. DNA or RNA hybridization techniques are exquisitely sensitive, and they have the advantage that they can be performed on fixed tissue samples. Molecular techniques for the detection of EBV also take advantage of the presence of repeated sequences within the genome, allowing the binding of multiple probe molecules to each genome. The *Bam*HI W fragment is frequently used for this purpose, because up to 10 copies of this sequence may be present within each genome. Recently, a similar philosophy led to the use of probes

**Table 3** EBV Detection Methods[a]

| Technique | Target | Sensitivity | Specificity | Localizing ability |
|---|---|---|---|---|
| IF | EBNA | + + + | + + + | + + + |
| | VCA | + | + + + | + + + |
| | EA | + | + + + | + + + |
| | MA | +/− | + | + |
| SH | DNA | + + + | + + + | − |
| NH | RNA | + + | + + + | − |
| ISH | DNA/RNA | + | + + | + + + |
| Culture | Live virus | + − + + + | + + + | − |

[a]ISH, in situ hybridization; IF, immunofluorescence; SH, Southern hybridization; NH, northern hybridization.

directed against EBER RNAs, which are present in extremely high copy number in latently infected cells.

The use of genomic probes also allows the investigator to study the structure of the virus genome and the expression of specific genes within the tissues of interest. Among the most common molecular techniques employed to date are Southern and northern analysis of nucleic acids extracted from samples. In these techniques, DNA or RNA is extracted and separated by molecular weight on a gel (genomic and viral DNA are first digested with restriction enzymes to facilitate the transfer process and provide information about the EBV genome structure). The nucleic acids are then transferred to a membrane and detected with complementary probes using autoradiography or immunochemistry. The main advantages of Southern and northern detection methods is their sensitivity (0.1–1 copy of EBV genome per cell) and specificity (provided the probe is chosen carefully and does not react with cellular DNA or RNA).

For localization of the EBV genome to specific cells, in situ hybridization is used. In situ hybridization is similar to the previously described nucleic acid hybridization techniques, except that it is performed in intact tissues, either fixed or frozen. The tissue of interest is tightly affixed to a slide, and labeled probe is incubated with the tissue. Unbound probe is washed off, and the presence of viral nucleic acids is detected with autoradiography or chemically.

The most sensitive technique for the detection of EBV nucleic acids is the polymerase chain reaction (PCR). In this technique, synthesized primers are used to amplify genomic or RNA sequences within samples of extracted nucleic acids. This technique is exquisitely sensitive and can be used to detect EBV DNA at one genome copy in 1 cell per 100,000 or even more cells. Bearing in mind that circulating B lymphocytes, which have a wide tissue distribution, may harbor latent EBV genomes, one must be cautious about the presence of low copy numbers of EBV DNA or RNA discovered using this technique!

## PROTOTYPE EBV-INDUCED ILLNESS: INFECTIOUS MONONUCLEOSIS

### Clinical Manifestations

Infectious mononucleosis is best described as a self-limited lymphoproliferative disorder. The classic syndrome of infectious mononucleosis is usually seen in adolescents and young adults (42). The signs and symptoms may vary depending on the age of the patient; children can have few or no symptoms, but older adults can have a severe illness with more complications. In a large population, the age at which primary infection occurs is dependent upon the living conditions and the socioeconomic status of the region. EBV infections in developing countries occur at an early age, but EBV infection is usually delayed until the teenage years in more developed countries (43).

The onset of symptoms in IM is usually abrupt. The initial symptoms include malaise, fatigue, fevers, sweats, and chills. These early symptoms are soon followed by the development of anorexia, pharyngitis, and dysphagia. Pharyngitis is the most characteristic symptom and is seen in 80–85% of patients with IM.

The early physical signs seen in IM usually include cervical adenopathy (posterior cervical nodes most commonly), splenomegaly (in 50–60% of patients), hematomegaly (15–25%), and jaundice (5–10%). Severe pharyngitis appears during the first week of the illness, and tonsillar hyperplasia and pharyngeal edema may occur. Palatal petechiae are relatively common and occur in the presence of a normal platelet count.

## Laboratory Diagnosis

Laboratory abnormalities in IM are common. The hematologic hallmark of IM is an absolute lymphocytosis (>4000 $mm^{-3}$) that begins 1 week into the illness and peaks at 2–3 weeks. The degree of lymphocytosis usually reaches 0–70% of the white blood cell count (WBC). Atypical lymphocytes comprise at least 10% of the total WBC and are present in all young adults with IM. These cells represent the T cell response to EBV and are comprised of activated suppressor and cytotoxic cells. The atypical lymphocyte appears large, contains vacuolated or basophilic cytoplasm, and has an indented nuclei with dense chromatin. Atypical lymphocytes may be seen in other illnesses, including cytomegalovirus (CMV) mononucleosis, viral hepatitis, rubella, rubeola, mumps, toxoplasmosis, and herpes simplex virus (HSV) infections.

Diagnostic tests for IM include a positive heterophil antibody response and, even more specific, an anti-VCA IgM antibody. Antibodies against early antigens develop early in the illness, but anti-EBNA antibodies do not appear until months after onset.

## Pathology

The pathologic changes seen in IM are dramatic. The lymph node architecture is distorted by cellular expansion of the sinuses and intrasinusodal areas. B and T cell immunoblasts are the predominant cell type infiltrating the lymph nodes. Reed-Sternberg–like cells, often present in lymph nodes obtained from patients with IM, can be histologically indistinguishable from those seen in

Hodgkin's disease. Necrosis and increased vascularity are also common within lymph nodes.

Pathologic changes in other organs are common. The splenic white pulp, trabeculae, blood vessels, and capsule may be infiltrated or distorted by an immunoblastic infiltration. Splenic enlargement may lead to a greater likelihood of rupture of the spleen with trauma. Lymphocytes and immunoblasts infiltrate the portal areas of the liver and extend to the area between the lobules and sinusoids, causing elevations in serum liver function tests. The bone marrow also contains a lymphocytic and lymphoblastic infiltrate in most cases, and monocytoid cells and lymphoblasts often form small clusters. Because these infiltrates are morphologically similar to lymphomas and leukemias, the interpretation of bone marrow aspirates and biopsies can be hazardous during IM. The presence of granulomas composed of fibroblasts, plasma cells, and reticular cells in the marrow of patients with IM has also been described.

## Hematologic Manifestations

Peripheral blood changes in all lineages are common with IM and may lead to complications, including infection, anemia, and bleeding (2,44,45). During the first week of the acute illness mild leukopenia occurs in 10–20% of individuals, but leukocytosis resulting from the lymphocytosis previously described usually occurs in the second week. Uncommonly, a leukemoid reaction that can mimic acute leukemia, with total WBC values of 30,000–80,000 $\mu l^{-1}$, is observed but usually resolves over 1–2 weeks. A syndrome similar to juvenile chronic myelogenous leukemia (JCML) has been described in IM. This illness is manifested by hepatosplenomegaly, leukocytosis, thrombocytopenia, and increased levels of fetal hemoglobin. It can be differentiated from JCML by bone marrow karyotype (the karyotype in EBV-associated disease is usually normal) and by the demonstration of serologic evidence of recent EBV infection.

Mild neutropenia is a common finding during the first 4 weeks of IM. The incidence of moderate neutropenia (500–1000 $mm^{-3}$) was 10% in a recent review of children with IM. The bone marrow usually shows adequate numbers of neutrophilic precursors at this stage, whereas in severe neutropenia (< 500 granulocytes $mm^{-3}$) the marrow contains a few myeloid cells. Deaths as a result of severe neutropenia are rare and generally occur later in the illness (3–4 weeks). The mechanism of neutropenia is currently unknown; antineutrophil antibodies of unknown pathologic significance are present and may play a role. However, a variety of mechanisms have been proposed (see Table 4), among them nonspecific inhibition of myeloid precursors by suppressor cells or lymphokines, direct infection of progenitor cells with or without im-

**Table 4** Potential Mechanisms of EBV-Induced Hematologic Changes

| Mechanism | Effector |
|---|---|
| Nonspecific immunity | Interferons |
| | Suppressor T cells |
| Specific response to infected progenitor cell | Antibody |
| | EBV cytotoxic T cell |
| Phagocytosis of progenitors | Monocyte |
| Cross-reactive epitopes between cell and viral proteins | Cytotoxic T cell |
| | Antibody |
| Direct viral toxicity to progenitor cell | Virus or products |
| Superinfection with another virus | Second virus or products |

mune destruction of the cells, and the development of antibodies against shared epitopes of the virus and the myeloid cell.

Anemia is uncommon during acute IM (occurring in 1–3% of cases) and when seen is usually due to autoimmune hemolysis. Hemolysis develops during the first 1–2 weeks after the onset of symptomatic IM and usually resolves within 4–8 weeks. Spherocytes and increased osmotic fragility are characteristic, and among patients developing an autoimmune anemia, 70% have a positive Coomb's test. A variety of antibodies have been reported, anti-i being the most commonly described. The anti-i antibody is usually a cold-reacting, low-titer IgM antibody of variable thermal amplitude. An IgG antibody to the i antigen may be found in some cases, in which case the hemolysis is mediated by an IgM antibody directed against the IgG anti-i antibody. The frequent presence of the anti-i antibody (which is usually not associated with overt hemolysis) is not yet explained and may represent nonspecific production of autoreactive antibody by B cells stimulated by EBV. The presence of other red blood cell autoantibodies, including anti-N, anti-I, and the Donath-Landsteiner antibody, have been described in IM. EBV infections may accelerate red blood cell (RBC) destruction in cases of hereditary red cell defects, such as hereditary elliptocytosis, pyruvate kinase deficiency, hereditary spherocytosis, and paroxysmal nocturnal hemoglobinuria (PNH).

Chronic anemias occurring after IM are rare, although cases of chronic pure red cell aplasia caused by T cell-mediated bone marrow suppression have been described (46). One case (Baranski and Young, unpublished data) with large quantities of EBV in the bone marrow detected by in situ hybridization and immunofluorescence had an incomplete response to intravenous acyclovir treatment and eventually a complete response to cyclosporin A therapy (see Fig. 3).

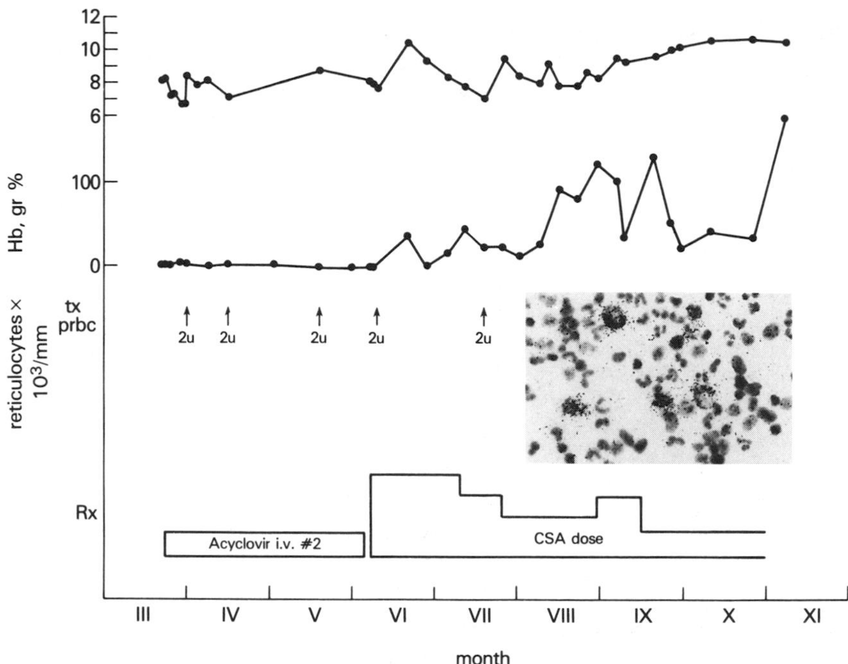


**Figure 3** Response of a patient with EBV-related pure red cell aplasia to immunosuppressive therapy with acyclovir and cyclosporine A. The patient initially presented with no signs or symptoms of IM. In situ hybridization studies of the patient's bone marrow demonstrated EBV genome within approximately 10% of the cells examined (insert). A bone marrow aspirate obtained before treatment was probed with an $^{35}$S-labeled EBV *Bam*HI W DNA fragment. The cells containing EBV DNA are identified by silver grains within the photoemulsion overlying the cells. The patient had a response to a previous course of intravenous acyclovir before course 2, seen here. There was no response to course 2 of acyclovir (months IV and V), and cyclosporine A (CSA) was started on month VI. There was a rapid response to CSA consisting of a rise in reticulocytes and hemoglobin and a marked decrease in transfusion requirements.

Platelet abnormalities are also relatively common during EBV infection. Mild thrombocytopenia ($<150{,}000\ mm^{-3}$) is the rule, but severe thrombocytopenia leading to hemorrhagic complications occurs in occasional cases. Thrombocytopenia usually occurs in the second or third week of the clinical illness and resolves spontaneously. Since splenomegaly is common (50% of IM cases) and the bone marrow usually shows increased megakaryocytes during the thrombocytopenic period, the mechanism of thrombocytopenia is presumed to be increased platelet destruction. Production of antiplatelet antibodies has been documented.

Idiopathic thrombocytopenic purpura, disseminated intravascular coagulation (DIC), and the hemolytic uremic syndrome (HUS) are rarely reported complications of IM, usually occurring during the convalescent phase of the illness.

## EBV-INDUCED APLASTIC ANEMIA

The clinical association of a specific virus with aplastic anemia (AA) has been best documented with EBV (44). The pancytopenia usually occurs within a month of IM and has a variable course. The etiology is not well understood, but several lines of evidence suggest that an immune mechanism is likely to be responsible for the marrow damage occurring in these patients. A current summary of published bone marrow biopsy-confirmed cases of EBV-associated aplastic anemia are presented in Table 5.

EBV-associated AA does not always follow the classic course of infectious mononucleosis. In one series of six patients, three had typical IM, one had a nonspecific viral illness, and two had no preceding symptoms. In all these patients EBV was detected within the bone marrow by immunofluorescence, Southern hybridization, and/or in situ hybridization, but EBV was not detectable in peripheral blood cells. EBV was not detected in the marrow aspirates of an individual with IM, in normal controls, in other patients with AA, or in patients with other hematologic diseases (54). These data indicate that patients with EBV-associated aplastic anemia have a particularly high concentration of EBV in the bone marrow, although the reason for this is unclear. Analysis of virus isolates in two patients with aplastic anemia and from patients with pancytopenia have shown genomic deletions similar to those seen in the nontransforming strain of EBV derived from the cell line P3HR-1 (40,54), now found in the wild. Moreover, supernatants of primary marrow cultures from two of the patients with AA were able to induce early antigen expression in Raji cells, a characteristic of nontransforming EBV strains. This evidence raises the possibility that the EBV infection in EBV-associated aplastic anemia patients is predominantly lytic, either because of the virus strain or because the patient's cells are more permissive for productive infection. However, although EBV replication may be ongoing in these patients, only one patient recovered while undergoing acyclovir therapy. The apparently limited value of acyclovir therapy is not surprising, even if infection is primarily lytic, since patients with acute infectious mononucleosis, chronic mononucleosis, and patients with the X-linked lymphoproliferative syndrome during primary EBV infection have also failed to benefit from acyclovir.

We have shown that EBV can infect erythroid progenitor cells in vitro without altering the number or size of the colonies, raising the possibility that marrow failure seen with EBV infections may not simply result from exuberant lytic infection. In these studies bone marrow cells were depleted of B cells and B cell precursors using immunoadherence to plastic, infected with EBV, and cultured in vitro in semisolid bone marrow cultures in the presence of hematopoietic growth factors. The hematopoietic colonies were removed individually and examined for the presence of B cells, EBV genome, and EBV antigens. The hematopoietic colonies contained $<0.2\%$ B or pre-B cells detected by fluorescent-activated cell sorting (FACS) analysis. EBV was present within 1.2–5.1% of erythroid colony cells by EBNA immunofluorescence. Occasional cells stained positive for VCA and had EBV DNA detected by in situ hybridization. Pooled colonies contained EBV DNA as determined by dot hybridization and Southern analysis. Cells pooled from erythroid colonies were stained with a fluorescein-labeled monoclonal antibody to glycophorin (an erythroid lineage-specific antigen defining the M/N blood group), sorted on a fluorescence-activated cell sorter, and analyzed by immunofluorescence and DNA hybridization. The glycophorin-positive cells contained 1.2–2.4% cells that stained for EBNA. Cells within this group also contained EBV DNA detected by Southern hybridization. The glycophorin-positive cells contained a small number of monocytes, but these monocytes (readily identified in these preparations by their morphology) did not stain for EBNA, and purified monocytes were not infected by EBV in separate experiments. In similar experiments, purified CD34-positive cells (a marker for hematopoietic progenitor cells) were infected with EBV, cultured, and analyzed as before. Erythroid colonies derived from the CD34-positive cells also contained EBV DNA and EBNA antigen. EBV infection of bone marrow did not cause a significant decrease in erythroid colony number or size (26).

Several lines of evidence suggest that EBV-associated aplastic anemia may be immune mediated. First, as described earlier, EBV induces abnormalities in the immune system, including altered helper-suppressor T lymphocyte ratios, T cell activation, T suppressor cell proliferation, and enhanced lymphokine production. Similar abnormalities have been described in other patients with aplastic anemia (54). Figure 4 shows the abnormal peripheral blood lymphocyte phenotype of a patient (case 12, Table 5) who developed aplastic anemia 8 weeks after acute IM. This patient had a predominance of activated Leu-$2^+$ ($CD8^+$) cells in her peripheral blood at the time she presented, 24% of which were activated as determined by HLA-DR expression. Second, some patients with EBV-associated aplasia have responded to antithymocyte globulin (ATG), which likely acts as an immunosuppressant (55). Third, T cells from the marrow of patients with aplastic anemia and pure red cell aplasia can inhibit autologous hematopoiesis in vitro (46,56). Lastly, EBV-specific cytotoxic lymphocytes can inhibit autologous hematopoiesis in vitro when bone marrow is exposed to EBV before adding the T-cells (54).

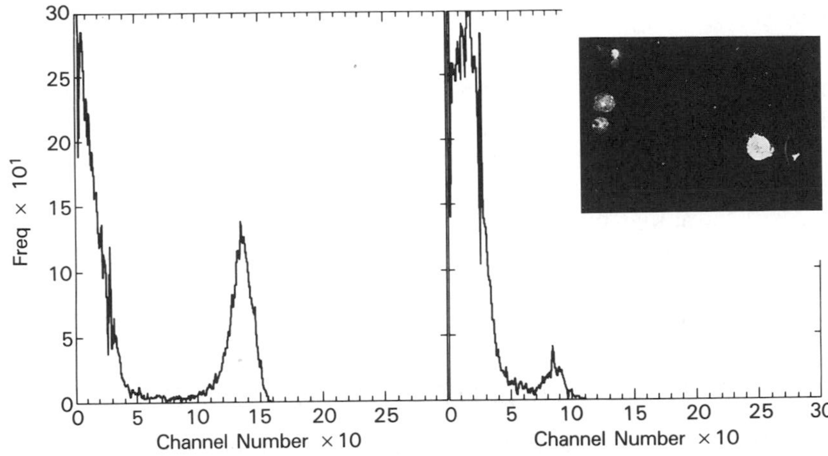


**Figure 4** Peripheral blood lymphocyte phenotype of a patient with aplastic anemia occurring 1 month after acute IM. The insert is a photomicrograph of a bone marrow cell staining positive for EBNA by indirect immunofluorescence. Left: fluorescence histogram of patient lymphocytes stained for Leu-2 (CD8). Most of the peripheral blood lymphocytes (91%) stain for Leu-2. Of these, 24% bear HLA-DR, a marker of cell activation. Right: fluorescence histogram of peripheral blood lymphocytes stained for Leu-3 (CD4): 8% of the cells stain positive for Leu-3. The CD4/CD8 ratio in this case is very low. Activated lymphocytes are not detected in the peripheral blood of normal individuals using this technique.

**Table 5** Known Cases of EBV-Associated Aplastic Anemia[a]

| Case | Age | Sex | Time from onset (weeks) | Treatment | Outcome | Reference |
|---|---|---|---|---|---|---|
| 1 | 12 years | F | 3 | Prednisone | Alive/CR | 47 |
| 2 | 17 years | F | 4 | ATG | Alive/CR | 48 |
| 3 | 3 years | M | 2 | None | Dead | 49 |
| 4 | 7 years | M | 2 | Prednisolone | Dead | 50 |
| 5 | 20 years | M | 4 | Prednisone | Alive/CR | 51 |
| 6 | 7 years | M | 4 | None | Alive/CR | 52 |
| 7 | 11 years | F | 6 | methylprednisone | Died | 52 |
| 8 | 12 years | F | 1 | None | Died | 53 |
| 9 | 29 years | M | 2 | ATG/ACV | Died | 54 |
| 10 | 25 years | M | 8 | ATG/ACV/AND | Died | 54 |
| 11 | 13 years | M | 3 | ATG | Alive/CR | 54 |
| 12 | 15 years | F | 8 | ATG/ACV/CyA Methylprednisone | Died | 54 |
| 13 | 18 months | M | Not applicable | ATG | Alive/CR | 54 |
| 14 | 22 years | M | 12 | ATG | Alive/CR | 54 |

[a]ATG, antithymocyte globulin; ACV, Acyclovir; AND, androgens; CyA, cyclosporine A; CR, complete remission.

The presence of EBV is required for the inhibition of hematopoiesis seen in this model (Baranski and Young, unpublished observations).

Taken together, the evidence suggests that the presence of EBV alone is probably not sufficient to inhibit marrow growth. T cells are probably required to cause marrow dysfunction both in vitro and in vivo. Therefore, immunosuppression seems to be the best treatment of EBV-associated AA at the present time. Acyclovir may be useful in conjunction with immunosuppressive therapy in an attempt to prevent uncontrolled replication of EBV.

## X-LINKED LYMPHOPROLIFERATIVE SYNDROME

In the mid-1970s three families were described in which male children developed severe complications following their primary EBV infection, often leading to death from infection with associated hypogammaglobulinemia, marrow hyperplasia, or lymphoma. Since the initial description of the X-linked lymphoproliferative (XLP) syndrome, over 161 cases have been described in 44 unrelated kindreds (45,57). Studies of restriction fragment polymorphisms in XLP patients have linked the disease to the q24–q27 region of the X chromosome. Using this polymorphism, one can identify individuals who carry the gene and perform prenatal diagnosis of individuals affected with the disease.

Of patients with this disorder, 75% present with severe fatal IM, and the remainder of the patients present with lymphoma alone (15%) or with hypogammaglobulinemia alone (10%). Of the individuals with fatal IM, 25% die with marrow aplasia, 15% develop uncontrolled lymphoproliferation, and 10% have or subsequently develop hypogammaglobulinemia. Overlap exists, as patients surviving the acute IM may later develop lymphomas or hypogammaglobulinemia.

Patients with XLP often present with high fevers, abnormal liver tests, and an atypical lymphocytosis at the time of diagnosis. Most patients die within 2–3 weeks from progressive liver failure, bleeding, sepsis, or massive lymphoproliferation. The diagnosis can usually be established with standard serologic assays: patients with XLP usually make heterophil antibodies, IgM anti-VCA antibodies, and antibodies to EA.

At autopsy, the majority of patients with XLP have immunoblastic infiltration of most lymphoreticular organs. The immunoblasts appear to be both B and T cells, similar to the cells seen in a normal individual with IM. Most XLP patients also have lymphoid infiltration of the central nervous system (CNS); heart, lungs, and liver. A proportion of patients may have lymphocyte depletion, often accompanied by histiocytic infiltration, within the splenic pulp and lymph node follicles. In contrast, patients undergoing autopsy at later stages of the acute infection usually have necrosis of the liver, lymph nodes, and splenic white pulp. The bone marrow is infiltrated by atypical lymphocytes, lymphoblasts, and plasma cells during the acute EBV infection. A marked histiocytic infiltration with erythrophagocytosis follows, and eventually severe depletion of marrow elements and stromal damage occur (58).

Lymphoproliferative disorders in patients with XLP are often similar to those seen in herpesvirus-induced polyclonal lymphoproliferations in animals (59). Most lymphomas are immunoblastic lymphomas, although histology consistent with Burkitt's lymphoma (but without the characteristic 8;14 chromosomal translocation) or lymphoplasmacytoid immunoblastic lymphoma is also seen. These lymphoproliferative disorders are similar to those described in immunosuppressed transplant recipients. It seems probable that the early, nonspecific component of the immune system that normally limits the proliferation of EBV-infected cells in acute IM is defective in these patients, leading to a polyclonal lymphoproliferative disorder.

Individuals with XLP have normal immunity before their first EBV infection. A number of groups have studied the immunologic competence of XLP patients in many pedigrees. A few patients were evaluated before their initial EBV infection and then again during acute IM. Most patients demonstrate normal T and B lymphocyte numbers and normal proliferative responses to pokeweed mitogen, phytohemagglutinin (PHA), and concanavalin A before infection. They also have normal responses to soluble antigens and alloantigens, normal quantitative immunoglobulins, and normal B cell responses to antiimmunoglobulin. In one patient studied before the initial EBV infection, NK function was also intact.

During EBV infection, patients have suppressed responses to mitogens and antigens, similar to other patients with acute IM. They also demonstrate normal or increased cytotoxicity to EBV-infected targets, elevated suppressor-helper T cell ratios, and normal interferon production.

XLP patients who survive the primary EBV infection subsequently suffer from impaired immunity, which lasts indefinitely. They often have decreased IgG production in the face of normal B lymphocyte numbers, depressed lymphocyte responses to antigens and mitogens, decreased NK cell function, and poor primary and secondary immune responses to vaccines. In contrast, lymphocyte phenotyping reveals normal numbers of B and T lymphocytes. Suppressor/cytotoxic T cells are increased in relation to the helper cells, and EBV-specific memory cells are often deficient. Hypogammaglobulinemia is probably induced by circulating suppressor cells capable of inhibiting antibody production by autologous B cells.

In summary, children with XLP appear to have functionally normal immune systems until they are exposed to EBV. If they survive the primary EBV infection, they develop deficient T cell immune responses, which lead ultimately to death from opportunistic infections or lymphoproliferative disorders.

Treatment of patients with XLP during primary EBV infection is supportive only. Acyclovir treatment has not benefited. Current data suggest that the consequences of EBV infection in XLP patients are not due to productive infection: acyclovir only inhibits virus replication—it has no theoretical benefit. Immunoglobulin replacement and antibiotic therapy are effective for preventing infection in hypogammaglobulinemic patients. Bone marrow transplantation using HLA-matched marrow from a sister has improved immune function in two patients with XLP. Both patients had nearly normal immune function after transplant, including the production of anti-EBNA antibodies. A third patient who underwent bone marrow transplantation died of adenovirus-induced hepatitis soon after. Standard chemotherapeutic treatment of the B cell lymphomas can cure the malignancies.

## SPORADIC FATAL IM

Death due to EBV lymphoproliferative disorders also occurs sporadically (58,59). Some of the patients in families who develop overwhelming lymphoproliferation during an acute EBV infection have been girls. These individuals die of uncontrolled lymphoproliferation and hypertrophy of the liver, spleen, and lymph nodes. The lymph node architecture is distorted by proliferating lymphoid cells, and the node capsules may also be infiltrated. Necrosis of affected organs may follow. The bone marrow may be involved, and large numbers of abnormal lymphoid cells that stain for EBNA may circulate in the peripheral blood. Surface immunoglobulin staining of these peripheral cells often demonstrates both light-chain types, consistent with polyclonal activation of B lymphocytes infected with EBV. No patients have had chromosomal abnormalities characteristic of Burkitt's lymphoma.

As in XLP, individuals with sporadic fatal IM have multiple immune defects, including poor T cell responses and the inability to make antibodies to EBNA. Sporadic fatal IM appears to result from failure of the nonspecific component of the immune system to control the initial proliferation of B cells, resulting in death from lymphoproliferation, pancytopenia, or infection.

## VIRUS-ASSOCIATED HEMOPHAGOCYTIC SYNDROME

Risdall used the term "virus-associated hemophagocytic syndrome" (VAHS) to describe a group of patients with viral infections, benign generalized histiocytic proliferation, and hemophagocytosis (60). Since this original description, many cases of this illness have been described in both immunosuppressed and previously normal individuals. The illness has been linked to adenovirus, EBV (45,57,60,61), CMV, varicella virus, and herpesvirus infections. Risdall's original description of the syndrome included 19 patients. Of these, 2 had serologic evidence of recent EBV infection. One patient in Risdall's series had normal immunity before the EBV infection. The majority of Risdall's other patients had VAHS secondary to CMV infection. Predisposing conditions include leukemias, allografting, and immunologic diseases. The allograft recipients who have been described were predominantly renal transplant recipients who underwent splenectomy and antilymphocyte globulin treatment.

Patients usually present with a syndrome characterized by high fever, malaise, myalgia, rash, and extreme fatigue. Physical findings usually include generalized lymphadenopathy and hepatosplenomegaly. Laboratory studies may demonstrate elevated liver function tests, coagulopathies (prolonged partial thromboplastin, prothrombin, and thrombin times), increased fibrin degradation products, hypofibrinogenemia, and pancytopenia. Leukopenia is always present, and most patients have an anemia and/or thrombocytopenia as well. The reticulocyte count may initially be high but decreases as the disease progresses.

The appearance of the bone marrow is dependent on the stage of the disease at the time samples are obtained. Bone marrow aspirate smears early in the course of the disease are hypercellular with prominent erythrophagocytosis. Later the bone marrow becomes progressively hypocellular and histiocytes predominate. Megakaryocyte numbers are usually normal or increased. Lymph nodes are often infiltrated by immunoblasts, which may distort the nodal architecture. Eventually, the lymph nodes are depleted of lymphocytes and erythrophagocytic histiocytes infiltrate the sinusoids. The liver portal tracts are infiltrated with immunoblasts and histiocytes. The histiocytes present in the liver also frequently demonstrate erythrophagocytosis.

DNA hybridization techniques (predominantly Southern hybridization) have revealed EBV genomes within the lymph nodes, lung, liver, and lymphoblastoid cells of patients with EBV-related VAHS (61). Using a technique that can discriminate between circular and episomal DNA, one patient was shown to have replicating EBV genomes (linear form) within the lymph nodes. A second patient had multiple viral particles demonstrated by electron microscopy within liver and lymph node cells. In one study, in which DNA obtained from the lymph nodes was tested for immunoglobulin and T cell receptor rearrangements, the cells present were polyclonal.

The underlying immune defects in patients with EBV-associated VAHS are poorly understood. Immunosuppression with high-dose corticosteroids appears to be a major predisposing factor. Some data are available from two patients with no apparent immunodeficiency who were studied during their EBV-related VAHS (61). Both patients had normal numbers of T cells in the peripheral blood, but the helper-suppressor ratio was low because of an increase in cytotoxic/suppressor cells. Neither patient had the circulating atypical lymphocytes characteristic of IM. One patient showed increased numbers of NK cells as determined by Leu-7 antibody staining. The lymphocytes present in the lymph nodes of another patient consisted exclusively of activated T lymphocytes, with 43% bearing cytotoxic/suppressor markers and 19% expressing helper/inducer markers. Lymphocyte proliferation with lectins, was studied: one patient had a poor response to all mitogens, which returned to normal when the patient recovered, and the other had a poor response to concanavalin A alone. Natural killer cell function was normal in one patient studied. One patient had no detectable cytotoxicity for an EBV-infected lymphoblastoid cell line, in contrast to patients with XLP who have increased killing of EBV-infected target cells.

The natural course of EBV-induced VAHS is variable. Immunosuppressed patients have fared poorly, suggesting that discontinuation of immunosuppressive therapy should be of benefit. Indeed, patients treated with immunosuppressive therapy have not survived VAHS. The evidence for active EBV replication in patients with this disorder suggests that acyclovir therapy may be useful, as demonstrated in two patients with EBV-associated VAHS who recovered uneventfully without recurrences (61).

## EBV AND MALIGNANT NEOPLASIA

During infectious mononucleosis, EBV-infected B cells proliferate, eventually leading to a host immune response capable of regulating this proliferation. The virus remains in a latent state within the host B cells for life; therefore, the potential for unlimited proliferation of immortalized B cells exists in all EBV-infected individuals. Normally an HLA class I-dependent cytotoxic T cell population prevents the rapid outgrowth of these cells. This section describes the lymphoproliferative disorders associated with other congenital immunodeficiencies, those occurring spontaneously, such as Burkitt's lymphoma or nasopharyngeal carcinoma, or malignancies associated with acquired clinical immunosuppression, including HIV infections and chemical immunosuppression in allograft recipients. Table 6 lists the known EBV-associated neoplastic diseases. (For a comprehensive review, see Ref. 59).

### Lymphoproliferative Syndromes in Congenital Immunodeficiency Diseases

A number of congenital immunodeficiency syndromes besides XLP have been associated with a high risk of malignancy. Ataxia telangiectasia, com-

**Table 6** Neoplastic Diseases Associated with EBV

| |
|---|
| Lymphoid malignancies |
| Burkitt's lymphoma |
| Polymorphic B cell malignancies |
| T cell lymphomas |
| Carcinomas |
| Nasopharyngeal carcinoma |
| Salivary gland tumors |
| Adenoid-cystic carcinoma (Sjögren's syndrome) |
| Undifferentiated lymphoepithelial lesion |
| Palatine tonsil carcinoma |
| Supraglottic carcinoma (epithelial) |
| Thymic carcinoma |
| Cervical carcinoma (epithelial) |

mon variable immunodeficiency, and Wiskott-Aldrich syndrome carry a 15–25% risk of lymphoma or leukemia throughout the lifetime of the affected individual. Severe combined immunodeficiency is also associated with lymphoproliferation, and in this disease, lymphomas associated with thymic transplantation have been described. The majority of cancers in patients with congenital immunodeficiency are non-Hodgkin's lymphomas, usually classified as immunoblastic lymphoma, and these tumors frequently involve the brain, also a characteristic of HIV and allograft-related lymphomas. These similarities suggest a common pathogenesis, a defect in the immunologic regulation of EBV-immortalized B cells. EBV DNA has been demonstrated within an abdominal lymphoma in a patient with ataxia telangiectasia and within the tumors from children with severe combined immunodeficiency syndrome.

## Lymphoproliferation in Allograft Recipients

Many cases of EBV-associated lymphoproliferative disorders have been described in allograft recipients (62). Over 20% of malignancies seen in renal allograft recipients are lymphomas, most of which are immunoblastic in morphology. These tumors occur in renal transplant recipients at a rate at least 350 times that in the general population, and they have a high rate of CNS involvement. The tumors are usually B cell in origin and polyclonal as defined by surface immunoglobulin phenotype.

As in other immunodeficiencies, a spectrum of lymphoproliferative disorders occurs. Renal transplant patients have been described who developed an acute syndrome similar to fatal infectious mononucleosis. These individuals present with a sore throat, fever, and lymphadenopathy. EBV DNA was found within the lymphoid cells in two of three patients with the acute syndrome. Patients may also present with a local, more indolent lymphoproliferative disorder. Most tumors in allograft recpients are polyclonal or oligoclonal, although gradual progression to a monoclonal tumor occurs. Cytogenetic abnormalities are uncommon in patients presenting with an acute syndrome, but patients with localized disease frequently have random cytogenetic changes within the tumor cells.

Lymphoproliferative syndromes induced by EBV have been described in recipients of allografts other than kidneys, most commonly in heart and bone marrow recipients. Bone marrow transplant recipients are at high risk for EBV-induced lymphoproliferative disease if the donor marrow is T cell depleted or if they are treated with potent immunosuppressive monoclonal antibodies directed against T cells. In one small series, the use of acyclovir decreased the rate of EBV-driven lymphoproliferative disorders.

The treatment of choice for lymphoproliferative disorders occurring in allograft recipients is to discontinue immunosuppressive drugs. Chemotherapy, or a combination of intravenous gammaglobulin and interferon-$\alpha$, may benefit those patients whose disease progresses following withdrawal of immunosuppressive drugs.

## Lymphoproliferation in HIV Infections

A high incidence of non-Hodgkin's lymphomas in patients with the acquired immunodeficiency syndrome (AIDS) was first noted in the early 1980s. The most common tumor in such patients is the small noncleaved lymphoma, which contains the same cytogenetic abnormalities seen in small noncleaved cell lymphomas in the general population. These tumors are frequently monoclonal and contain rearrangements within the c-*myc* gene like those documented in sporadic Burkitt's lymphoma. Only 40% contain EBV DNA, and therefore EBV is not responsible for the lymphoproliferation in all cases.

Patients with human immunodeficiency virus (HIV) often have chronic lymphadenopathy that may progress to frank lymphoma. The T cell response to EBV is impaired in patients with AIDS and AIDS-related complex (ARC), which leads to an increase in circulating B cells containing EBV. Oral hairy leukoplakia, a complication of AIDS, has been associated with EBV lytic infection, which recent evidence suggests is a consequence of repeated infection of the cells on the side of the tongue by EBV released from epithelial cells. The anatomic localization suggests that the viral particles may be present in saliva emanating from the parotid ducts.

## Lymphoproliferation in Collagen Vascular and Granulomatous Diseases

Many collagen vascular diseases are associated with lymphoproliferation and lymphoid tumors. These diseases are commonly treated with immunosuppressive drugs, and it is not clear to what extent this participates in the pathogenesis. EBV DNA has been detected within the salivary glands of patients with Sjögren's syndrome, but the lymphomas arising in other patients with autoimmune disorders are usually of T cell origin. Of interest is that EBV has been associated with T cell lymphomas (see next section).

## Burkitt's Lymphoma

Although EBV was described within cell lines derived from Burkitt's lymphoma in 1964, the role of EBV in the pathogenesis of this tumor is still unknown (59,63). Burkitt's lymphoma is a monomorphic proliferation of lymphoid cells of specific histologic appearance (it is a subtype of small noncleaved cell lymphoma) that accumulate in large tumor masses within the jaw (predominantly in African patients) or abdomen; Burkitt's lymphoma can involve almost any organ or tissue of the body. The tumor cells are B lymphoblasts bearing either $\kappa$ or $\lambda$ surface IgM. The tumors are monoclonal, as defined by immunoglobulin light chains, glucose-6-phosphate dehydrogenase (G6PD) isoenzyme phenotypes, EBV clonality (when present), and molecular rearrangements.

Burkitt's lymphoma cells bear a nonrandom chromosomal translocation involving the terminal region of chromosome 8 (the location of the c-*myc* protooncogene) and one of the immunoglobulin chain loci on chromosome 14 (85% of cases), 22 (10%), or 2 (5%). These translocations result in deregulation of the c-*myc* gene by damage to the c-*myc* regulating region and functional usurpation by immunoglobulin regulatory sequences. As such, they provide a critical component of the pathogenesis of this disease and clearly distinguish it from the tumors seen in congenitally or pharmacologically immunosuppressed patients. Endemic Burkitt's lymphomas (occurring in equatorial Africa) contain EBV DNA in 95% of cases, whereas sporadic tumors in Europe and the United States contain EBV DNA in only 15–25% of cases. Replicating virus particles are not seen in Burkitt's lymphoma. Since 5–10% of Burkitt's lymphoma in seropositive patients within the endemic areas do not contain EBV DNA, it is reasonable to assume that there is a low incidence of EBV-negative Burkitt's lymphoma throughout the world, but this is overshadowed by EBV-positive cases within the endemic area.

It seems probable that environmental factors predispose to tumors in the endemic zone. One such potential environmental factor is malaria. It has been postulated that immunosuppression caused by malaria may allow a higher level of proliferation of EBV-containing cell clones, thus increasing the possibility that a chromosomal translocation may develop in a single cells and give rise to neoplasia. In this scenario, EBV increases the pool of cells in which a cytogenetic abnormality might occur. In support of this hypothesis, malarial infections reduce T cell cytotoxicity directed against EBV-infected cells. In Burkitt's lymphoma occurring in HIV-positive patients, it is also likely that the risk of translocations is increased because of the expanded EBV-infected B cell pool. However, in AIDS patients a number of other mechanisms can also serve to increase the B cell pool: alternatively, the chromosomal translocation might occur first, with EBV required for subsequent neoplastic transformation of the target cell. This hypothesis fails to explain the existence of EBV-negative, translocation-positive tumors. The possibility that the tumor cells in some cases are infected after the development of the tumor is also rendered unlikely by the assertion that EBV in Burkitt's lymphoma is clonal, indicating that the tumor arises from a single EBV-infected cell.

It was recently shown that EBV latent gene expression in Burkitt's lymphoma differs from that in lymphoblastoid cell lines. In the latter, EBNA-2, EBNA-3, and LMP all appear to have an important role in cell transformation. In Burkitt's lymphoma, however, only EBNA-1 appears to be invariably expressed. Thus, whatever role EBV plays in Burkitt's lymphoma, the mechanism differs from that involved in blastic transformation of normal B lymphocytes (63).

Within the endemic area, Burkitt's lymphoma often develops years after the initial EBV seroconversion. Africans destined to develop EBV have higher levels of anti-VCA antibodies, presumably due to a higher body burden of virus. In one small series, it was shown that if the anti-VCA titer in an individual exceeds twice the population mean, the risk of Burkitt's lymphoma is 30-fold greater than in the remainder of the population.

Burkitt's lymphoma is invariably fatal unless treated with appropriate chemotherapy. Bone marrow transplantation (autologous or allogeneic) has been successfully used in a subset of patients who relapse or fail to achieve a complete remission after standard chemotherapy.

## EBV and Hodgkin's Disease

EBV DNA can be detected in some malignant lymph nodes of patients with Hodgkin's disease (HD), regardless of the presence of Ig gene rearrangements. In one study, 4 of 21 (19%) tissue specimens were positive for the EBV genome as detected by Southern hybridization (18). Surprisingly, 3 of 4 samples contained monoclonal EBV genome as determined by analysis of the EBV terminal repeats, and the fourth patient had three clones. A second study demonstrated the EBV genome in 7 of 42 (17%) cases of HD and in 1 of 22 patients with Ki-1 anaplastic large cell lymphoma (tumors containing cells morphologically similar to Reed-Sternberg cells) (64). All EBV genomes in this study were monoclonal, and all seven cases of HD containing EBV genome were of the nodular sclerosing subtype. In situ analysis revealed EBV genome within the Hodgkin and Reed-Sternberg cells from 2 of the 4 patients in the first study. A third family study demonstrated the presence of EBV DNA by Southern hybridization in tissue from 2 of 4 tumors derived from 4 brothers who died of lymphoma (3 HD and 1 non-Hodgkin's lymphoma) (65). Of these patients 2 had no detectable T cell immunity against EBV-infected cells and failed to make antibodies to EBNA. Since the initial reports, two larger studies of malignant tissue from patients with HD demonstrated the presence of EBV genome in 58% of patients (198 cases total) (66) and in 29% (28 cases total) of patients (17), respectively. These larger studies have demonstrated EBV genome within HD tumor tissue of multiple histologic subtypes.

The role of EBV in the development of some cases of Hodgkin's disease is unknown, and clearly not all cases contain EBV genomes. It is of interest that many patients with HD have elevated antibody titers to EBV but T cell immunity to EBV-infected cells may be decreased, suggesting either that they have poor immunity against EBV or a higher burden of EBV-infected cells, or both. The incidence of Hodgkin's disease in individuals who have had IM is higher than that seen in individuals who have not had IM.

## EBV and T Cell Lymphomas

Although EBV appears to be trophic for B cells, other cells are known to harbor EBV DNA and may be infected by EBV in vitro. The C3d receptor is presumed to be the main receptor for EBV, but cells that do not bear detectable C3d receptors (as determined by fluorescent-activated cell sorting analysis) can be infected with EBV. Some cells, such as T cells, may bear low levels of the C3d receptor not perceptible by FACS analysis. However, immature (thymic) T cells are known to express C3d receptors. T cells cultured from patients with acute lymphocytic leukemia (ALL) and T cell lymphoblastic lymphomas, both of thymic origin, do in fact contain EBV receptors on their cell membrane.

Several patients have recently been described in whom malignant T cells contain the EBV genome. In one study, three patients with chronic illnesses characterized by fever, pneumonia, dysgammaglobulinemia, hematologic abnormalities, and very elevated EBV antibody titers developed T cell lymphomas in lymph nodes, peripheral blood, and many other organs. These lymphomas were characterized immunologically as T cells, had T cell receptor rearrangements, and contained EBV DNA by Southern analysis. The EBV genome within the cells was found to be monoclonal by analysis of the terminal repeats (22).

In a second report, a child with a 3 month illness characterized by fever, lymphadenopathy, and coronary artery dilatation had recently been observed to have undergone EBV seroconversion. The peripheral blood contained excessive numbers of activated $CD4^+$ cells as determined by flow cytometry, and 36% of the peripheral blood cells contained EBNA. The $CD4^+$ cells were selected with a fluorescence-activated cell sorter and found to contain EBV DNA and expressed EBNA. None of these cells expressed B cell antigens or detectable C3d receptor. The investigators could not establish immortalized cell lines from the patient (67).

T cells containing EBV have also been described in lethal midline granuloma and nasopharyngeal lymphomas (68), chronic EBV infection (69), benign T cell lymphoproliferation (70), and $CD8^+$ T cell lymphoma (71).

There is now no doubt that some T cell lymphomas contain EBV, but the mechanism of infection and the frequency of such disorders remains to be determined.

## Nasopharyngeal Carcinoma

Nasopharyngeal carcinoma (NPC) is a neoplasm of epithelial cells that ranges histologically from an undifferentiated type to a tumor indistinguishable from other squamous cell carcinomas (2,19). In all histologic types, EBV DNA is present in the carcinoma cells. Patients with this tumor have markedly elevated titers of antibodies directed against EBV antigens. The serologic pattern differs fro that in normal individuals and in other diseases in that IgA and IgG titers to EA-D and VCA are particularly high. These antibodies are also elevated in individuals at high risk for NPC in endemic areas.

The incidence of NPC is particularly high in southern China and in Eskimos living in Alaska and Greenland. This geographic variability has not been explained, although a genetic predisposition has been postulated. In southern China the use of herbal medicines containing phorobol esters or the habit of eating dried fish has been linked to NPC. No chromosomal abnormalities or abnormal oncogene expression in NPC tumors has been reported.

The role of EBV in the development of NPC (and also of other tumors in the head and neck area) is unknown. Many patients with NPC demonstrate "reactivation" of EBV, as measured by EA antibody titers, before the development of NPC. Recently, selective expression of EBV latent genes was seen in NPC. LMP and EBNA-1 are both expressed, but other EBNA are not. The finding that mice transgenic for LMP develop a keratinizing syndrome and have increased expression of a specific keratin gene may be relevant to the pathogenesis of squamous cancers associated with EBV. LMP is also known to play a role in the immortalization of epithelial cells.

Treatment of NPC consists of irradiation and chemotherapy: local excision is not usually feasible owing to the tumor location. Interestingly, the titers of antibodies to EBV antigens fall with successful treatment of NPC.

## CONCLUSIONS

Epstein-Barr virus is a ubiquitous human herpesvirus that can induce a wide variety of hematologic abnormalities at the time of the initial infection or anytime during the life span of the host if the immune regulation of EBV-infected B cells is altered. Although initially thought to infect only B cells, sensitive molecular detection techniques have shown that the trophism of EBV is not limited to B cells. Once EBV infects a cell, it can replicate (lytic phase) or remain latent. B cells containing latent virus are capable of unlimited proliferation for life.

The exuberant immune response to EBV can be responsible for many of the clinical manifestations of acute IM. The immune response to EBV is initially nonspecific. Eventually, EBV-specific antibodies and HLA-restricted EBV-specific T cells predominate and persist for life. Immunosuppressive drugs and HIV infection can inhibit the T cell control of immortalized B cells, resulting in widespread lymphoproliferation. Congenital immunodeficiencies are also associated with EBV-induced lymphoproliferation or severe impairment of immunity following exposure to EBV.

Hematologic abnormalities during EBV infection are common. The etiology of these changes is not well understood; however, a variety of mechanisms, such as nonspecific marrow inhibition by activated T cells, antibodies, or lymphokines, specific inhibition of EBV-infected hematopoietic progenitors by antibodies or T cells, and hemophagocytosis, are postulated.

EBV-transformed cells can also give rise to monoclonal tumors, such as Burkitt's lymphoma and NPC, although the events leading to these diseases are not well understood. Burkitt's lymphoma developing within endemic regions of equatorial Africa contains EBV DNA in most cases. The environmental factor responsible for the development of tumors within the endemic area is unknown, although malaria has been postulated since it decreases T cell immunity to EBV-transformed B cells. The 8;14 chromosomal translocation found in Burkitt's lymphoma juxtaposes the c-*myc* protooncogene with an immunoglobulin chain regulatory region, resulting in deregulation of the c-*myc* gene. Burkitt's lymphoma containing the 8;14 chromosomal translocation in nonendemic regions does not usually contain EBV DNA.

EBV has been detected within the Reed-Sternberg cells of patients with Hodgkin's disease and T cell lymphoma cells. Further studies are needed to fully understand the pathogenesis of EBV-related T cell malignancies.

## REFERENCES

1. Editorial. Epstein-Barr virus silver anniversary. Lancet 1989; 1:1171–3.
2. Giller RH, Grose C. Epstein-Barr Virus: the hematologic and oncologic consequences of host-virus interaction. Crit Rev Hematol Oncol 1980; 9:149–95.

3. Farrell PJ. Epstein-Barr virus genome. Adv Viral Oncol 1989; 8:103–30.
4. Kieff E, Dambaugh T, Heller M, et al. The biology and chemistry of Epstein-Barr Virus. J Infect Dis 1982; 146:506–17.
5. Thorley-Lawson D. Basic virological aspects of Epstein-Barr Virus infection. Semin Hematol 1988; 25:247–60.
6. Tosato G. The Epstein Barr virus and the immune system. Adv Cancer Res 1987; 49:75–125.
7. Fingeroth J, Clabby M, Strominger J. Characterization of a T-lymphocyte Epstein-Barr virus/C3d receptor (CD21). J Virol 1988; 62:1442–7.
8. Sixbey JW, Vesterinen EH, Nedrud JG, Raab-Traub N, Walton LA, Pagano JS. Replication of Epstein-Barr virus in human epithelial cells infected in vitro. Nature 1983; 306:480–3.
9. Swendeman S, Thorley-Lawson DA. The activation antigen BLAST-2, when shed, is an autocrine BCGF for normal and transformed B cells. EMBO J 1987; 6:1637–42.
10. Zerbini M, Ernberg I. Can Epstein-Barr virus infect and transform all the B-lymphocytes of human cord blood? J Gen Virol 1983; 64:539–47.
11. Sixbey JW, Nedrud JG, Raab-Traub N, Hanes RA, Pagano JS. Epstein-Barr virus replication in oropharyngeal epithelial cells. N Engl J Med 1984; 310:1225–30.
12. Miller G. Niederman JC, Andrews LL. Prolonged oropharyngeal excretion of Epstein-Barr virus after infectious mononucleosis. N Engl J Med 1973; 288: 229–32.
13. Greenspan JS, Greenspan D, Lennette ET, et al. Replication of Epstein-Barr virus within the epithelial cells of oral "hairy" leukoplakia, an AIDS-associated lesion. N Engl J Med 1985; 313:1564–71.
14. Sixbey JW, Lemon SM, Pagano JS. A second site for Epstein-Barr virus shedding: the uterine cervix. Lancet 1986; 2:1122–4.
15. Prange E, Trautmann JC, Kreipe H, Claus S, Parwaresch MR. Epstein-Barr virus (EBV) and lymphoid tissues in infectious mononucleosis. Exp Hematol 1990; 18:590.
16. Lung ML, Lam WK, So SY, Lam WP, Chan KH, Ng MH. Evidence that the respiratory tract is a major reservoir for Epstein-Barr virus. Lancet 1985; 1:889–92.
17. Staal SP, Ambinder R, Beschorner WE, Hayward GS, Mann R. A survey of Epstein-Barr virus DNA in lymphoid tissue. Am J Clin Pathol 1989; 91:1–5.
18. Weiss LM, Strickler JG, Warnke RA, Purtilo DT, Sklar J. Epstein-Barr DNA in tissues of Hodgkin's disease. Am J Pathol 1987; 129:86–91.
19. Prasad U, Ablashi DV, Levine PH, Pearson GR. Nasopharyngeal carcinomal Kuala Lumpur: University Malaya Press, 1983.
20. Fox RI, Pearson G, Vaughan JH. Detection of Epstein-Barr virus-associated antigens and DNA in salivary gland biopsies from patients with Sjogren's syndrome. J Immunol 1986; 137:3162–8.
21. Armstrong G, Longo D, Faggioni A, Ablashi D, Pearson G, Slovin S. Detection and isolation of Epstein-Barr virus in lymphocytes from patients with chronic B-lymphocytic leukemia. In: Magrath I, O'Conor GT, Ramot B, eds. Pathogenesis of leukemias and lymphomas: environmental influences, Vol. 1. New York: Raven Press, 1984; 259–62.

22. Jones J, Shurin S, Abramowsky C, et al. T-cell lymphomas containing Epstein-Barr viral DNA in patients with chronic Epstein-Barr virus infection. N Engl J Med 1988; 318:733–41.
23. Wolf BC, Martin AW, Neiman RS, et al. The detection of Epstein-Barr virus in hairy cell leukemia cells by in situ hybridization. Am J Pathol 1990; 136:717–23.
24. Karpas A, Hayhoe FG, Greenberger J, Neumann H. Alkaline phosphatase in Epstein-Barr nuclear antigen-positive cell lines. Science 1978; 202:318–9.
25. McGuire LJ, Huang DP, Teoh R, Arnold M, Wong K, Lee JC. Epstein-Barr virus genome in thymoma and thymic lymphoid hyperplasia. Am J Pathol 1988; 131:385–90.
26. Baranski B, Moore J, Armstrong G, Magrath I, Young N. Epstein-Barr virus associated aplastic anemia: demonstration of virus in clinical bone marrow samples and in hematopoietic progenitor cells infected in vitro. Clin Res 1987; 35: 419A.
27. Rocchi G, Ragona G, Revoltella RP. EBV expression in human non-lymphoid hematopoietic cell lines. Prog Med Virol 1984; 30:129–38.
28. Morgan D, Ablashi DV. Detection of EBNA and rescue of transforming EBV in megakaryocyte cells established in culture. In: Levine PH, Ablashi DV, Pearson GR, Kotardis, eds. Epstein-Barr virus and associated diseases, international symposium on Epstein-Barr virus malignant associated diseases. Boston: Martinus Nijhoff, 1985; 402–7.
29. Pearson GR. The Epstein-Barr virus genome and phenotypic expression during lytic cycle. AIDS Res 1986; 2(Suppl 1):S49–56.
30. Miller G. The switch between latency and replication of Epstein-Barr virus. J Infect Dis 1989; 161:833–44.
31. Klein G. Viral latency and transformation: the strategy of Epstein-Barr virus. Cell 1989; 58:5–8.
32. Knutson JC, Sugden B. Immortalization of B lymphocytes by Epstein-Barr virus: what does the virus contribute to the cell? Adv Viral Oncol 1989; 8:151–72.
33. Sugden B. An intricate route to immortality. Cell 1989; 57:5–7.
34. Rowe M, Rowe DT, Gregory CD, et al. Differences in B cell growth phenotype reflect novel patterns of Epstein-Barr virus latent gene expression in Burkitt's lymphoma cells. EMBO J 1987; 6:2743–51.
35. Tosato G, Blaese RM. Epstein-Barr virus infection and immunoregulation in man. Adv Oncol 1985; 37:99–148.
36. Svedmyr E, Ernberg I, Seeley J, et al. Virologic, immunologic, and clinical observations on a patient during the incubation, acute, and convalescent phases of infectious mononucleosis. Clin Immunol Immunopathol 1984; 30:437–50.
37. Epstein MA, Randle BJ, Finerty S, Kirkwood JK. Not all potently neutralizing vaccine-induced antibodies to Epstein-Barr virus ensure protection of susceptible experimental animals. Clin Exp Immunol 1986; 63:485–90.
38. Pearson GR. Infectious mononucleosis: the humoral response. In: Schlossberg D, ed. Infectious mononucleosis, 2nd ed. New York: Springer-Verlag, 1989; 89–99.
39. Landry ML, Fong KY. Nucleic acid hybridization in the diagnosis of viral infections. Clin Lab Med 1985; 5:513–29.

40. Schooley RT, Carey RW, Miller G, et al. Chronic Epstein-Barr virus infection associated with fever and interstitial pneumonitis. Ann Intern Med 1986; 104: 636–43.
41. Alfieri C, Ghibu F, Joncas JH. Lytic, nontransforming Epstein-Barr virus (EBV) from a patient with chronic active EBV infection. Can Med Assoc J 1984; 131: 1249–52.
42. Cheesman SS. Infectious mononucleosis. Semin Hematol 1988; 25:261–8.
43. Straus SE, Fleishner GR. Infectious mononucleosis epidemiology and pathogenesis. In: Schlossberg D, ed. Infectious mononucleosis. New York: Springer-Verlag, 1989; 8–28.
44. Baranski B, Young N. Hematologic consequences of viral infections. Hematol Oncol Clin North Am 1987; 1:167–83.
45. Sullivan JL. Hematologic consequences of Epstein-Barr virus infection. Hematol Oncol Clin North Am 1987; 1:397–417.
46. Socinski MA, Ershler WB, Tosato G, Blaese RM. Pure red blood cell aplasia associated with Epstein-Barr virus infection: evidence for T-cell-mediated suppression of erythroid colony forming units. J Lab Clin Med 1984; 104:995–1006.
47. Lazarus KH, Baehner RL. Aplastic anemia complicating infectious mononucleosis: a case report and review of the literature. Pediatrics 1981; 67:907–10.
48. Shadduck RK, Windelstein A, Zeigler Z, et al. Aplastic anemia following infectious mononucleosis: possible immune etiology. Exp Hematol 1979; 7:264–70.
49. Case 31-1984. N Engl J Med 1984; 311:314–22.
50. van Doornik MC, van T Veer-Korthof ET, Wierenga H. Fatal aplastic anemia complicating infectious mononucleosis. Scand J Haematol 1978; 20:52–6.
51. Mir MA, Delamore IW. Aplastic anemia complicating infectious mononucleosis. Scand J Haematol 1973; 11:314–8.
52. Jain S, Sherlock S. Infectious mononucleosis with jaundice, anemia, and encephalopathy. Br Med J 1975; 8:907–10.
53. Ahronheim GA, Auger F, Joncas JH, Ghibu F, Rivard GE, Raab-Traub N. Primary infection by Epstein-Barr virus presenting as aplastic anemia. N Engl J Med 1983; 309:313–4.
54. Baranski B, Armstrong G, Truman JT, Quinnan GV, Straus SE, Young NS. Epstein-Barr virus in the bone marrow of patients with aplastic anemia. Ann Intern Med 1988; 109:695–704.
55. Baranski BG, Young NS. Autoimmune aspects of aplastic anemia. In Vivo 1988; 2:91–4.
56. Shadduck RK, Winkelstein A, Zeigler Z, et al. Aplastic anemia following infectious mononucleosis: possible immune etiology. Exp Hematol 1979; 7:264–71.
57. Sullivan JL. Epstein-Barr virus and lymphoproliferative disorders. Semin Hematol 1988; 25:269–79.
58. Weisenburger DD, Purtilo DT. Failure in immunologic control of the virus infection: fatal infectious mononucleosis. In: Epstein MA, Achong BG, eds. The Epstein-Barr virus: recent advances. New York: John Wiley and Sons, 1986; 129–161.

59. Magrath I. Infectious mononucleosis and malignant neoplasia. In: Schlossberg D, ed. Infectious mononucleosis. New York: Springer-Verlag, 1989; 143–71.
60. Risdall RJ, McKenna RW, Nesbit ME, et al. Virus-associated hemophagocytic syndrome. A benign histiocytic proliferation distinct from malignant histiocytosis. Cancer 1979; 44:993–1002.
61. Sullivan JL, Woda BA, Herrod HG, Koh G, Rivara FP, Mulder C. Epstein-Barr virus-associated hemophagocytic syndrome: virological and immunopathological studies. Blood 65:1097–104.
62. Cleary ML, Dorfman RF, Sklar J. Failure in immunological control of the virus infection: Post-transplant lymphomas. In: Epstein MA, Achong BG, eds. The Epstein Barr virus: recent advances. New York: John Wiley and Sons, 1986; 164–81.
63. Magrath I. The pathogenesis of Burkitt's lymphoma (in press). Adv Cancer Res.
64. Anagnostopolous I, Herbst H, Niedobitek G, Stein H. Demonstration of monoclonal EBV genomes in Hodgkin's disease and KI-1-positive anaplastic large cell lymphoma by combined Southern blot and in situ hybridization. Blood 1989; 74:810–6.
65. Donhuijsen-Ant R, Abken H, Bornkamm G, et al. Fatal Hodgkin and non-Hodgkin lymphoma associated with persistent Epstein-Barr virus in four brothers. Ann Intern Med 1988; 109:946–52.
66. Herbst H, Niedobitek G, Kneba M, et al. High incidence of Epstein-Barr virus genomes in Hodgkin's disease. Am J Pathol 1990; 137:13–8.
67. Kikuta H, Taguchi Y, Tomizawa K, et al. Epstein-Barr virus genome-positive T lymphocytes in a boy with chronic active EBV infection associated with Kawasaki-like disease. Nature 1988; 333:455–7.
68. Harabuchi Y, Yamanaka N, Kataura A, et al. Epstein-Barr virus in nasal T-cell lymphomas in patients with lethal midline granuloma. Lancet 1990; 335:128–30.
69. Bonagura VR, Katz BZ, Edwards BL, et al. Severe chronic EBV infection associated with specific EBV immunodeficiency and an EBNA$^+$ T-cell lymphoma containing linear, EBV DNA. Clin Immunol Immunopathol 1990; 57:32–44.
70. Yoneda N, Tatsumi E, Kawanishi M, et al. Detection of Epstein-Barr virus genome in benign polyclonal proliferative T-cells of a young male patient. Blood 1990; 76:172–7.
71. Richel D, Lepoutre JM, Kapsenberg JG, et al. Epstein-Barr virus in a CD8-positive T-cell lymphoma. Am J Pathol 1990; 136:1093–9.

# 6

# Human Cytomegalovirus

**Stephen St. Jeor**

*University of Nevada, Reno*
*Reno, Nevada*

**Jaroslaw P. Maciejewski**

*National Heart, Lung and Blood Institute*
*Bethesda, Maryland*

## STRUCTURE AND FUNCTION

### History and Description

The isolation of human cytomegalovirus (HCMV) from salivary glands was reported simultaneously in 1956 by Rowe et al. and Smith (1,2). Because of the large cells containing intranuclear inclusions associated with HCMV infections, the virus was designated cytomegalovirus, and clinical disease caused by HCMV infections was referred to as cytomegalic inclusion disease. Based on its morphologic appearance, HCMV was classified as a herpesvirus (3,4). The HCMV genome is the largest of any of the herpesvirus, consisting of a linear double-stranded DNA molecule with a molecular weight of $1.5 \times 10^8$ D or 240 kb (5,6). The genome has a high guanine and cytosine content, resulting in a density of 1.716 g/cm$^3$. The DNA exists as four distinct isomers present in equal molar amounts containing long and short unique sequences with both internal and terminal inverted repeats (3,4). The long and short unique sequences can invert in relationship to each other to create the four isomers. Electron microscopic examination of purified virus shows typical herpesvirus particles with an electron-dense icosahedral core containing 162 capsomeres surrounded by a large pleomorphic lipid envelope (3,4). In addition to infectious virus, electron micrographs reveal large numbers of empty

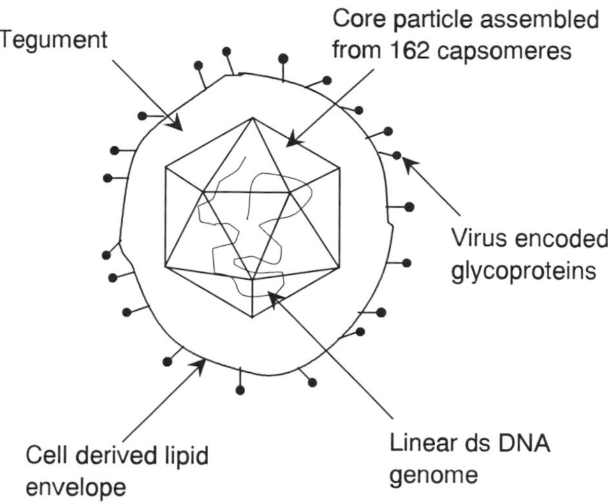


**Figure 1** Typical HCMV virion.

particles containing either no DNA or partial genomes. The lipid envelope is derived from the host cell and contains virus-coded glycoproteins that are important in recognition by the immune response of the host (3). Figure 1 is an artist's concept of a typical HCMV virus.

## Replication

The HCMV genome has been sequenced and found to contain over 200 open reading frames (7). Relatively few of the gene products have been identified, and the function of the majority of the proteins is unknown. As with other herpesviruses, gene expression is temporally regulated into immediate early (IE), early (E), and late (L) periods. The IE genes are transcribed by the host polymerase in the absence of protein synthesis within the first 2 h following infection (3,8,9). The exact function of the IE gene products is unknown, but they appear to be regulatory and are able to transactivate a number of cellular and virus genes. HCMV E genes are transactivated by IE gene products, and their expression begins within 2 h following infection. Transcription of the E genes requires de novo protein synthesis but not DNA replication (4,10). In general, the E genes code for products involved in the replication of virus, such as a distinct HCMV specific DNA polymerase and DNA binding proteins (3,4). Late gene expression is transactivated by both IE and E gene products and occurs concomitantly with virus DNA replication (3,4).

The majority of the late gene products code for virus structural proteins (3,4).

### Cell Specificity and Its Effect on HCMV Replication

The type of infection produced by HCMV varies with the animal species from which the cell was derived as well as the type of cell infected. *Productive* infections, which result in the replication of infectious progeny, occur only in the animal species from which the virus was initially isolated and primarily in diploid fibroblasts. *Abortive* infections are those in which infection is initiated but transcription is limited to expression of the IE genes. Abortive HCMV infections occur in a number of cell types from a variety of animal species. HCMV can enter virtually any cell type, but there is a block in virus gene expression. *Latent* infections commonly occur following either an acute or subclinical infection. Infections by virtually all herpesviruses results in a lifetime latent infection of the host. Here transcription of the virus genome is limited and no virus is produced until an external stimulus activates transcription of the virus genome and synthesis of virus progeny is initiated.

Infection of lymphocytes by HCMV may be an example of an abortive or latent infection since only IE virus gene products are normally detected. However, in the presence of interleukin-2 the virus replicates in human T cells (11). At present little information is available concerning the mechanism of HCMV latency; however, herpes simplex virus (HSV) may serve as a model for examining latent infections by herpesviruses. When neurons are infected with HSV a latent infection is established. The infection is characterized by production of a single latency-associated transcript (LAT) (12). When the virus is activated from this latent state, normal virus transcription occurs.

This highly restricted host range is the primary difference between cytomegaloviruses and lytic members of the herpesvirus group. Under in vitro conditions, infections by cytomegalovirus are limited to diploid fibroblasts, yet surprisingly, in vivo HCMV can be isolated from a variety of other cell types, including monocytes, macrophages, granulocytes, and endothelial cells (13–15).

In contrast to the majority of herpesviruses, which shut off host macromolecular synthesis, HCMV infection induces cell DNA and RNA replication during both productive and abortive infections (16–19). In productive infections, virus and cell DNA replication occur concomitantly (17). Since induction of cell macromolecule synthesis is a characteristic of DNA tumor viruses, it has been postulated that HCMV may have oncogenic potential (20). The mechanism of virus induction of cell macromolecule synthesis is unclear. Supernatants from HCMV-infected cells contain a growth factor-like substance that induces DNA replication in resting fibroblasts (21). The IE antigen of HCMV may play a role in the activation of certain cellular genes; IE is a strong transactivator of genetic elements, including the long terminal repeats of HIV and the simian virus 40 (SV40) origin of DNA replication (22–24). The increased macromolecule synthesis in HCMV-infected cells is specific: certain genes (heat-shock genes, specific oncogenes, and certain interleukin genes) could be induced, but others were not affected by HCMV replication (16,25,26). The function of cellular macromolecular synthesis in HCMV replication is unknown but may be important in the regulation of latent or productive HCMV infections.

## EPIDEMIOLOGY

### Incidence of Infection

Cytomegalovirus infection is endemic in virtually the entire population. Because many HCMV infections are subclinical or can mimic other virus infections, it has been difficult to associate mild clinical symptoms with HCMV infections. Based on seropositivity, the incidence of HCMV appears to vary with the age and socioeconomic status of the population. In the United States, the incidence of HCMV infection in adults, as measured by the presence of antibody, is approximately 50% (27–29), but this may represent an underestimate. A recent study in England, which used the polymerase chain reaction to determine the percentage of normal blood donors who carry leukocytes containing HCMV DNA, reported that the leukocytes from 98% of normal male blood donors over 50 years of age were positive for HCMV DNA (27). Considering the high incidence of HCMV in normal donors, it is surprising that the transmission rate does not approach 100% in recipients of blood from male donors over 50 years old. Male homosexuals represent a group who are highly susceptible to HCMV infection. In the United States, the incidence of HCMV antibody in male homosexuals approaches 100%. The incidence of HCMV infection in people living in developing countries is higher at a much younger age than in the United States. In a study of a random sample of people from Uganda, the incidence of HCMV antibody, as determined by complement fixation tests, was 100% (unpublished observations).

### Oral Transmission

There are several different routes by which HCMV infections are acquired. A relatively high incidence of transmission of HCMV to day-care workers indicates that the virus is transmitted by an aerosol or oral route (25,30). Since infants congenitally infected with HCMV often develop a persistent infection in which virus is shed in the urine for extended periods of time, the contaminated urine may serve as a source of virus. HCMV is present in lymphatic tissue in the upper respiratory tract, and contaminated saliva may also serve as a source of virus. HCMV has been isolated from leukocytes present in human milk (31), and in populations that have a high incidence of HCMV at a relatively early age, breast-feeding has been a suspected route of transmission; the relatively neutral pH found in the stomach of nursing infants would not destroy the virus and thus allow vertical transmission.

## Sexual Transmission

Evidence indicating the HCMV is sexually transmitted includes the report that the virus has been isolated from the urogenital tract and, at least in the case of murine cytomegalovirus, can replicate in spermatogenic cells (32,33). The reported high incidence of HCMV in prostitutes and male homosexuals further supports the supposition that HCMV may be sexually transmitted (34–36).

## Parenteral Transmission

HCMV can be transmitted parenterally by transfusions of cellular components of blood and by organ transplantation. There is an average infection rate of 13% after transfusions to immunocompetent recipients, most infections being asymptomatic (37). Leukocytes must play an important role in the transmission of human cytomegalovirus (28,29,38,39). Several studies have reported the detection of HCMV in fresh peripheral blood cells (14, 28,40,41). Diosi and coworkers, using cocultivation of leukocytes with human fibroblasts, detected HCMV in 2 of 37 apparently normal healthy blood donors (28). Taken together these data indicate that (1) A viremia is associated with HCMV infections, (2) the virus is present in the leukocyte fraction and not free in serum, (3) viremia may persist for months following infection, (4) virus can be transmitted by whole-blood transfusion to normal repicients, and (5) HCMV may be present in a latent state in peripheral blood cells.

## Congenital HCMV Infections

HCMV is one of the most important causes of clinically significant congenital infections of newborn infants (32,42,43). Infection can be caused by either a primary infection during pregnancy or by activation of latent virus; recent studies indicate that HCMV infections of the developing fetus are most severe when caused by a primary infection rather than by activation of latent virus (31,44). HCMV infections occur not only during fetal development but may develop after birth either from virus present in the birth canal or by transmission from infected maternal cells present in breast milk.

### Transmission in Immunologically Impaired Hosts

An important factor in the development of HCMV infections is the immune status of the host. With the use of intensive immunosuppression for organ transplantation and the emergence of the acquired immunodeficiency syndrome (AIDS), HCMV has emerged as a significant problem in infectious disease management. Although the role of the immune response in protection against HCMV infections has only recently begun to be understood, it is clear that the presence of a normal antibody response is not sufficient to protect against reinfection or activation of HCMV (45). Immunosuppressed individuals not only can be reinfected but may be infected with multiple strains of HCMV (45). Patients with the highest risk of mortality from cytomegalovirus infection are seronegative recipients of a transplant who receive tissue from seropositive donors, patients receiving chemotherapy, and low-birth-weight premature infants.

## PATHOGENESIS

Since the first isolation of HCMV from salivary glands, the virus has been found in numerous tissues, including peripheral blood leukocytes, kidney, brain, and lung (13,15,32). Although the majority of HCMV infections are subclinical, diverse syndromes are associated with HCMV infections, ranging from a mild febrile illness associated with a viremic phase to life-threatening pneumonia. Table 1 lists many of the clinical syndromes associated with HCMV and illustrates the various diseases seen in different patient populations.

### Subclinical Infections

Manifestations of HCMV infections are dependent on the immune status of the infected individual. In adults in the United States, the incidence of antibody to HCMV varies from 50 to 75% or greater, yet a clinical history of HCMV infection can be obtained in less than 1% of the population. Occasionally, a self-limited, heterophil-negative mononucleosis-like syndrome associated with malaise, myalgia, sore throat, and fever occurs at the time of seroconversion. Lymphadenopathy, splenomegaly, and more serious complications, such as pneumonitis, hepatitis, meningoencephalitis, and myocarditis, are rare. HCMV infections in healthy adults result in seroconversion. Following infection the virus remains in a latent state for the rest of the life of the individual but can be reactivated if the immune response is depressed.

**Table 1** Clinical Manifestations of Human Cytomegalovirus Infections

| |
|---|
| Patients with normal immune responses |
| Subclinical infections |
| Infectious mononucleosis |
| Hepatosplenomegaly |
| Latent infections |
| Subclinical hepatitis |
| Patients with impaired immune responses |
| Interstitial pneumonia (bone marrow transplant patients) |
| Hepatitis |
| Infectious mononucleosis, heterophil negative |
| Chlorioretinitis |
| Disseminated systemic infections |
| Persistent infections resulting in viruria and/or viremia |
| Congenital and neonatal infections |
| Generalized systemic infections |
| Pneumonia, gastroenteritis |
| Failure to thrive |
| Central nervous system involvement |
| Inner ear infections, deafness |
| Mental retardation |
| Persistent infections of multiple organs associated with viruria and/or viremia |

## Congenital HCMV Infections

It was recognized as early as 1950 that the presence of large giant cells with intranuclear inclusions are associated with congenital HCMV infections, which often result in severe defects (42,43). HCMV congenital infections result in chorioretinitis, calcification of the cerebrum, microcephaly, hematologic disorders, and pneumonia (32,42,43). The effect of fetal development on the severity of infection is less clear: infection early in development is more likely to result in severe, often multiple defects, but when exposure occurs after the first trimester the consequences are less certain. Figure 2 is an electron micrograph of a section of kidney from an infant who died shortly after birth of HCMV disease. The arrows point to the distinct HCMV particles containing a dark-staining core surrounded by a lipid envelope. Virus was recovered from the liver, brain, kidney, and lungs of this infant.

Identification of the exact time during pregnancy when infection occurs can be difficult, since in normal adults HCMV disease is usually subclinical (in contrast, rubella virus infections are often associated with a distinct rash that alerts both patient and physician to the possibility of a virus infection) (42).

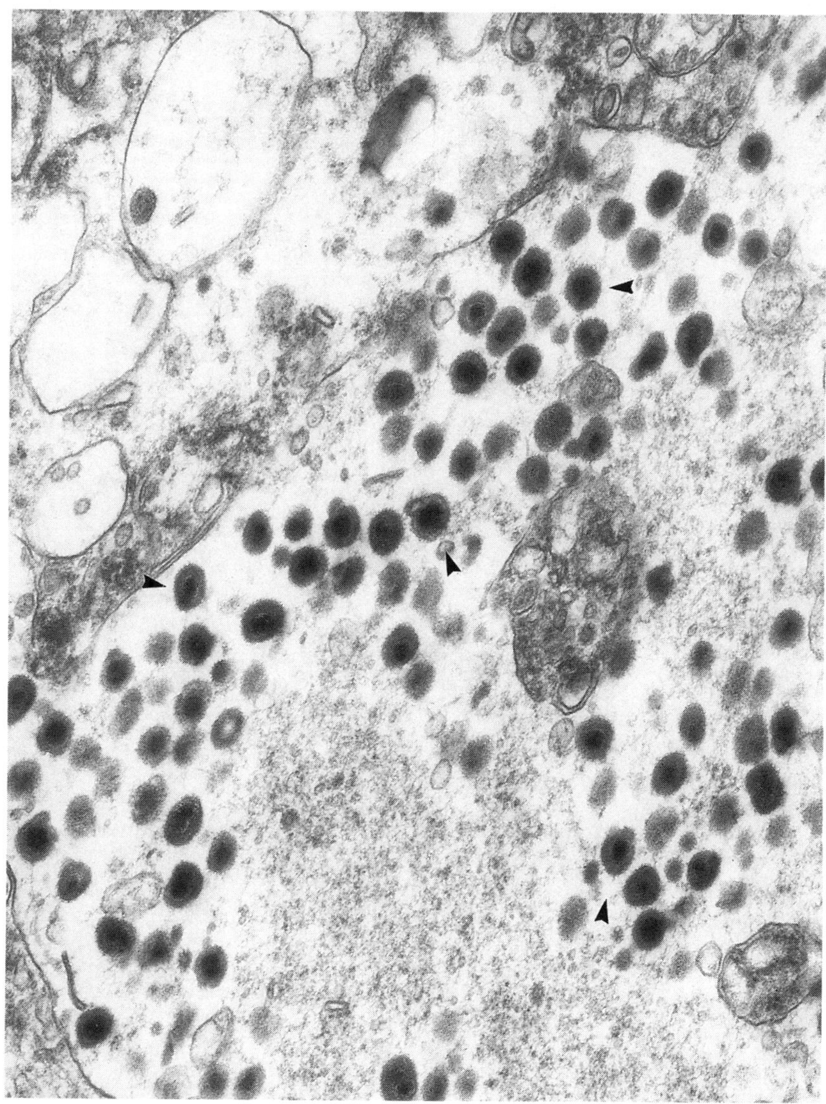

**Figure 2** Electron micrograph of kidney from an infant who died after birth of HCMV disease.

The severity of the infection is undoubtedly related to the level of fetal development up to the time of exposure and whether the infection was a primary exposure or caused by reactivation of latent virus (44). Infection that results from activation of latent virus has less severe consequences to the fetus than primary infection (44). Children who are exposed to HCMV either at birth or in utero often shed virus for several years (14,43,44). The presence of HCMV in an infant is not invariably associated with congenital defects; when children in a hospital nursery were examined for viruria, as many as 1% were shedding HCMV with no apparent congenital malformations (43, 46). Persistently infected children appear to mount a normal antibody response but are unable to eradicate the virus. This may be caused by a defect in T cell immunity or by immunologic tolerance caused by the infection occurring early in immunologic development and clonal selection eliminating specific T cell clones (47).

## Opportunistic HCMV Infections in the Immunocompromised Host

Individuals at greatest risk of developing severe cytomegalovirus disease are those with impaired immune responses (certainly the susceptibility of the fetus to HCMV infection is based on the development of the immune response late in gestation). HCMV infections following iatrogenic or acquired immunosuppression are important clinical problems, particularly with the increased use of organ transplants, the use of potent immunosuppressive drugs, and the emergence of the acquired immunodeficiency syndrome. In allograft recipients, HCMV infection is not only frequently associated with the functional impairment of the grafted organ but may also trigger the allograft rejection, as in the case of HCMV glomerulitis in the renal transplantation. Alternatively, treatment of the rejection crisis increases the risk of HCMV infection. The intensity of immunosuppressive therapy correlates with the incidence of HCMV infections.

There is an apparent difference between the manifestations of HCMV observed in bone marrow transplant patients compared to that in people with AIDS. HCMV pneumonitis is common in transplant patients but rarely associated with AIDS. This may be because bone marrow transplant patients are more severely immunosuppressed than people with AIDS. Additionally, whole-body radiation may make the lung more susceptible to pneumonia because of resultant tissue damage (Riddell, personal communication).

Because of the high incidence of HCMV in individuals with AIDS as well as in male homosexuals, HCMV has been hypothesized as a cofactor in its development (34–36). Epidemiologic studies indicate an excellent correlation between the presence of HCMV and the development of AIDS (34,48). Experimental evidence supporting the role of HCMV as a cofactor in AIDS comes from in vitro studies demonstrating that the major IE gene product of HCMV can function as a strong trans activator of a number of other genes, including the long terminal repeat (LTR) of HIV (22,23,49). In addition, HCMV and HIV may simultaneously infect the same cell, providing an opportunity for intracellular trans activation of latent HIV. HCMV suppression of the immune response may shorten the time between HIV exposure and the development of clinical manifestations of AIDS.

## CLINICAL DIAGNOSIS

HCMV infection is usually defined by virus isolation and/or positive serology. HCMV disease is defined by the occurrence of specific manifestations, such as interstitial pneumonia, gastrointestinal disease, hepatitis, or the HCMV syndrome. Asymptomatic infections are defined as HCMV infection in the absence of HCMV disease.

In acute HCMV infection, leukocytosis and lymphocytosis with >20% variant lymphocytes are present. Early in the infection an increase in the number of natural killer cells can be observed. Later HCMV infection is associated with an increase in $CD8^+$ and $CD8^+$, HLA-$DR^+$ cells and a $CD4^+$ lymphopenia. In HCMV infection of the immunocompromised host, the results of laboratory tests strongly depend on the primary disease. Symptoms related to graft rejection or other opportunistic infections may be difficult to differentiate from HCMV infection. In transplant patients and in infants, HCMV infection may be associated with neutropenia and thrombocytopenia. A definitive diagnosis of HCMV infection can be made only by isolating the virus or by demonstrating a rise in specific antibody titer. Historically, the diagnosis of HCMV was dependent on the presence of diagnostic large multinucleated cells containing intranuclear inclusions (owl's eye cell) detected most easily in the urine during an HCMV kidney infection. A number of commercially available serologic tests are now available, including enzyme-linked immunosorbant assay (ELISA) and fluorescent antibody assays that can be used for the detection of both IgG and IgM antibody to HCMV. Antibodies to late antigens persist at high titer long after disappearance of the viremia.

Three major types of HCMV infection may occur: (1) primary infection with viremia, viruria, and an IgM increase followed by a switch to IgG; (2) reactivation with increased IgG titer, but often only HCMV shedding is detectable; and (3) reinfection with a different strain of HCMV with viremia and a possible IgM response.

Patients with acute HCMV infections shed virus in the urine. Isolation of virus by cell culture is a long procedure, often requiring 4–6 weeks, and secondary contamination by both bacteria and fungi is sometimes a problem. IE antigen expression was recently used as a marker of virus infectivity. Human fibroblasts are infected with clinical samples and screened 24–72 h after inoculation for IE expression by fluorescence. Direct detection of HCMV IE gene expression in peripheral blood leukocytes with monoclonal antibodies can also be used for diagnosis and monitoring of HCMV infections. In primary HCMV infections, antigenemia usually occurs 7–10 days before seroconversion. The rapid IgG response typical of secondary infection may still lag 10 days behind the onset of HCMV antigenemia. A correlation exists between the level of HCMV antigenemia and the severity of the HCMV infection. In diagnosing congenital HCMV infections by serologic methods, it is essential that either the presence of IgM-specific antibody be demonstrated or that HCMV-specific IgG levels either remain constant or increase with time following infection. When a congenital HCMV infection is suspected, virus isolation or IE HCMV antigen expression is the preferred test.

Perhaps the most promising test for the detection of virus DNA is by polymerase chain reaction (PCR). Since the entire DNA sequence of the virus is known, there are several regions of the genome that can be used for amplification by PCR. [However, some regions of the HCMV genome are known to share homology with human DNA (3,4).] PCR should prove to be the most sensitive method for the detection of virus DNA.

## INTERACTIONS WITH THE HEMATOPOIETIC SYSTEM

Murine cytomegalovirus (MCMV) has been used as a model to investigate the effect of HCMV on hematopoiesis. Irradiated mice infected with MCMV failed to reconstitute bone marrow (50). Furthermore, MCMV interferes with the formation of granulocytes and megakaryocytes (51–53). In the murine model the inability of immunosuppressed infected animals to generate hematopoietic stem cells is the primary reason for failure of animals to survive.

Patients with active HCMV infections often have hematologic manifestations, such as thrombocytopenia, hemolytic anemia, and hepatosplenomegaly (51–53). The degree of hematologic involvement is related to the immune status of the host: in patients with a normal immune response, HCMV infections are generally subclinical, but patients with impaired immune responses are more likely to exhibit hematologic dyscrasias. Infants congenitally infected with HCMV can develop anemia and thrombocytopenia (32, 43,44). Among several manifestations of HCMV disease in bone marrow transplant patients, HCMV infection-associated aplasia occurred in 5 of 60 transplanted patients; the incidence among the transplanted patients with viremia was 11% (54). After renal transplantation, acute HCMV infection usually produced only prolonged fever, but leukopenia occurred in about 30% of cases and predicted a fatal outcome (55). HCMV viremia, viruria, and antigenemia are extremely common after bone marrow transplantation. Within 5 weeks of transplantation, in 83% of cases HCMV was detected by gene amplification (56). Although HCMV infections in bone marrow transplant recipients have been credited with graft failure, the recent reports studying large transplantation series have been conflicting. In analyzing pretransplant HCMV infections, no effect on the rate of recovery of neutrophils and platelets was found (57). The most frequent manifestation of HCMV disease was fatal interstitial pneumonia (57,58). In other series of autologous and allogeneic transplant recipients, a delayed recovery, especially of platelets, has been reported (50,51,54,59). Thrombocytopenic complications may be caused by direct infection of megakaryocyte by HCMV. Megakaryocytes containing typical HCMV inclusions have been described (51,52). In addition to other manifestations of HCMV disease in bone marrow transplant, an HCMV syndrome with prolonged fever and at least a 50% reduction in either absolute neutrophil count or platelet count associated with viruria and viremia is common (58). Graft-versus-host disease or host-versus-graft disease in bone marrow recipients also are frequently associated with active HCMV infection.

Evidence supporting the ability of HCMV to infect cells of the hematopoietic system includes the following: (1) HCMV can be transmitted by blood obtained from apparently healthy donors, indicating that the virus is either latent in blood cells or produces a persistent subclinical infection (28,38, 39,60), (2) HCMV can persist in the blood for months after infection and is clearly present in the leukocyte fraction (14). Patients receiving multiple units of blood often develop a fever associated with an infectious mononucleosis-like syndrome. This syndrome is associated with an increase in complement fixation antibody against HCMV, and virus can be isolated from the peripheral blood (28,29,38,39). Such HCMV infections are normally self-limited and the patient recovers. In immunocompromised patients and neonates, transfusion-acquired HCMV infections can be life threatening (61,62). Screening blood donors for HCMV antibody status has decreased the transmission of virus in this patient population (61,62), as has the use of leukocyte-depleted blood (63).

Despite the isolation of HCMV from circulating blood cells, which specific cell type is infected with HCMV, whether the virus is present in a latent or persistent state, and how virus expression in hematopoietic cells is regulated remain open questions.

## Lymphocytes

During HCMV infection, the number of cytotoxic T cells in peripheral blood increases (64). The constitutive production of interferon-$\gamma$ (IFN-$\gamma$) and tumor necrosis factor by lymphocytes seen in recipients after bone marrow transplantation is greatly enhanced by in vitro incubation of blood mononuclear cells with infected autologous marrow fibroblasts (65). Since HCMV-infected cells show enhanced expression of LFA-3 (66), HCMV infection of grafted tissue may trigger the rejection, a mechanisms that could be responsible for the high coincidence of HCMV infection and graft failure or rejection.

In the murine system, $CD8^+$ cells protect animals against the lethal MCMV infection (11,67,68). A similar effect could be observed in human graft recipients (56,69). $CD8^+$-mediated cytolytic activity for HCMV-infected targets is present in normal seropositive persons but cannot be detected in marrow transplant patients who succumb to HCMV pneumonia (69).

Several lines of evidence indicate that lymphocytes may be important targets for HCMV in latent and active infection. T cells from patients with HCMV infections failed to respond normally to mitogens and antigens, suggesting that HCMV may be exerting a functional effect on T lymphocytes, possibly by direct infection (70). The mechanism of inhibition is unclear but is thought to be related to altered cytokine production or to the presence of a specific inhibitor of cytokine activity in HCMV-infected cells (25,26, 71,72). Olding et al. reported that murine cytomegalovirus could be isolated from the B lymphocytes of infected animals following in vitro mitogen activation (73). Human lymphoblastoid cell lines of both T and B origin and human peripheral lymphocytes are susceptible to infection with HCMV (74,75), but often only immediate early gene products are expressed as in an abortive infection. In HCMV-infected lymphocytes and lymphoblastoid cells, although the total number of HCMV genomes increases the level of infectious virus fails to rise above input levels. Recently, Braun and Reisser reported that HCMV would replicate in human lymphocytes if the cells were maintained in the presence of interleukin-2 (11).

## Granulocytes

HCMV was localized in blood cells of viremic patients following transplantation in both the polymorphonuclear and mononuclear fraction, with the highest titer of virus present in the polymorphonuclear cells (76). As with lymphocytes, granulocytes could be abortively but not productively infected with HCMV (77). In vivo, HCMV antigen was present in the granulocytes of viremic patients and the presence of antigen correlated with an active viremia (78) but may represent phagocytosis of HCMV antigens during acute viremia. Since HCMV can be detected in short-lived granulocytes only during the viremic phase of infection, polymorphonuclear cells are unlikely to play a role in maintaining HCMV latency.

## Mononuclear Phagocytes

Macrophages and monocytes are important in the pathogenesis of both HIV and HCMV (79–82). The characteristics of these cells that contribute to virus pathogenesis include the following: (1) monocytes differentiate into macrophages and colonize virtually all body tissues; (2) monocyte-derived macrophages exist in tissues from months to years and are therefore ideal for harboring latent virus; (3) monocytes and macrophages are affected by a number of cytokines that may alter their susceptibility to virus infection; and (4) in turn, monocytes, and macrophages produce cytokines that affect the immune response, which may mediate HCMV effects (25).

The data concerning the effects of HCMV on the production of major monokines appear conflicting. Some studies were performed in transformed cells that retain specific markers of monocytes-macrophages; others were performed with freshly isolated cells infected either in vivo or in vitro. For example, in some studies HCMV blocked interleukin-1 (IL-1) production, but other investigators suggested that infected cultures contained an inhibitor of IL-1 activity (25). Although inhibition of IL-1 activity was reported to be caused by mycoplasma (83), other studies using mycoplasma-free strains have reproduced the presence of putative IL-1 inhibitor (25,84). In contrast, the IE gene of HCMV transfected into monocytes upregulated IL-1 activity (72,85), an effect consistent with the known action of the IE gene as a strong

**Table 2** Effect of HCMV on Cellular Immunity[a]

| Investigators (ref.) | IL-1 | IL-2 | Inhibitor | Mitogen response |
|---|---|---|---|---|
| Rinaldo et al. (70) | NT | NT | NT | Inhibits |
| Rodgers et al. (83) | Down | NT | Yes | NT |
| Kapasi and Rice (84) | Down | Down | No | Inhibits |
| Moses and Garnett (25) | Down | NT | Yes | NT |
| Turtinen et al. (26) | Up | NT | NT | NT |
| Iwamoto et al. (71) | Up[b] | NT | NT | NT |
| Dudding et al. (110) | Up[b] | NT | NT | NT |

[a]Up or down indicates HCMV either up- or downregulates the level of cytokines; NT, not tested.

[b]A cloned IE gene of HCMV was used in these studies.

activator of transcription. Upon activation with lipopolysaccharide, HCMV-infected cells also produced increased levels of tumor necrosis factor (TNF) and IL-1 (26). HCMV infection may also inhibit the ability of monocytes to respond to cytokines, such as IL-1 and IL-2 (25,83,84). The functional effects of HCMV on the mononuclear phagocytes are summarized in Table 2.

In vitro, monocytes are susceptible to infection with HCMV, but until recently the infection was thought to be abortive because only IE mRNA and IE gene products were detected (77,86). However, more recent studies using in situ hybridization techniques have demonstrated that both IE and late mRNA were present in monocytes from AIDS patients (77). In studies using fluorescence-activated cell sorting and polymerase chain reaction, monocytes were shown to be the predominant blood cell type harboring HCMV (60). In our experiments, mononuclear phagocytes infected in vitro with HCMV supported virus replication, although the level of virus production was 1000-fold less than in human fibroblasts (Fig. 3). Infection of macrophages with HCMV resembled a latent or persistent rather than productive infection. In contrast, HCMV infection of human fibroblasts results in a much higher production of virus and a more rapid decline in virus infectivity. Recently, Ibanez and colleagues demonstrated that HCMV could replicate in differentiated macrophages (87).

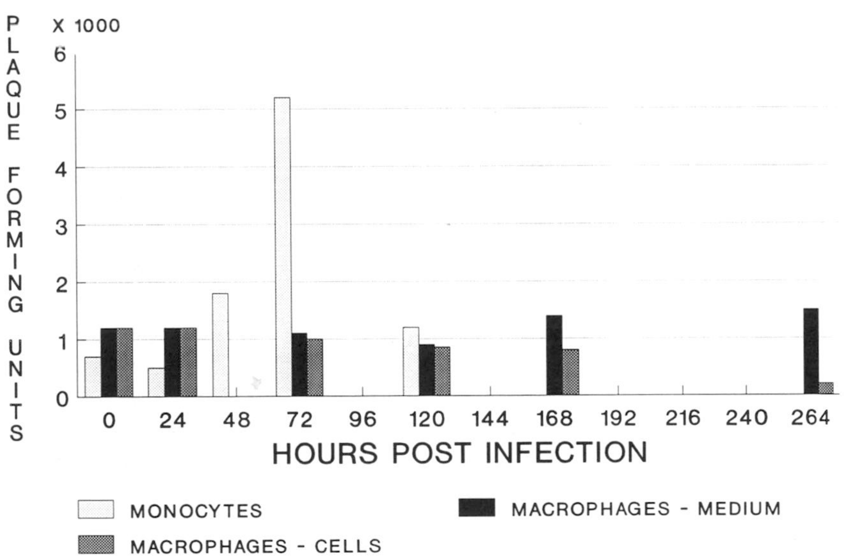


**Figure 3** Replication of human cytomegalovirus in human monocytes and macrophages.

The demonstration of the importance of macrophages in the pathogenesis of HIV has renewed interest in the significance of these cells in viral infections (80,81). HIV gene expression in macrophages is modulated by the presence of monokines (80). Investigations using murine cytomegalovirus as a model for virus latency implicate macrophages as important in latent infections. When mice were infected with murine cytomegalovirus, it could be isolated from macrophages but not lymphocytes of infected animals 3 months after initial challenge (79,88). HCMV-infected macrophages have altered cell surface expression of specific phenotypic markers as well as depressed phagocytic activity (88). In vitro, HCMV can infect both monocytes and macrophages, and infected monocytes can differentiate into macrophages with virus mRNA detectable for at least 3 weeks following inoculation (unpublished data). Because macropohages can remain viable in tissues for many months to years, they could serve as a potential reservoir for HCMV (79,89,90).

The state of HCMV in peripheral blood during nonviremic periods is unknown. HCMV can be detected by PCR in virtually all adult males over 50 years of age (27), but because the rate of transmission in patients who receive a single unit of blood is much lower than expected, about 0.7%, the presence of virus alone may not be sufficient to produce disease (91). HCMV may be latent in most circulating blood cells and rarely activated by transfusion; alternatively, a high level of virus may be required for transmission. The ability to isolate infectious HCMV by cocultivation of leukocytes with human fibroblasts indicates that at least a subpopulation of these cells can support HCMV replication.

## Hematopoietic Progenitors

Although there is an agreement that infection of bone marrow progenitors by HCMV suppresses hematopoiesis, the mechanism by which this occurs is unclear. In vitro, HCMV interferes with colony formation by hematopoietic progenitors (72,92–94). The effects of HCMV have been attributed to several factors, including direct infection of progenitors, infection of supporting stromal cells, indirectly resulting in progenitor cell death, interference with the ability of precursor cells to respond to cytokines, and induction of factors that inhibit hematopoiesis or HCMV suppression of cytokine production required for hematopoiesis. HCMV infection of bone marrow stromal cells (92,93) and interruption of cytokine production may be important pathophysiologic mechanisms.

Laboratory strains and clinical isolates of HCMV can infect bone marrow stromal cells in vitro, and infected stromal cells have a reduced capacity to support the proliferation of primitive myeloid progenitor cells (92,

93). Apperley et al. reported that infection of bone marrow mononuclear cells or clonogenic progenitor cells with either clinical isolates or laboratory strains of HCMV had no effect on colony morphology or cell proliferation, nor could HCMV mRNA be detected in these cells (92), but infected stromal cells demonstrated a reduced capacity to support proliferation of primitive myeloid progenitor cells (92). Simmons et al. also reported the HCMV-infected stromal cells had a reduced capacity to support the proliferation of hematopoietic progenitor cells, possibly as a result of selective inhibition of the synthesis of granulocyte colony-stimulating factor (G-CSF) by these cells (93). They also showed that 40% of clinical isolates, but not laboratory-adapted strains, could directly inhibit colony formation by purified bone marrow progenitors. In contrast, Sing and Ruscetti reported that both clinical isolates and the Towne laboratory strain of HCMV interfered with the ability of normal bone marrow cells to form hematopoietic colonies when stimulated by granulocyte-macrophage colony-stimulating factor (GM-CSF) or G-CSF; the laboratory strain did not affect multipotential (colony-forming units–granulocytes-erythroid cells-monocytes-macrophages, CFU-GEMM) or erythroid (blast-forming units, BFU-E) colony-forming cells, but a fresh clinical isolate demonstrated inhibitory effects on these cells (94). HCMV-specific mRNA and IE antigens could be detected in colonies derived from infected progenitors. Rakusan et al. reported that both the AD169 strain and various clinical isolates of HCMV inhibited the formation of granulocyte-macrophage colonies of bone marrow and blood cells, but with large variations in the potency of the different clinical isolates in suppressive activity (72). In our laboratory, a recombinant of HCMV (RC256) was used to demonstrate the susceptibility to infection by HCMV of nonadherent bone marrow progenitor cells (95). RC256 contains the *lac*Z gene of *Escherichia coli*, which codes for galactosidase (X-gal) activity under the control of the HCMV early promoter; when a chromogenic substrate (X-gal) is added to the cells expressing LacZ, the resultant color allows a single infected cell to be identified (95). Nonadherent cells from normal human bone marrow were infected with RC256, dispersed, and cultured in methylcellulose with appropriate hematopoietic factors. After addition of X-gal to infected cultures, intense blue colonies were detected (Fig. 4), showing that HCMV can infect hematopoietic progenitor cells and infected cells are capable of forming myeloid colonies. HCMV moderately reduced myeloid colony formation, but the colonies expressing *lac*Z activity appeared morphologically normal (96). Using the recombinant RC256 we could directly show that $CD34^+$ bone marrow progenitors can be infected with HCMV. The percentage of HCMV-infected cells was higher within the purified $CD34^+$ population than in unseparated bone marrow, indicating that early progenitor cells are more likely targets for HCMV than mature cells. In vitro studies show that HCMV, in

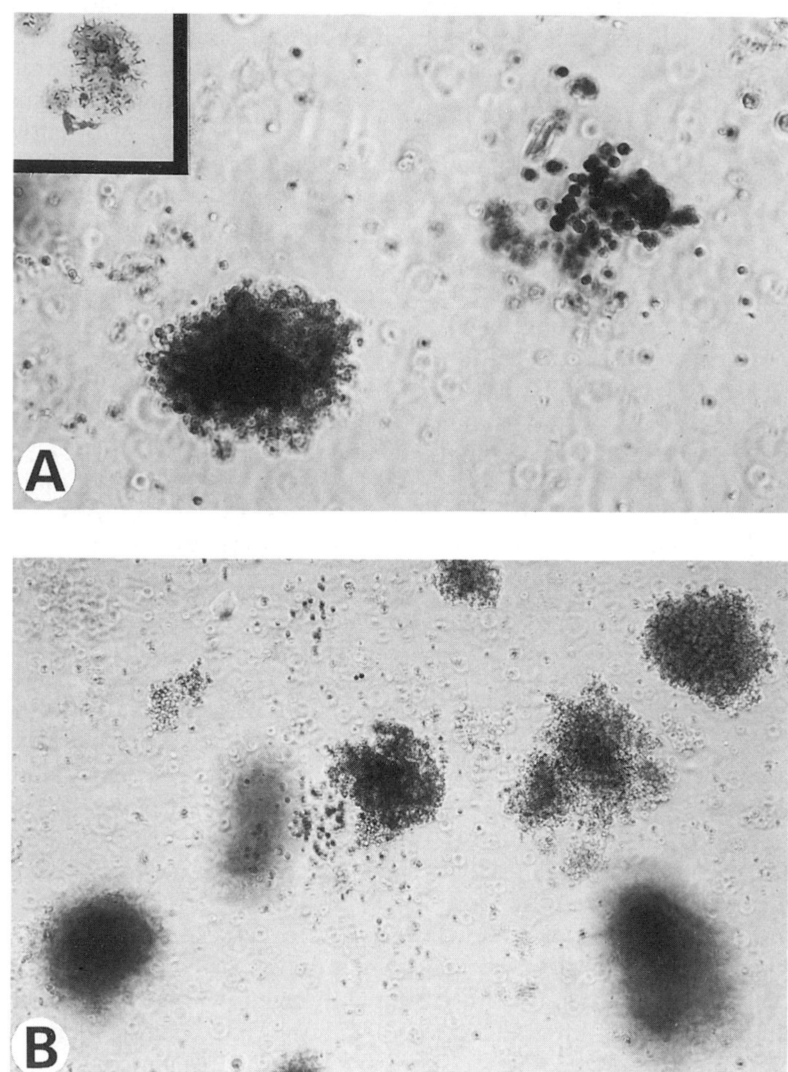


**Figure 4** Hematopoietic colonies infected with a strain of HCMV containing the gene for $\beta$-galactosidase.

addition to stromal fibroblasts, can infect bone marrow progenitor cells. Apparently, marrow progenitors can survive infection, are capable of proliferation and differentiation, and probably maintain latent virus. It remains unclear whether these cells can serve as a source of dissemination or reactivation of HCMV in vivo.

## THE HEMATOPOIETIC SYSTEM AND HCMV LATENCY

There are both epidemiologic and experimental data to support the hypothesis that HCMV may be latent in hematopoietic cells (38,40,76,78,97). However, determining the site of HCMV latency has proven to be difficult. For example, epidemiologic studies indicate HCMV can be transmitted by whole blood, but it has been difficult to directly detect HCMV in units of blood suspected of transmitting virus (29,38,39). Schrier et al. demonstrated that HCMV IE gene products were present in B lymphocytes, but the virus failed to productively infect these cells (41). Since HCMV can be isolated more readily by cocultivation of viable leukocytes on permissive fibroblasts than if cell lysates are used for virus isolation (70), this implies that HCMV may be present in a noninfectious form and require a cellular function for activation. HCMV can infect early hematopoietic progenitor cells, and the virus can be detected in the differentiated progeny generated through the proliferation of infected precursor cells (96); by inference HCMV may persistently infect bone marrow progenitor cells in vivo. Progeny released from the bone marrow may enter the blood and disseminate the virus to a variety of tissues.

A number of possibilities may explain the mechanisms of HCMV latency. Virus may be present in a latent state in a subpopulation of blood cells and virus production activated following blood transfusion. Alternatively, HCMV may be present in a small proportion of cells as a persistent infection, in which virus is constantly being produced. Because so few cells are infected, infectious virus is difficult to isolate. The high percentage of virus-positive blood donors, as determined by PCR (27), indicates that either HCMV DNA is present in a high copy number in a few cells or a relatively high percentage of the cells must contain at least a single genome.

## THERAPEUTIC APPROACHES

### Prevention

Because of the incidence of HCMV in the population, there is a high potential for its transmission by blood products. Transfusion-acquired HCMV infections in immunocompetent patients only rarely give rise to serious disease, however, seronegative immunocompromised patients are at significant risk of developing clinically significant cytomegalovirus infections. The incidence of HCMV disease caused by blood products can be reduced significantly by the use of seronegative HCMV donors (62). In pediatric patients much lower rates of transmission occur when both the donor and recipient of blood are antibody negative. The relevance of the presence of HCMV nucleic acid as detected by PCR in peripheral blood cells must be determined before routing screening of donors by PCR can be advised. Depletion of leukocytes from blood also reduces transmission of HCMV (98) and has the advantage of not requiring donor screening.

## Vaccine Development

HCMV vaccines have been developed using both attenuated and killed virus preparations (82,99). An attenuated vaccine derived from the Towne strain of HCMV was used to vaccinate normal individuals and patients before transplantation (99,100). The immune response to HCMV was boosted without adverse clinical symptoms, and latent virus was not detected following vaccination. Because attenuated strains of HCMV may have an oncogenic potential (20), the use of subunit vaccines has been of interest. Neutralizing antibodies have been produced in guinea pigs against a cloned HCMV glycoprotein (IgG) that was expressed in Chinese hamster ovary cells, demonstrating the feasibility of this approach in vaccine development (82).

Evidence that antibody against HCMV is protective has come from a number of studies (101,102). Immune or hyperimmune globulin, although it did not significantly reduce the incidence of HCMV infection, decreased the morbidity and mortality associated with HCMV infections. The efficacy of immune IgG may be enhanced by the simultaneous use of gancyclovir (101). However, cell-mediated immunity may be much more important than antibodies in protection against HCMV infections (85,103). Induction of cell-mediated immunity can protect mice against challenge with murine cytomegalovirus (68,103). The development of adoptive immunity cloning-expanded T cells in humans is a plausible approach to immunization. The proteins and epitopes that may be important in the development of adoptive immunity are probably different from those involved in humoral immunity and are only now being defined.

## Chemotherapy

The most promising drugs currently used to treat HCMV infections are gancyclovir, 9-(1,3-dihydroxy-2-proxy)methylguanine (DHPG) (104–106), and foscarnet (107). Gancyclovir is used in a variety of clinical conditions, and current clinical trials are designed to determine the range of clinical situations in which gancyclovir can effectively be used (63). A concern with the use of gancyclovir is its hematologic cytotoxicity (63), but this does not appear to threaten the use of this drug.

Additionally, the emergence of gancyclovir-resistant HCMV strains is a potential problem with therapy (104). Recent studies of AIDS patients indicated that approximately 20% of patients receiving gancyclovir continue to shed virus during therapy; in half of these patients these are drug-resistant strains (104).

Foscarnet is a pyrophosphate analog that inhibits HCMV in vitro by blocking a virus-specific DNA polymerase (108). In clinical trials, foscarnet has demonstrated efficacy in the treatment of HCMV retinitis in people with AIDS. Foscarnet can be used in conjunction with zidovudine, which is a distinct advantage in AIDS therapy. Unfortunately, maintenance therapy is required since relapse occurs when therapy is discontinued (108). Although foscarnet-resistant mutants have not been clinically described, they have been isolated in tissue culture, indicating potential for the development of resistant mutants. The drug is administered by intravenous drip because of the short half-life. Adverse effects include renal toxicity and anemia. It is clear that the presence of resistant strains and the cytotoxicity associated with the use of gancyclovir and foscarnet mandate the development of additional drugs that are effective in the treatment of HCMV infections.

### Immunotherapy

The adoptive transfer of T cells appears promising in the treatment of HCMV infections. Greenberg and colleagues selected HCMV-specific T cell clones from recipients before grafting, proliferated the clones in vitro, and infected them back into the recipient (85). The procedure reduced the morbidity and mortality associated with HCMV infections following bone marrow transplantation.

## REFERENCES

1. Rowe WP, Hartley JW, Waterman S, et al. Cytopathogenic agent resembling human salivary gland virus recovered from tissue cultures of human adenoids. Proc Soc Exp Biol Med 1956; 92:418–24.
2. Smith MG. Propagation in tissue cultures of a cytopathogenic virus from human salivary gland virus (SGV) disease. Proc Soc Exp Biol Med 1956; 92:424–30.
3. Mach M, Stamminger T, Jahn G. Human cytomegalovirus: recent aspects from molecular biology. J Gen Virol 1989; 70:3117–46.
4. Stinski M. Fields virology, 2nd ed. New York: Raven Press, 1990; 1959–80.

5. DeMarchi JM, Blankenship ML, Brown BD, Kaplan AS. Size and complexity of human cytomegalovirus DNA. Virology 1978; 89:643–6.
6. Geelen J, Walig C, Wertheim P, van der Noorda J. Human cytomegalovirus DNA. I. Molecular weight and infectivity. J Virol 1978; 26:813–16.
7. Chee MS, et al. Analysis of the protein coding content of the sequence of human cytomegalovirus strain AD169. Curr Top Microbiol Immunol 1990; 154: 126–69.
8. Malone CL, Vesole DH, Stinski MF. Transactivation of a human cytomegalovirus early promoter by gene products from the immediate-early gene IE2 and augmentation by IE1: mutational analaysis of the viral proteins. J Virol 1990; 64:1498–506.
9. Stenberg RM, Stinski MF. Autoregulation of the human cytomegalovirus major immediate early gene. J Virol 1985; 56:676–82.
10. Wathen MW, Stinski MF. Temporal patterns of human cytomegalovirus transcription mapping the viral RNAs synthesized at immediate early, early and late times. J Virol 1982; 41:462–77.
11. Braun W, Reiser HC. Replication of human cytomegalovirus in human peripheral blood T-cells. J Virol 1986; 60:29–36.
12. Sedarati F, Izumi KM, Wagner EK, Stevens JG. Herpes simplex virus type 1 latency-associated transcription plays no role in establishment or maintenance of a latent infection in murine sensory neurons. J Virol 1989; 63(10):4455–8.
13. Kinney JS, Onorato IM, Stewart JA. Cytomegalovirus infection and disease. Pediatrics 1985; 151:772–4.
14. Lang DJ, Noren B. Cytomegalovirus following congenital infection. J Pediatrics 1968; 73(6):812–9.
15. Weller TH. The cytomegaloviruses: ubiquitous agents with protean clinical manifestations. N Engl J Med 1971; 285:203–14.
16. Santomenna LD, Colberg-Poley AM. Induction of cellular hsp70 expression by human cytomegalovirus. J Virol 1990; 64:2033–40.
17. St Jeor SC, Hutt R. Cell DNA replication as a function in the synthesis of human cytomegalovirus. J Gen Virol 1977; 37:65–73.
18. St Jeor SC, Rapp F. Replication of cytomegalovirus in cells pretreated with 5-iodo-2′-deoxyuridine. J Virol 1973; 11:686–90.
19. Tanaka S, Furukawa T, Plotkin SA. Human cytomegalovirus stimulates host cell RNA synthesis. J Virol 1975; 15:297–304.
20. Albrecht T, Rapp F. Malignant transformation of hamster embryo fibroblasts following exposure to ultraviolet irradiated human cytomegalovirus. Virology 1973; 53–61.
21. Gonczol E, Plotkin SA. Cells infected with human cytomegalovirus release a factor(s) that stimulates cell DNA synthesis. J Gen Virol 1984; 65:1833–7.
22. Davis MG, Kenney SC, Kamine J, Pagano JS, Huang ES. Immediate early region of HCMV trans-activates the promoter of human immunodeficiency virus. Proc Natl Acad Sci U S A 1987; 84:8642–6.
23. Nelson JA, Gnann JW Jr, Ghazal P. Regulation and tissue specific expression of human cytomegalovirus. Curr Top Microbiol Immunol 1980; 1–44.
24. Pari GS, St Jeor SC. Effect of human cytomegalovirus on replication of SV40 origin and the expression of T antigen. Virology 1990; 177:1–5.

25. Moses AU, Garnett HM. The effect of human cytomegalovirus on the production and biologic action of interleukin-1. J Infect Dis 1990; 162:381–8.
26. Turtinen LW, Assimacopoulos A, Haase AT. Increased monokines in cytomegalovirus infected myelomonocytic cell cultures. Microb Pathog 1989; 7:135–45.
27. Bevan JS, Daw BA, Day JR, Ala FA, Walker MB. Polymerase chain reaction for detection of human cytomegalovirus infection in a blood donor population. Br J Haematol 1991; 78:94–9.
28. Diosi P, Moldovan E, Tomescu M. Latent cytomegalovirus infection in blood donors. Br Med J 1969; 4:660–2.
29. Kaariaimen L, Klemola E, Paloheimo J. Rise of cytomegalovirus antibodies in an infectious mononucleosis like syndrome after transfusion. Br Med J 1966; 1:1270–2.
30. Pass RF, Kinney JS. Child care workers and children with protean clinical manifestations. N Engl J Med 1985; 75:971–3.
31. Stagno S, Reynolds DW, Pass RF, Alford CA. Breast milk and the risk of cytomegalovirus infection. Med Intell 1980; 302:1073–6.
32. Alford CA, Britt WJ. Cytomegalovirus. In: Fields virology, 2nd ed. New York: Raven Press, 1990; 1981–2010.
33. Dutko FJ, Oldsteon MB. Murine cytomegalovirus infects spermatogenic cells. Proc Natl Acad Sci U S A 1979; 76:2988–91.
34. Drew LW, Mills J, Hauer LB, Miner RC, Rutherford GW. Declining prevalence of Kaposi's sarcoma in homosexual AIDS patients parallelled by fall in cytomegalovirus transmission. Lancet 1988; 1:66.
35. Drew WL, Mills J, Levy J, et al. Cytomegalovirus infection and abnormal T-lymphocyte subset ratios in homosexual men. Ann Intern Med 1085; 103:61–3.
36. Drew WL, Sweet ES, Miner RC, Mocarski ES. Multiple infections by cytomegalovirus in patients with acquired immunodeficiency syndrome documentation by Southern blot hybridization. J Infect Dis 1984; 150:952–3.
37. Turgeon ML. Transfusion acquired infectious disease. In: Turgeon, ML, ed. Fundamentals of immunohematology—theory and technique. Philadelphia: Lea & Febiger, 1989; 371–411.
38. Amstrong D, Ely M, Steger L. Post-transfusion cytomegalovirus and persistence of cytomegalovirus in blood. Infect Immun 1971; 3(1):159–63.
39. Foster KM, Jack I. A prospective study of the role of cytomegalovirus in post-transfusion mononucleosis. N Engl J Med 1969; 280:1311–6.
40. Dankner WM, McCutchan JA, Richman DD, Hirata K, Spector SA. Localization of human cytomegalovirus in peripheral blood leukocytes by in situ hybridization. J Infect Dis 1990; 161:31–6.
41. Schrier RD, Nelson JA, Oldstone M. Detection of human cytomegalovirus in peripheral blood lymphocytes in a natural infection. Science 1984; 230:1048–51.
42. Gilstrap LC, Sebastian F. Cytomegalic virus infection in pregnancy. In: Infections in pregnancy. New York: Alan R. Liss, 1990; 151–63.
43. Wigglesworth JS, Singer DB. Textbook of fetal and perinatal pathology. Oxford: Blackwell Scientific, 1991; 525–91.
44. Stagno S, Pass BF, Cloud G, et al. Primary cytomegalovirus infection in pregnancy: incidence, transmission to fetus and clinical outcome. JAMA 1986; 256: 1904–8.

45. Spector SA, Hirata KK, Neuman TR. Identification of multiple cytomegalovirus strains in homosexual men with acquired immunodeficiency syndrome. J Infect Dis 1984; 150:953–6.
46. Spector SA, Schmidt K, Ticknor W. Cytomegaloviruria in older infants in intensive care nurseries. J Pediatr 1982; 14:81–7.
47. Oldstone MBA. Viral persistence and immune dysfunction. Hosp Practice 1990; 81–98.
48. McDougal JK, Olson KA, Smith PP, Collier AC. Detection of cytomegalovirus and AIDS-associated retrovirus in tissues of patients with AIDS, Kaposi's sarcoma and persistent lymphadenopathy. Antibiot Chemother 1987; 38:99–112.
49. Ghazal P, Young J, Giulietti E, et al. A discrete cis element in the human immunodeficiency virus long terminal repeat mediates synergistic trans activation by cytomegalovirus immediate early proteins. J Virol 1991; 65:6735–42.
50. Mutter W, Reddehase MF, Busche FW, Buhring HJ, Koszinowski WH. Failure in generating hemopoietic stem cells is the primary cause of death from cytomegalovirus disease in the immunocompromised host. J Exp Med 1988; 167: 1645–58.
51. Chesney PJ, Taber A, Gilbert EMF, Shahidi MY. Intranuclear inclusions in megakaryocytes in congenital cytomegalovirus infection. J Pediatr 1979; 92: 957–8.
52. Verdonck LF, VanHeugten H, deGast GC. Delay in platelet recovery after bone marrow transplantation: impact of cytomegalovirus infection. Blood 1985; 66: 921–5.
53. Winston DJ, Ho WG, Lin CH, Budinger MD, Champlin RE, Gale RP. Delay in platelet recovery after bone marrow transplantation: impact of cytomegalovirus infection. Am J Med 1984; 106:128–33.
54. Einsele H, Steidle M, Saal J, Ehninger G, Muller CA. Symptomatic HCMV infection is associated with altered immunreconstitution after BMT. In: Landini MP, ed. Progress in cytomegalovirus research, 1991; 295–8.
55. Rubin RH, Cosimi AB, Tolkoff-Rubin NE, Russel PS, Hirsch MS. Infectious disease syndromes attributable to cytomegalovirus and their significance among renal-transplant recipients. Transplantation 1977; 24:458–64.
56. Einsele H, Steidle M, Vallbracht A, Saal JG, Ehninger G, Muller CA. Early occurrence of human cytomegalovirus infection after bone marrow transplantation: occurrence of cytomegalovirus disease and effect on engraftment. Blood 1991; 77:1114–1110.
57. Reusser P, Fischer LD, Buckner DC, Thomas DE, Meyers JD. Cytomegalovirus infection after autologous bone marrow transplantation: occurrence of cytomegalovirus disease and effect on engraftment. Blood 1990; 75:1888–94.
58. Ljungman P, Bjorkstrand B, Ehrnst A. Forsgren M, Lounqvist B. CMV infection after autologous bone marrow transplantation. In: Landini MP, ed. Progress in cytomegalovirus research. Amsterdam: Excepta Medica, 1991; p. 15–9.
59. Wingard JR, Yen-Hung CD, Burns WH, et al. Cytomegalovirus infection after autologous bone marrow transplantation with comparison to infection after allogeneic bone marrow transplantation. Blood 1988; 71:14323.
60. Taylor-Wiedman J, Sissons JG, Borysiewiecz LK, Sinclair JH. Monocytes are a major site of persistence of human cytomegalovirus in peripheral blood mononuclear cells. J Gen Virol 1991; 72(9):2059–64.

61. Bowden BA, et al. Cytomegalovirus immune globulin and seronegative blood products to prevent primary cytomegalovirus infection after marrow transplantation. N Engl J Med 1986; 314:1006–10.
62. Yeager AS, Grumet FC, Hafleigh EB, Arvin AM, Bradley JS, Prober CG. Prevention of transfusion-acquired cytomegalovirus infections in newborn infants. J Pediatr 1981; 98(2):281–7.
63. DeArnond B. Clinical trials of gangciclovir. Transplant Proc 1991; 23:171-3.
64. Duncombe AS, Meager A, Grant PH, et al. Interferon and tumor necrosis factor production after bone marrow transplantation is augmented by exposure to marrow fibroblasts infected with cytomegalovirus. Blood 1990; 76:1046–53.
65. Carney WP, Rubin RH, Hoffman BA, Hansen WP, Healey HR, Hirsch S. Analysis of T lymphocyte subsets in cytomegalovirus mononucleosis. J Immunol 1981; 126:2114–6.
66. Hutchinson K, Eren E, Grundy JE. Expression of ICAM and LFA-3 following cytomegalovirus infection. In: Landini MP, ed. Progress in cytomegalovirus research. Amsterdam: Excepta Medica, 1991; 267–71.
67. Gussow D, Clackson T. Direct clone characterization from plaques and colonies by the polymerase chain reaction. Nucleic Acids Res 1989; 17(10):4000–4000.
68. Reddehase MJ. Bone marrow dysfunction in irradiated cytomegalovirus-infected mice. Transplant Proc 1991; 23:8–11.
69. Reusser P, Riddell SB, Meyers JD, Greenberg PD. Cytotoxic T-lymphocyte response to cytomegalovirus after human allogeneic bone marrow transplantation: pattern of recovery and correlation with cytomegalovirus infection and disease. Blood 1991; 78:1373–80.
70. Rinaldo CR Jr, Black PH, Hirsch MS. Interaction of cytomegalovirus with leukocytes from patients with mononucleosis due to cytomegalovirus. J Infect Dis 1977; 136(5):667–78.
71. Iwamoto GK, Monick MM, Clark BD, Auron PE, Stinski MF, Hunninghake GW. Modulation of interleukin 1 beta gene expression by the immediate early genes of human cytomegalovirus. J Clin Invest 1990; 85:1853–7.
72. Rakusan TA, Juneja HS, Fleischmann WR Jr. Inhibition of hemopoietic colony formation by human cytomegalovirus in vitro. J Infect Dis 1989; 159(1):127–30.
73. Olding LB, Jensen FC, Oldsteon MBA. Pathogenesis of cytomegalovirus infection I. Activation of virus from bone marrow derived lymphocytes by in vitro allogeneic reaction. J Exp Med 1975; 141:561–72.
74. Joncas JH, Menezes J, Huang HS. Persistence of CMV genome in lymphoid cells after congenital infection. Nature 1975; 258:432–3.
75. Tocci MJ, St Jeor SC. Persistence and replication of the human cytomegalovirus genome in lymphoblastoid cells of B and T origin. Virology 1979; 96:664–8.
76. Fiala M, Payne JE, Perne TV, et al. Epidemiology of cytomegalovirus infection after transplantation and immunosuppression. J Infect Dis 1975; 132(4): 421–33.
77. Einhorn L, Ost A. Cytomegalovirus infection of human blood cells. J Infect Dis 1984; 149(2):207–14.
78. Revello MG, Percivalle E, Zavattoni M, Parea M, Grossi P, Gerna G. Detection of human cytomegalovirus immediate early antigen in leukocytes as a marker of viremia in immunocompromised patients. J Med Virol 1989; 29:88–93.

79. Hayashi K, Saze K, Uchida Y. Studies of latent cytomegalovirus infection: the macrophage as a virus-harboring cell. Microbiol Immunol 1985; 29(7):625–34.
80. Kalter DC, Nakamura M, Turpin JAr. et al. Enhanced HIV replication in macrophage colony-stimulating factor-treated monocytes. Immunol 1991; 146(1): 298–306.
81. Kitano K, Abboud CN, Ryan DH, Quan SG, Baldwin GC, Golde DW. Macrophage-active-colony-stimulating factors enhance human immunodeficiency virus type 1 infection in bone marrow stem cells. Blood 1991; 77:1699–705.
82. Spaete RR. A recombinant subunit vaccine approach to HCMV vaccine development. Transplant Proc 1991; 23:90–6.
83. Rodgers BCr, Scott DM, Mundin J, Sissons JGP. Monocyte-derived inhibitor of interleukin 1 induced by human cytomegalovirus. J Virol 1985; 55(3):527–32.
84. Kapasi K, Rice GPA. Cytomegalovirus infection of peripheral blood mononuclear cells: Effects on interleukin-1 and -2 production and responsiveness. J Virol 1988; 62:3603–7.
85. Greenberg P, Goodrich J, Riddell S. Adoptive immunotherapy of human cytomegalovirus infection: potential role in protection from disease progression. Transplant Proc 1991; 23:97–101.
86. Rice GPA, Schrier RD, Oldstone MBA. Cytomegalovirus infects human lymphocytes and monocytes: virus expression is restricted to immediate early gene products. Proc Natl Acad Sci USA 1984; 81:6134–8.
87. Ibanez CE, Schrier R, Ghazal P, Wiley C, Nelson JA. Human cytomegalovirus productively infects primary differentiated macrophages. J Virol 1991; 65:6581–8.
88. van Bruggen I, Price P, Robertson TA, Papadimitriou JM. Morphological and functional changes during cytomegalovirus replication in murine macrophages. Leuko Biol 1989; 46:508–20.
89. Seljelid R, Fandrem J, Smedsrod B. The macrophage as a multifunctional effector cell. 1990; 257–76.
90. St. Jeor SC, Maciejewski J, Young N. Replication of human cytomegalovirus in macrophages and monocytes and the effect of cytokines on virus gene expression, 3rd/ed. Amsterdam: Elsevier, 1991; 303–6.
91. Prince AM, Szmuness W, Millian SJ, David DD. A serologic study of cytomegalovirus infections associated with blood transfusions. N Eng J Med 1971; 284: 1125–31.
92. Mittal SK, Field HJ. Analysis of the bovine herpesvirus type 1 thymidine kinase (TK) gene from wild-type virus and TK-deficient mutants. J Gen Virol 1989; 70:901–18.
93. Simmons P, Kaushansky K, Torok-Storb B. Mechanisms of cytomegalovirus-mediated myelosuppression: perturbation of stromal cell function versus direct infection of myeloid cells. Proc Natl Acad Sci 1990; 87:1386–90.
94. Sing GK, Ruscetti FW. Preferential suppression of myelopoiesis in normal human bone marrow cells after in vitro challenge with human cytomegalovirus. Blood 1990; 75(10):1965–73.
95. Spaete RR, Mocarski ES. Insertion and deletion mutagenesis of the human cytomegalovirus genome. Proc Natl Acad Sci USA 1987; 84:7213–7.

96. Maciejewski J, Bruening E, Young NS, St. Jeor SC. Cytomegalovirus infection of human bone marrow progenitor cells. Implications for HCMV persistence and latency. Blood 1991; 80(1):170–8.
97. Negro F, Bonino F, Di Bisceglie A, Hoofnagle JH, Gerin JL. Intrahepatic markers of hepatitis, delta virus infection: a study by in situ hybridization. Hepatology 1989; 10:916–20.
98. De Graan-Hentzen YCE, Gratama JW, Mudde GC, et al. Prevention of primary cytomegalovirus infection in patients with hematologic malignancies by intensive white cell depletion of blood products. Transfusion 1989; 29:757–60.
99. Plotkin SA. Cytomegalovirus vaccine development-past and present. Transplant Proc 1991; 23:85–9.
100. Plotkin SA, Starr SE, Friedman HM, Gonczol E, Weibel RE. Protective effects of towne cytomegalovirus vaccine against low-passage cytomegalovirus administered as a challenge. Infect Dis 1989; 159(5):860–5.
101. Snydman DR. Prevention of cytomegalovirus-associated diseases with immunoglobulin. Transplant Proc 1991; 23:131–5.
102. Winston DJ, Ho WG, Lin CH et al. Intravenous immunoglobulin for prevention of cytomegalovirus infections and interstitial pneumonia after bone marrow transplantation. Ann Intern Med 1987; 106:12–8.
103. Lawson CMr, O'Donoghue H, Reed WD. The role of T cells in mouse cytomegalovirus myocarditis. Immunology 1989; 67:132–4.
104. Biron KK, Gancyclovir-resistant human cytomegalovirus clinical isolates: resistance mechanisms and in vitro susceptibility to antiviral agents. Transplant Proc 1991; 23:162–7.
105. Meyers JD. Critical evaluation of agents used in the treatment and prevention of cytomegalovirus infection in immunocompromised patients. Transplant Proc 1991; 23:139–43.
106. Schmidt GM. Treatment of CMV infections and disease in transplantation. Transplant Proc 1991; 23:126–30.
107. Balfour HH. Management of cytomegalovirus disease with antiviral drugs. Rev Infect Dis 1990; 12:s849–60.
108. Chrisp P, Clissold SP. Foscarnet: a review of its antiviral activity. Pharmacokinetic properties and therapeutic use in immunocompromised patients with cytomegalovirus retinitis. Drugs 1991; 41:104–29.
109. Webster A, Lee CA, Cook DG, et al. Cytomegalovirus infection and progression towards AIDS in haemophiliacs with human immunodeficiency virus infection. Lancet 1989; 2:63–5.
110. Dudding L. Cytomegalovirus stimulates expression of monocyte-associated mediator gene. J Immunology 1989; 143(10):3343–52.

# IV

# FLAVIVIRUSES

# 7

# Dengue Virus and Hematopoiesis

**Stephen J. Rosenfeld, Jonathan R. Hibbs, and Neal S. Young**

*National Heart, Lung and Blood Institute*
*Bethesda, Maryland*

## INTRODUCTION

Dengue is a mosquito-borne disease with worldwide distribution. Depending on virulence factors and host immune status, infection can manifest as a severe but nonfatal viral syndrome or a rapidly progressive and frequently fatal hemorrhagic fever. Thrombocytopenia and neutropenia are prominent clinical features and accompany suppression of all hematopoietic lines. Potential mechanisms of hematosuppression include both direct viral infection of progenitors and immune-mediated destruction, providing an accessible model for marrow failure in other contexts.

## VIROLOGY

Dengue virus replicates in the mosquito host, qualifying it as an arbovirus. It belongs to the family Flaviviridae, genus *Flavivirus*, a group that takes its name from the yellow fever virus (Latin *flavus*, yellow). Four serotypes exist, designated dengue 1–4; these determine the specificity of the host antibody response.

The dengue virion consists of an envelope that is derived from the host cell, a nucleocapsid, and a linear positive-stranded RNA genome. The genome is organized with the structural genes C, pre-M, and E on the 5′ end and the nonstructural proteins on the 3′ end, all within a single open reading frame

A

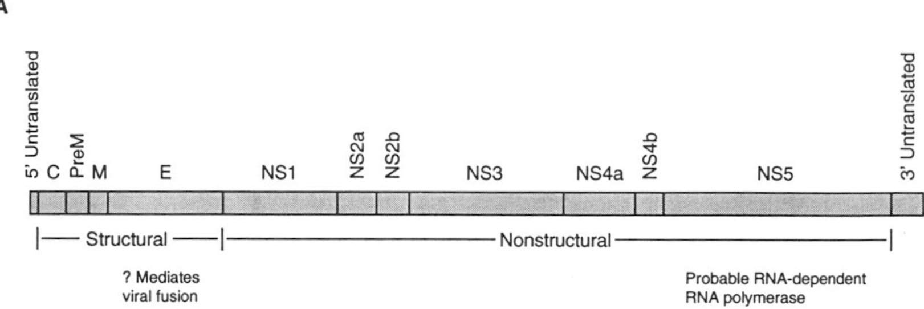


B

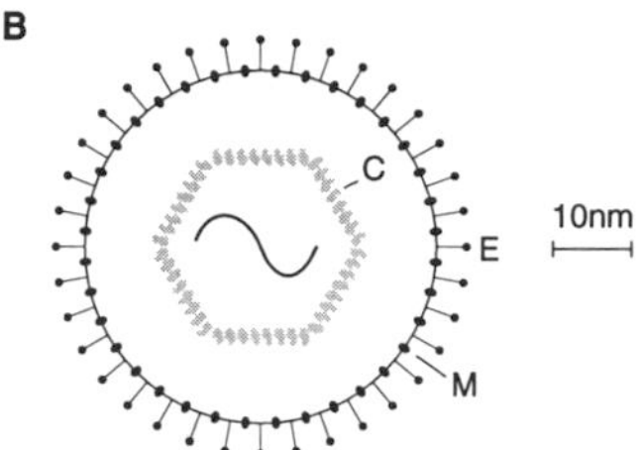


**Figure 1** Organization of the dengue genome. Dengue virus has a linear single-stranded RNA genome of approximately 11 kb. Structural proteins are expressed from the 5′ end and nonstructural proteins from the 3′ end. The genomic RNA is first used as the message for translation of viral proteins; later it serves as a template for RNA replication by a virally encoded RNA-dependent RNA polymerase.

(Fig. 1). Replication is mediated by a virally encoded RNA-dependent RNA polymerase and does not involve a DNA intermediate. Viral proteins are produced by translation of the genome into a single polyprotein that is cleaved either during translation or posttranslationally by host signalases and virally encoded proteinases (1).

The structural proteins of dengue have been studied extensively. Structural protein C is a 13–16 kD protein that forms the viral capsid. Pre-M is a glycoprotein that is only found on the envelope of intracellular virus. During release from the cell, pre-M is cleaved to the mature protein M. Structural protein E is an envelope protein that probably mediates receptor binding and fusion of the viral envelope with the host cell membrane. A highly conserved region around amino acid 100 encodes the presumed fusion-related sequence Gly-Leu-Phe-Gly (2).

The viral nonstructural proteins are less well characterized. Nonstructural protein 1 (NS1) forms a dimer that is expressed on the plasma membrane of infected cells. NS2a is required for the proper processing of NS1. The amino-terminal third of NS3 encodes the protease activity responsible for proper cleavage of NS2b and NS3. NS5 contains the common polymerase sequence Gly-Asp-Asp and encodes the viral RNA-dependent RNA polymerase (2,3).

The assembled virion is a spherical particle with a diameter of 40–50 nm. Spikes (5–10 nm) consisting of structural protein E project from the lipid envelope and contain hemagglutination and neutralization epitopes (1,3). The envelope encloses a 25–30 nm nucleocapsid made up of structural protein C. Like other enveloped RNA viruses, dengue is relatively fragile. Infectivity is lost after virus is heated to 50 °C, treated with ultraviolet light, or exposed to detergents or trypsin (3).

The life cycle of dengue involves alternate replication stages in the mosquito vector and the human host. The virus is taken up by a female mosquito during a blood meal on an infected human. Dengue replicates in the insect's gut and reaches the salivary glands after a temperature-dependent extrinsic incubation period. It is at this stage that the insect's bite can transmit the virus to humans (4). Details of the second replicative stage can be inferred from experimental infection of nonhuman primates (5). Virus is inoculated intracutaneously when an infected mosquito feeds. After infection and replication in cells near the site of inoculation, the virus spreads first to the lymphatics and then to the blood. During the viremic phase virus can be demonstrated in multiple organs, including the lung, liver, spleen, and skin. The intracellular phase of the viral life cycle is likely to be similar to that of other enveloped RNA viruses. It is initiated when virus binds to specific cell surface receptors and is internalized in clathrin-coated pits (6,7). Decreasing pH in the endosome triggers fusion of the viral envelope with the membrane of the endosome, and the nucleocapsid is released into the host cell cytoplasm. Fusion is followed by uncoating of the viral RNA, translation and production of viral proteins, and replication of RNA. Assembly of viral progeny take place in the perinuclear region of the cytoplasm. Progeny virus is found in membrane-bound vesicles (8); virions are released after fusion of these vesicles with the plasma membrane or after the infected cell is lysed. The new virions are then available for further infection within the host or for transmission by a mosquito.

## CLINICAL SYNDROMES

Infection with dengue virus presents as either classic dengue fever (DF) or dengue hemorrhagic fever and dengue shock syndrome (DHF/DDS; Table 1). The initial phase of the infection is identical in both syndromes. The abrupt onset of high fever is seen 2–7 days after virus is deposited intracutaneously by a mosquito. Fever may reach 103–106°F and is accompanied by a severe frontal or retroorbital headache. The pulse is inappropriately slow for the

**Table 1** Clinical Manifestations of Dengue Fever and Dengue Hemorrhagic Fever[a]

| Finding | Classic dengue | Dengue hemorrhagic fever |
|---|---|---|
| Fever | + + + + | + + + + |
| Positive tourniquet test | + + | + + + + |
| Petechiae or ecchymoses | + | + + |
| Confluent petechial rash | 0 | + |
| Hepatomegaly | 0 | + + + + |
| Maculopapular rash | + + | + |
| Myalgia, arthralgia | + + + | + |
| Lymphadenopathy | + + | + + |
| Leukopenia | + + + + | + + |
| Thrombocytopenia | + + | + + + + |
| Shock | 0 | + + |
| Gastrointestinal bleeding | 0 | + |

[a]Symptoms of classic dengue fever were reported in white adults, and dengue hemorrhagic fever symptoms were compiled largely from indigenous children in Thailand (61). Differences in these populations may account for some of the differences in the clinical manifestations observed.

degree of temperature elevation. Myalgia may be severe, leading to the appellation "breakbone fever." A generalized macular rash may appear transiently in the early febrile period, and nausea, vomiting, anorexia, and generalized lymphadenopathy are common late in the febrile stage. Fever lasts 2–7 days, and defervescence may be accompanied or followed by the appearance of a second maculopapular rash. A temperature spike with the second rash gives the disease its characteristic saddle-shaped fever curve. In uncomplicated dengue fever convalescence may be slow, with a long period of depression, anorexia, and asthenia (9–11).

In individuals who develop DHF/DSS, defervescence marks the beginning of the life-threatening phase of the illness. Weakness, irritability, and lethargy accompany the signs of impending shock, including tachycardia, narrowed pulse pressure, and cool and clammy extremities. Peripheral and circumoral cyanosis can develop. A transudative pleural effusion is common, and pericardial and peritoneal effusions may be present as well. Laboratory studies reveal thrombocytopenia, complement consumption, the development of disseminated intravascular coagulation, and a metabolic acidosis. The hematocrit is increased by hemoconcentration. Shock may last 24–36 h, and mortality with supportive care can be as high as 10–40% (12).

Both forms of dengue are characterized by hemorrhagic manifestations. In dengue fever these are restricted to the signs and symptoms of thrombocytopenia, including epistaxis, petechiae, purpura, menorrhagia, and limited gastrointestinal bleeding. Thrombocytopenia is more severe in individuals suffering from DHF/DSS, leading to gross spontaneous ecchymoses and severe gastrointestinal hemorrhage. In addition, a tourniquet placed on the arm produces distal petechiae (positive tourniquet test), indicating increased capillary fragility.

The diagnosis of dengue in its severe or epidemic forms is usually straightforward, but the differential diagnosis of milder cases or cases that occur in relative isolation is wide, ranging from influenza to yellow fever. The diagnosis can be made by (1) isolating virus from blood, (2) demonstrating dengue-specific IgM 2–6 weeks after infection, or (3) demonstrating a fourfold rise in dengue-specific IgG between acute and convalescent sera (13).

## HISTORY AND EPIDEMIOLOGY

Outbreaks of hemorrhagic fever were documented in the eighteenth and nineteenth centuries as burgeoning world commerce carried mosquito vectors to new areas and naive populations. The first virologically confirmed reports of DF (9,10) and DHF/DSS (14,15) described epidemics in the Philippines, and dengue epidemics have occurred in most nations in Southeast Asia and the Pacific throughout this century. Within the past 5 years dengue epidemics have occurred in mainland China (16), India (17,18), Indonesia (19), Singapore (20), and Taiwan (21). Dengue was once pandemic in the Western Hemisphere as well, but vector control programs nearly eradicated the mosquito vector at midcentury (22). Unfortunately, the continued public health investment required for vector control has not been maintained, and resurgent insect populations have been accompanied by increasingly frequent reports of dengue epidemics, especially in the Caribbean Basin. Most reported cases of dengue in North America are imported (23), but the vector is now well established in the southeastern United States (24). There is no reason to expect that the virus will not soon follow.

The annual incidence of dengue is difficult to estimate. More than 80% of acutely infected individuals have nonspecific symptoms or are asymptomatic (25), and more than one-third of all clinically identified "dengue fever" cases are due to agents other than dengue virus (26). It has been calculated that over 100 million cases of dengue virus infection occur annually, and DHF/DSS has caused more than 1.5 million hospitalizations and 30,000 deaths over the past 20 years (27). Increasingly frequent reports of dengue epidemics are consistent with a worldwide secular trend toward increased incidence (27–29).

Increased risk of dengue infection is associated with factors that increase the likelihood of vector exposure, such as the absence of screens or mosquito nets (30). Open containers of water near the household provides breeding sites for *Aedes aegypti* (31–33), one of the two mosquito species responsible for most cases of dengue, and are also associated with an increased incidence of infection (4,32,34,35). Probably for these reasons, socioeconomic status correlates inversely with incidence of dengue (36,37), although in hyperendemic areas, such as Bangkok, higher socioeconomic status offers little protection from infection (38). Socioeconomic and nutritional status is directly correlated with the incidence of DHF/DSS (39), suggesting that host factors associated with general good health are important in development of the shock syndrome (see later).

## HEMATOLOGIC ASPECTS OF INFECTION

The effects of dengue infection on the peripheral blood counts are characteristic and were used by early observers to differentiate classic dengue fever from yellow fever and malaria. Early accounts described a decline in neutrophil number early in the infection, producing an absolute leukopenia and relative lymphocytosis (40,41). An absolute lymphocytosis accompanied by mild eosinophilia was reported during convalescence. In the 1920s and 1930s, the impact of dengue on U.S. troops stationed in the tropics prompted two classic studies of controlled infection (9,10). In both studies volunteers were isolated in mosquito-free wards long enough to preclude externally acquired infection and then exposed to controlled "doses" of infected mosquitos. Both trials confirmed leukopenia and relative lymphocytosis, but neither reported eosinophilia among the participants. The decline in mature granulocytes was accompanied by an increase in immature forms, and large vacuolated mononuclear cells appeared late in the febrile stage or during early recovery. These may have been what would now be described as atypical lymphocytes.

Because of the generally benign course of classic dengue fever, there are few studies of the bone marrow during infection. A description of serial bone marrow biopsies performed on an infected U.S. Peace Corps volunteer at days 4, 7, and 12 after the onset of fever revealed decreased precursors in all lineages. On day 4 both myelopoiesis and erythropoiesis appeared qualitatively normal, but cells belonging to both lineages were decreased in number. Megakaryocytes were quantitatively diminished but also showed degenerative features, such as loss of normal granularity and decreased cytoplasmic volume. By day 7 the bone marrow was hypercellular, with increased numbers in all lineages, primarily young megakaryocytes. On day 12 a moderate lymphocytic infiltrate was present and all hematopoietic lines were again decreased, although not to the extent seen on day 4 (42).

Changes in the peripheral blood in cases of DHF/DSS are more extreme than those seen in dengue fever. A study of children with DHF/DSS in Bangkok in 1960 reported early leukopenia with a proportional decrease in both granulocytes and lymphocytes, accompanied by the appearance of reactive lymphocytes (43). A larger series showed that leukopenia was characteristic of mild cases of DHF/DSS, but patients who progressed to shock or death typically developed a leukocytosis, with total leukocyte counts as high as 40,000 $mm^{-3}$ (44). Leukocytosis was the result of increases in both neutrophils and lymphocytes. Thrombocytopenia with circulating platelets below 100,000 $mm^{-3}$ was common, especially among patients with more severe disease. Studies of lymphocyte subsets have shown that the atypical lymphocytes seen during the early phase of infection are non-B, non-T. Circulating B cell numbers appear to stay constant or to increase during infection, but both $CD4^+$ and $CD8^+$ T cells decline. The number of atypical lymphocytes peaks on the day of shock, and the number of T cells reaches its nadir at the same time (45,46).

The bone marrow findings in DHF/DSS occur in three stages. Early in the infection the bone marrow is hypocellular. Megakaryocytes have been described as decreased or normal, and the erythroid lineage shows maturation arrest. This hypocellular first stage lasts from days 1 to 4. Megakaryocytes rebound first and usher in the hypercellular second stage, from days 5 to 8. All lineages are increased and may show megaloblastic changes. A lymphocytic infiltrate may also appear. The third, or recovery, stage begins after day 10, when marrow cellularity and morphology return to normal (44,47).

## PATHOPHYSIOLOGY

Most evidence suggests that the primary target cells for dengue infection are those derived from the mononuclear phagocyte lineage. The virus has been demonstrated in peripheral monocytes, Kupffer cells, pulmonary and thymic macrophages, and skin dendritic cells from infected patients (39). Involvement of the reticuloendothelial system explains the "flulike" symptoms of dengue fever, which likely result from the release of soluble mediators either directly from infected cells or as part of the immune response to infection. The capillary leak and ensuing shock of DHF/DSS may be the result of an exaggeration of the same process, with additional factors leading to dysregulation of cytokine release. There are two complementary theories to explain the nature of these factors: one relies on changes in host immune status and the other on changes in viral virulence.

The first explanation for DHF/DSS invokes antibody-dependent enhancement (ADE) of infection (48). A dengue infection leads to the production of both serotype-specific and cross-reactive pan-dengue antibodies. Type-specific antibodies provide lifelong protection, but cross-reactive antibodies are produced at a lower concentration and provide only short-lived protection. Protection against infection with another dengue serotype lasts only 3–6 weeks (12), after which the concentration of cross-reactive antibodies falls below the level required for neutralization. If the individual is now exposed to infection with a second serotype, antidengue antibodies bind to but do not inactivate the virus. The resulting immune complexes bind to the Fc receptors of the target cells and amplify the infection by providing an alternate entry route for the virus.

Clinical and epidemiologic data support the theory of antibody-dependent enhancement. The incidence of DHF/DSS is highest in areas of the world like Southeast Asia, where multiple dengue serotypes are endemic (4). In the Caribbean, where dengue is seen in periodic epidemic form, DHF/DSS cases have occurred primarily in the setting of a second epidemic with a new viral serotype (49), usually dengue 2 (4). The incidence of DHF/DSS in infants correlates with the presence of maternal antidengue antibodies: the number of DHF/DSS cases increases from birth to 1 year of age as maternal antibody concentrations decline below neutralizing levels and then decreases as concentrations fall below the threshold required for antibody-dependent enhancement (4). A prospective study in Bangkok showed that, in school-age children, the presence of antibodies with in vitro enhancing ability was correlated with approximately six times the risk of developing DHF/DSS (50). Antibody-dependent enhancement of infection can be demonstrated both in vitro and in vivo in the laboratory. Higher levels of viremia are seen in monkeys in the setting of a second infection with a new serotype, and antibody can enhance infectivity of dengue as well as many other viruses in cell culture (51). In addition to enhancing viral entry into target cells, formation of immune complexes can have other deleterious effects on the host. Complement consumption occurs during infection, and all complement components with the exception of C9 fall precipitously during severe DHF/DSS (52).

Despite the convincing nature of these data, in several epidemics cases of DHF/DSS were reported in the setting of primary infections. An epidemic on the Pacific island of Niue in the 1970s exposed a population to dengue who had not seen the virus for 25 years. Cases of DHF/DSS were reported in persons too young to have been exposed in earlier epidemics (53). Similar cases of DHF/DSS were reported from Greece in the late 1930s, but serologic data from these cases are controversial (39,54). It is possible that strain-related virulence factors may play a role in the development of DHF/DSS in the absence of antibody enhancement.

The importance of viral factors was confirmed by a study of dengue 2 isolates from patients with dengue fever and DHF/DSS (55). Fresh human monocytes were exposed to a fixed amount of virus in the presence of optimizing concentrations of nonneutralizing antibodies, and infection productivity was assessed by measuring progeny virus in the supernatant and counting the number of infected cells. Under identical conditions, virus isolates from patients with DHF/DSS were able to generate significantly more progeny virions. Attempts to find molecular correlates for these differences in virulence have been unsuccessful thus far (56).

## MECHANISMS OF HEMATOSUPPRESSION

The cytopenias seen with dengue infection appear to be the result of decreased production, although consumption may play an additive role in thrombocytopenia and neutropenia. Bone marrow function can be depressed by soluble mediators of inflammation, such as interferon-$\gamma$ (57). Release of this cytokine has been demonstrated from virus-specific T cell clones isolated from the peripheral blood of donors exposed to dengue. In addition to producing interferon-$\gamma$, these clones proliferated in response to virus and lysed infected target cells (58).

In addition to being innocent bystanders of an overactive immune response, recent in vitro data suggest that hematopoietic lineages other than monocytes may be primary targets of dengue infection. In cultures of freshly harvested human bone marrow, dengue 4 primarily infected erythroid progenitors (8). Infection was not cytolytic and did not qualitatively impair colony formation, but infected colonies appeared morphologically abnormal. The virus was able to infect multiple hematopoietic cell lines, including the erythroleukemia cell line K562 (Fig. 2). Infection was maintained indefinitely in continuous culture, with infected cells showing only a mild decrease in growth rate. The ability of dengue to infect hematopoietic cells varies among serotypes. Dengue 2 is less efficient than dengue 4 at infecting erythroid cells but infects cell lines of both myelomonocytic and lymphocytic lineage (59). Lineage specificity may have pathophysiologic significance, because dengue 2 is associated with DHF/DSS to a greater extent than other serotypes (4).

There are several mechanism by which a direct bone marrow infection could be suppressive. In vivo infection may be directly cytolytic, although there is no evidence of this in vitro. Infected cells may be lysed by activated cells of the immune response. Dengue-related antigen is easy to detect on the cell membrane of infected cells, including cells of hematopoietic lineage (unpublished data), and these cells may become targets in the effort to clear the virus. Before such lytic events, infection may compromise the ability of hematopoietic cells to proliferate and differentiate, leading to the observed maturation arrest and megaloblastic changes. Such a loss of "luxury" functions (60) cannot be detected in cell culture but may occur in vivo.

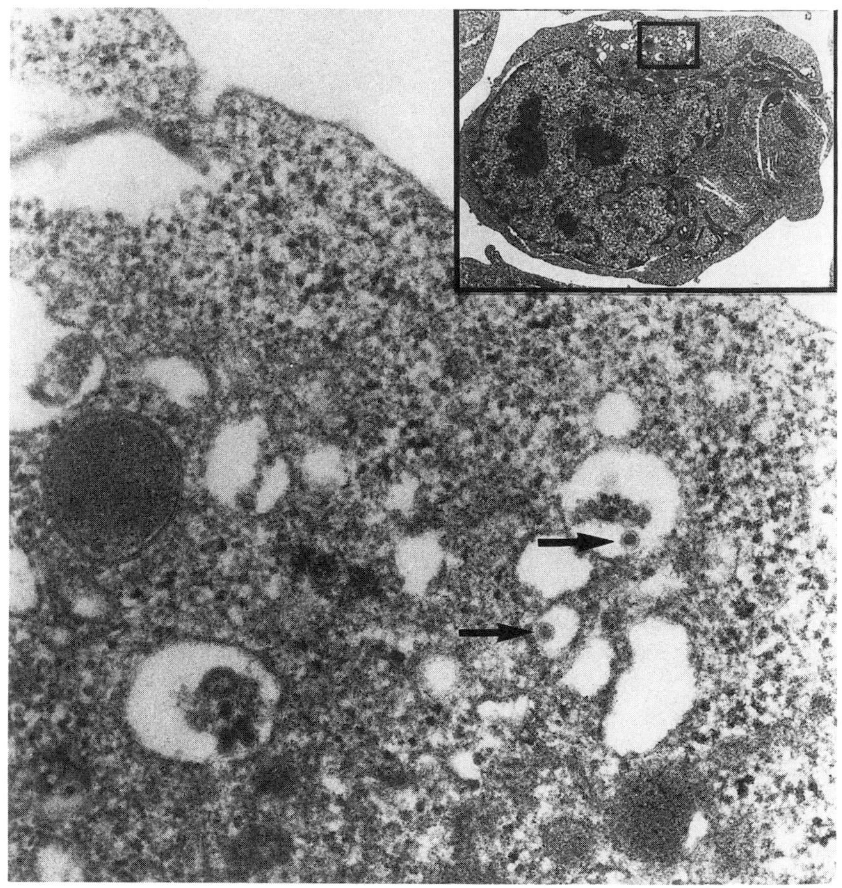

**Figure 2** Electron micrograph of a K562 cell infected with dengue 4. The inset shows the infected cell with a box surrounding the enlarged area. The arrows indicate two discrete virus particles; other particles are visible in the cytoplasm and vesicles of the infected cell.

## SUMMARY

The constancy of the hematopoietic effects of dengue set it apart from other viruses that can sporadically affect the bone marrow, such as cytomegalovirus, Epstein-Barr virus, and human immunodeficiency virus. Its ability to suppress all lineages simultaneously separates dengue from such viruses as B19 parvovirus that predictably suppress a single lineage. Suppression may involve direct infection of progenitors, immune-mediated cytolysis, and indirect immune-mediated suppression through humoral factors. These characteristics make dengue a unique example of pathogen-bone marrow interaction and a potential model for studying idiopathic bone marrow failure.

## ACKNOWLEDGMENTS

Electron micrographs were generously provided by Anne Field, Public Health Laboratory Service Virus Reference Laboratory, London NW9 5HT, United Kingdom.

## REFERENCES

1. Rice CM, Strauss EG, Strauss JH. Structure of the *Flavivirus* genome. In: Schlesinger S, and Schlesinger MJ, The Togaviridae and Flaviviridae. New York: Plenum Press, 1986; 279–326.
2. Brandt WE. From the World Health Organization. Development of dengue and Japanese encephalitis vaccines. J Infect Dis 1990; 162:577–83.
3. Brinton MA. Replication of the flaviviruses. In: Schlesinger S, Schlesinger MJ, ed. The Togaviridae and Flaviviridae. New York: Plenum Press, 1986; 327–74.
4. Halstead SB. Selective primary health care: strategies for control of disease in the developing world. XI. Dengue. Rev Infect Dis 1984; 6:251–64.
5. Marchettc NJ, Halstead SB, Falkler WA Jr, Stenhouse A, Nash D. Studies on the pathogenesis of dengue infection in monkeys. 3. Sequential distribution of virus in primary and heterologous infections. J Infect Dis. 1973; 128:23–30.
6. Gollins SW, Porterfield JS. Flavivirus infection cnhancement in macrophages: an electron microscopic study of viral cellular entry. J Gen Virol 1985; 66:1969–82.
7. Ng ML, Lau LC. Possible involvement of receptors in the entry of Kunjin virus into Vero cells. Arch Virol 1988; 100:199–211X.
8. Nakao S, Lai CJ, Young NS. Dengue virus, a flavivirus, propagates in human bone marrow progenitors and hematopoietic cell lines. Blood 1989; 74:1235–40.
9. Siler JF, Hall MW, Hitchens AP. Dengue, Phil J Sci 1926; 29:1–304.
10. Simmons JS, St John JH, Reynolds FHK. Experimental studies of dengue. Phil J Sci 1931; 44:1-251.
11. Massachusetts General Hospital. Weekly clinicopathological exercises. Case 40–1989. A 40-year-old man with headache, fever, rash, and thrombocytopenia after a Caribbean trip. N Engl J Med 1989; 321:957–65.
12. Halstead SB. Dengue: hematologic aspects. Semin Hematol 1982; 19:116–31.
13. Hospedales CJ. Dengue fever in the Caribbean. West Indian Med J 1990; 39: 59–62.
14. Hammon WM, Rudnick A, Sather GF, ed. Studies on Philippine hemorrhagic fever: relationship to dengue viruses. In: Proceedings of the ninth Pacific scientific congress. Bangkok: Pacific Scientific Congress, 1957; 67–72.
15. Hammon WM, Rudnick A, Sather GE. Viruses associated with epidemic hemorrhagic fevers of the Philippines and Thailand. Science 1960; 131:1102–3.

16. Qiu FX, Chen QQ, Ho QY, Chen WZ, Zhao ZG, Zhao BW. The first epidemic of dengue hemorrhagic fever in the People's Republic of China. Am J Trop Med Hyg 1991; 44:364–70.
17. Chouhan GS, Rodrigues FM, Shaikh BH, et al. Clinical and virological study of dengue fever outbreak in Jalore city, Rajasthan 1985. Indian. J. Med. Res. 1990; 91:414–48.
18. Srivastava VK, Suri S, Bhasin A, Srivastava L, Bharadwaj M. An epidemic of dengue haemorrhagic fever and dengue shock syndrome in Delhi: a clinical study. Ann Trop Paediatr 1990; 10:329–34.
19. Samsi TK, Wulur H, Sugianto D, Bartz CR, Tan R, Sie A. Some clinical and epidemiological observations on virologically confirmed dengue hemorrhagic fever. Paediatr Indones 1990; 30:293–303.
20. Goh KT, Ng SK, Chan YC, Lim SJ, Chua EC. Epidemiological aspects of an outbreak of dengue fever/dengue haemorrhagic fever in Singapore. Southeast Asian J Trop Med Public Health 1987; 18:295–302.
21. Liu HW, Ho TL, Hwang CS, Liao YH. Clinical observations of virologically confirmed dengue fever in the 1987 outbreak in southern Taiwan. Kao Hsiung Hsueh Ko Hsueh Tsa Chih 1989; 5:42–9.
22. Ehrenkranz NJ, Ventura AK, Cuadrado RR, Pond WL, Porter JE. Pandemic dengue in Caribbean countries and the southern United States—past, present and potential problems. N Engl J Med 1971; 285:1460–9.
23. Centers for Disease Control. Imported dengue—United States, 1990. MMWR. 1991; 40:519–20.
24. Slosek J. *Aedes aegypti* mosquitoes in the Americas: a review of their interactions with the human population. Soc Sci Med 1986; 23:249–57.
25. Burke DS, Nisalak A, Johnson DE, Scott RM. A prospective study of dengue infections in Bangkok. Am J Trop Med Hyg 1988; 38:172–80.
26. Dietz VJ, Gubler DJ, Rigau-Perez JG, et al. Epidemic dengue 1 in Brazil, 1986: evaluation of a clinically based dengue surveillance system. Am J Epidemiol 1990; 131:693–701.
27. Halstead SB. Pathogenesis of dengue: challenges to molecular biology. Science 1988; 239:476–81.
28. WHO. Dengue haemorrhagic fever: diagnosis, treatment and control. Geneva: World Health Organization, 1986.
29. Gubler DJ. Dengue and dengue hemorrhagic fever in the Americas. PR Health Sci J 1987; 6:107–11.
30. Dantes HG, Koopman JS, Addy CL, et al. Dengue epidemics on the Pacific Coast of Mexico. Int J Epidemiol 1988; 17:178–86.
31. Schultz GW. Cemetery vase breeding of dengue vectors in Manila, Republic of the Philippines. J Am Mosq Control Assoc 1989; 5:508–13.
32. Gilbertson WE. Sanitary aspects of the control of the 1943–1944 epidemic of dengue fever in Honolulu. Am J Publ Health 1991; 35:261–70.
33. Usinger RL. Entomological phases of the recent dengue epidemic in Honolulu. Public Health Rep 1944; 58:423–30.
34. Koopman JS, Prevots DR, Vaca Marin MA, et al. Determinants and predictors of dengue infection in Mexico. Am J Epidemiol 1991; 133:1168–78.

35. Kaplan JE, Eliason DA, Moore M, et al. Epidemiologic investigations of dengue infection in Mexico, 1980. Am J Epidemiol 1983; 117:335–43.
36. Figueiredo LT, Cavalcante SM, Simoes MC. Dengue serologic survey of schoolchildren in Rio de Janeiro, Brazil, in 1986 and 1987. Bull Pan Am Health Organ. 1990; 24:217–25.
37. Waterman SH, Novak RJ, Sather GE, Bailey RE, Rios I, Gubler DJ. Dengue transmission in two Puerto Rican communities in 1982. Am J Trop Med Hyg 1985; 34:625–32.
38. Halstead SB, Scanlon JE, Umpaivit P, Udomsakdi S. Dengue and chikungunya virus infection in man in Thailand, 1962–1964. IV. Epidemiologic studies in the Bangkok metropolitan area. Am J Trop Med Hyg 1969; 18:997–1021.
39. Halstead SB. The Alexander D. Langmuir Lecture. The pathogenesis of dengue. Molecular epidemiology in infectious disease. Am J Epidemiol 1981; 114:632–48.
40. Carpenter DN, Sutton RL. Dengue in the isthmian canal zone. Including a report on the laboratory findings. JAMA 1905; 1905:214–6.
41. Vedder EB. The leukocytes in dengue. NY Med J 1907; 86:203–6.
42. Bierman HR, Nelson ER. Hematodepressive virus disease of Thailand. Ann Intern Med 1965; 62:867–84.
43. Nelson ER, Bierman HR, Chulajata R. Hematologic findings in the 1960 hemorrhagic fever epidemic (dengue) in Thailand. Am J Trop Med Hyg 1964; 12:642–9.
44. Nelson ER, Tuchinda S, Bierman HR, Chulajata R. Haematology of Thai haemorrhagic fever (dengue). Bull World Health Organ 35:43–4.
45. Wells RA, Scott RM, Pavanand K, Sathitsathein V, Cheamudon U, Macdermott RP. Kinetics of peripheral blood leukocyte alterations in Thai children with dengue hemorrhagic fever. Infect Immun 1980; 28:428–33.
46. Sarasombath S, Suvatte V, Homchampa P. Kinetics of lymphocyte subpopulations in dengue hemorrhagic fever/dengue shock syndrome. Southeast Asian J Trop Med Public Health 1988; 19:649–56.
47. Na-Nakorn S, Suingdumrong A, Pootrakul S, Bhamarapravati N. Bone-marrow studies in Thai haemorrhagic fever. Bull World Health Organ 1966; 35:54–5.
48. Halstead SB, O'Rourke EJ. Dengue viruses and mononuclear phagocytes. I. Infection enhancement by non-neutralizing antibody. J Exp Med 1977; 146: 201–17.
49. Kouri GP, Guzman MG, Bravo JR, Triana C. Dengue haemorrhagic fever/dengue shock syndrome: lessons from the Cuban epidemic, 1981. Bull World Health Organ 1989; 67:375–80.
50. Kliks SC, Nisalak A, Brandt WE, Wahl L, Burke DS. Antibody-dependent enhancement of dengue virus growth in human monocytes as a risk factor for dengue hemorrhagic fever. Am J Trop Med Hyg 1989; 40:444–51.
51. Halstead SB, Shotwell H, Casals J. Studies on the pathogenesis of dengue infection in monkeys. II. Clinical laboratory responses to heterologous infection. J Infect Dis 1973; 128:15–22.
52. Bokisch VA, Top FH. Jr, Russell PK, Dixon FJ, Muller-Eberhard HJ. The potential pathogenic role of complement in dengue hemorrhagic shock syndrome. N Engl J Med 1973; 289:996–1000.

53. Barnes WJ, Rosen L. Fatal hemorrhagic disease and shock associated with primary dengue infection on a Pacific island. Am J Trop Med Hyg 1974; 23:495–506.
54. Rosen L. Dengue in Greece in 1927 and 1928 and the pathogenesis of dengue hemorrhagic fever: new data and a different conclusion. Am J Trop Med Hyg 1986; 35:642–53.
55. Kliks S. Antibody-enhanced infection of monocytes as the pathogenetic mechanism for severe dengue illness. AIDS Res Hum Retroviruses 1990; 6:993–8.
56. Blok J, Samuel S, Gibbs AJ, Vitarana UT. Variation of the nucleotide and encoded amino acid sequences of the envelope gene from eight dengue-2 viruses. Arch Virol 1989; 105:39–53.
57. Zoumbos NC, Gascön P, Djeu JY, Trost SR, Young NS. Circulating activated suppressor T lymphocytes in aplastic anemia. N Engl J Med 1985; 312:257–65.
58. Kurane I, Meager A, Ennis FA. Dengue virus-specific human T cell clones. Serotype crossreactive proliferation, interferon gamma production, and cytotoxic activity. J Exp Med 1989; 170:763–75.
59. Kurane I, Kontny U, Janus J, Ennis FA. Dengue-2 virus infection of human mononuclear cell lines and establishment of persistent infections. Arch Virol 1990; 110:91–101.
60. Oldstone MB, Rodriguez M, Daughaday WH, Lampert PW. Viral perturbation of endocrine function: disordered cell function leads to disturbed homeostasis and disease. Nature 1984; 307:278–81.
61. Halstead SB, Udomsakdi S, Singharaj P, Nisalak A. Dengue chikungunya virus infection in man in Thailand, 1962–1964. 3. Clinical, epidemiologic, and virologic observations on disease in non-indigenous white persons. Am J Trop Med Hyg 1969; 18:984–96.

# 8

# Hepatitis Viruses and Bone Marrow Depression

**Pascal Bouffard and Jerome B. Zeldis**

*University of California, Davis, Medical Center*
*Sacramento, California*

## INTRODUCTION

Viral hepatitis is a well-defined syndrome usually caused by one of five viruses (hepatitis viruses A–E) that primarily infect the liver. Three of these five viral agents have been implicated in transient and severe depression of hematopoiesis. A variable period of time after infection, viremia and virus in the liver and bile are detectable. Soon thereafter, the patient mounts both humoral and cellular immunologic responses to the infection and transient bone marrow depression is observed. The reticulocyte count usually declines, as well as the number of circulating platelets and neutrophils. The bone marrow depression is usually mild and is not clinically significant. Concurrently or soon afterward, the aminotransferases often rise and the patient may or may not become jaundiced, depending on the extent of the liver injury. In animal studies, both hepatitis A and B viral antigens and nucleic acid are detected in the bone marrow. Hematologic abnormalities are observed during the course of all causes of viral hepatitis, especially hepatitis A (2), hepatitis B (2,3), and hepatitis non-A, non-B (NANB) (4), and hepatitis C virus (HCV).

Viral hepatitis is a minor cause of severe aplastic anemia, accounting for approximately 2.5% of all cases of aplastic anemia (5). In one series, 0.22% of patients with clinically diagnosed viral hepatitis developed aplastic anemia (6). The severe bone marrow depression may occur concomitantly with the onset of clinical hepatitis or can occur up to 10 months later (4,7).

Although males are more likely to develop bone marrow failure following hepatitis ($p < 0.05$), females are less likely to survive ($p > 0.025$) (7). The overall mortality among 174 patients with aplastic anemia associated with viral hepatitis was 85.1% in a series published in 1974 (7). With the application of supportive therapies, such as erythropoietin and granulocyte-macrophage colony-stimulating factor (GM-CSF), and the use of immunosuppressive therapy, such as antithymocyte globulin (ATG) and cyclosporine A, the survival of hepatitis-associated aplastic anemia has improved (8).

Hepatitis viruses directly suppress hematopoietic progenitor assays, but the mechanisms by which hepatitis infections affect hematopoiesis remain to be elucidated. Some possibilities include an immunologic attack on the bone marrow, a direct inhibitory effect of the viruses on particular bone marrow elements, or a direct effect on the complex interactions between progenitor and stromal cells (Fig. 1). It is likely that the interactions of each hepatitis virus with the hematopoietic system are different.

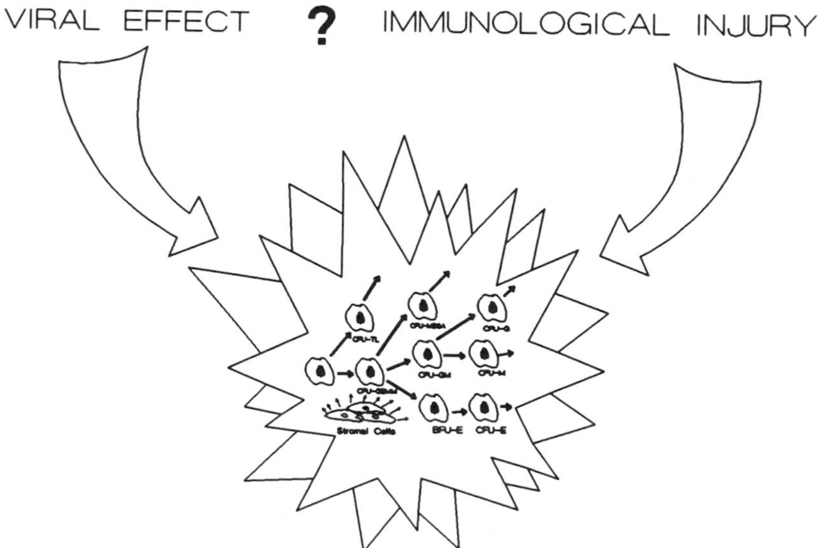


**Figure 1** Despite the in vitro evidence that hepatitis A, B, and C viruses inhibit bone marrow progenitor cell colony formation, the temporal sequence of hematopoietic depression makes it likely that immunologic mechanisms may have a role in this phenomenon as well.

Although not a human pathogen, the coronavirus mouse hepatitis virus 3 (MHV-3) can cause aplastic crises in mice. This agent grows to high titers in the mouse bone marrow (9). MHV-3 infects and diminishes the number of $mu^+$ B lymphocytes and pre-B cells but not their progenitors (pre-pre-B cells) (10). MHV-3 infection of macrophages induces interferon-$\gamma$ release. This can be partially abrogated by prostaglandin $E_2$ (11). Similarly, MHV-3 infection of T cells promotes the secretion of a prothrombin-cleaving activity (procoagulant) (12). The aplasia that results from MHV-3 infection may therefore be a combination of cytotoxic effects of the virus on bone marrow cells and the release of inhibitory cytokines from activated T cells and macrophages.

## HEPATITIS A VIRUS AND HUMAN HEMATOPOIETIC DISORDERS

The hepatitis A virus (HAV) is an enterically transmitted picornavirus that infects human hepatocytes (13). HAV may be directly cytotoxic to hepatocytes, but host-mediated immunologic responses contribute to its pathogenesis (14). The virion is composed of a linear, 7.48 kb single-stranded RNA genome and a capsid containing multiple copies of four proteins (15–18). The hepatitis is almost invariably self-limited and usually anicteric. HAV is a rare cause of fulminant hepatitis.

HAV infects chimpanzees (19), owl monkeys (20), and several species of South American marmoset monkeys (21). Disease in nonhuman primates resembles that in humans but is usually milder. Viral antigens are detected in serum, liver, bile, spleen, kidneys, and feces 2 weeks after infection. Early studies of the tissue distribution of HAV in marmosets revealed the bone marrow as a potential site of infection, but the bone marrow contained many orders of magnitude less virus than the liver (Provost, personal communication). Whether this represents contamination or true infection remains to be determined. Both primate and human cell lines can propagate HAV (13). Unlike other picornaviruses, the virus grows slowly and often needs a physical agent to disrupt the cells for virus to be released.

HAV infection has been associated with severe pancytopenia (22). At the time of the immune responses to HAV infection, hematopoietic abnormalities are observed, including granulocytopenia, moderate anemia with low reticulocyte count, and thrombocytopenia (7). Hepatitis A viral infection was implicated in a severe aplastic anemia that underwent spontaneous remission in a 6-year-old child (1). Marrow transplantation was not attempted because of the concomitant hepatitis. During the course of the child's illness, he seroconverted to high titers of anti-HAV antibodies and the pancytopenia resolved. In another case of HAV-associated aplastic anemia diagnosed by seroconversion to anti-HAV IgM, the peripheral blood T lymphocytes reduced the number of colony-forming units in culture (CFU-C) of the patient's own bone marrow, a finding that implied that a cellular immune mechanism was responsible for the marrow aplasia (23).

Busch and colleagues showed that in vitro assays of hematopoiesis, such as the colony-forming units of granulopoiesis and monopoiesis (CFU-GM) and blast-forming units of erythropoiesis (BFU-E), were inhibited by tissue culture-derived HAV (Fig. 2) (24). Maximal inhibition occurred when the bone marrow mononuclear cells were incubated with virus for over 12 h. The inhibition of differentiation and proliferation of the bone marrow cells did not occur when heat-inactivated HAV (85 °C for 3 minutes) was used or when the virus was incubated with neutralizing anti-HAV antibodies before exposure to bone marrow mononuclear cells. Although CFU-GM colony formation was inhibited to the same extent as BFU-E and CFU-mixed, the number of monocyte colonies in both CFU-mixed and CFU-GM was less than that for the other cell types. This result is consistent with clinical observations that the monocyte count is less affected than that of polymorphonuclear leukocytes and reticulocytes. Potent hematopoietic suppressors, such as interferons $\alpha$, $\beta$, and $\gamma$ and tumor necrosis factor (TNF), were not involved in the in vitro inhibition of colony growth.

The mechanism by which HAV directly inhibits in vitro hematopoiesis has not yet been elucidated. Since the usual hematopoietic abnormalities are concurrent with an immune response to the virus, an immunologic cause besides a direct action of the virus may have a role in the bone marrow suppression that occurs during early stages of the infection. Alternatively, mediators of infection other than interferon and TNF can be released that temporarily affect hematopoiesis or stromal function.

## HEPATITIS B VIRUS AND HUMAN HEMATOPOIESIS DISORDERS

Hepatitis B virus (HBV) is a member of the hepadnavirus family. This partially double-stranded DNA virus replicates by reverse transcription of an RNA pregenome. The 42 nm diameter virion (Dane particle) consists of three envelope proteins (large, middle, and small hepatitis B surface antigen, HBsAg) embedded in a lipid membrane that surrounds a core structure. The 20 nm diameter spherical core consists of hepatitis B core antigen (HBcAg) and encapsulates the partially double-stranded 3.2 kb long DNA, a viral DNA polymerase, and a protein kinase (25–27). The virus contains a number of regulatory elements, including enhancer sequences, a glucocorticoid-respon-

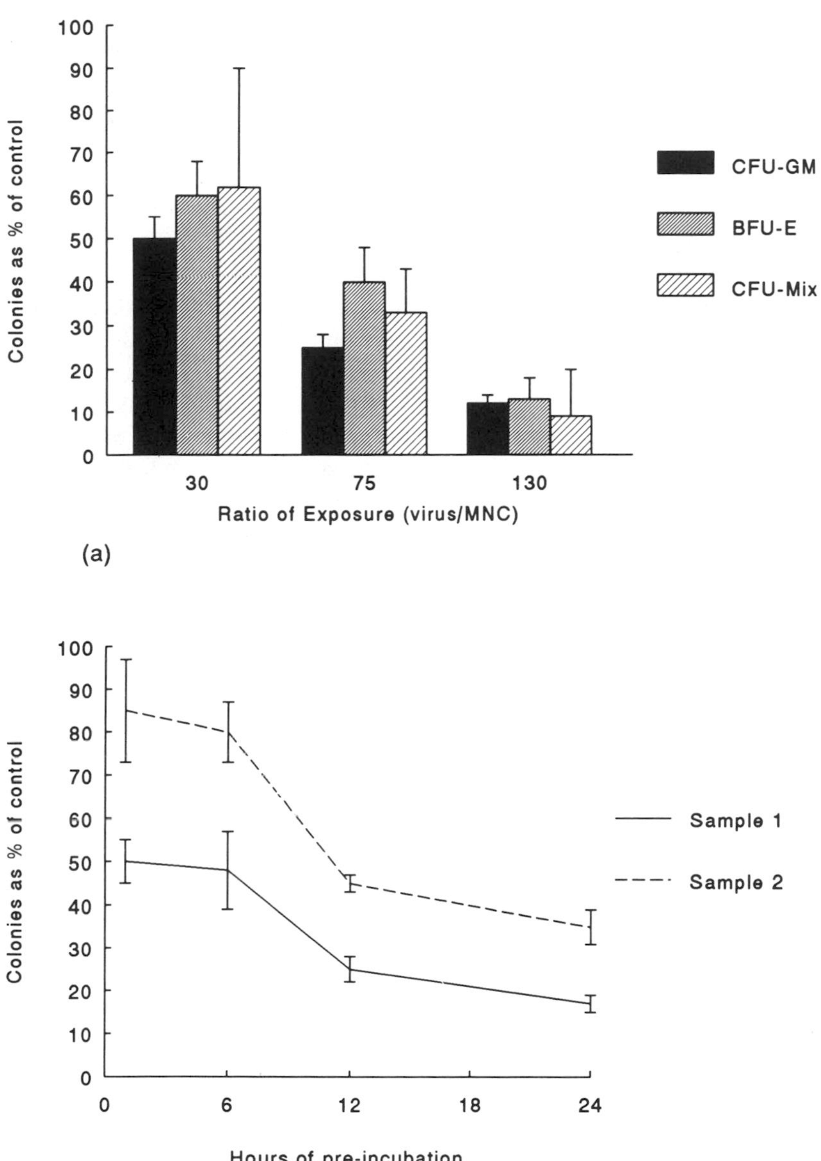


**Figure 2** (a) The ratio of exposure of HAV to mononuclear cells (MNC) correlates with the inhibition of bone marrow progenitor cell colony formation. (b) The duration of exposure of bone marrow mononuclear cells to virus correlates with the inhibition of bone marrow progenitor cell colony formation. (Adapted from Ref. 247.)

sive element, and a nonstructural viral protein (HBxAg) that is a transcriptional activator (28). Antibodies to HBV surface epitopes neutralize infection.

The hepatocyte necrosis that occurs during HBV infection may result from a cytotoxic T cell response to viral antigens, such as HBcAg and HBeAg, on the surface of infected cells (29,30). Rarely, accumulation of viral proteins may cause a direct cytopathic effect, as is seen in HBV-infected orthotopic liver transplant recipients and also in transgenic mice that produce a nonsecretable form of HBsAg (31).

HBV infection is usually mild or subclinical, but fulminant hepatitis can occur (32). The outcome of HBV infection is usually either self-limited or persistent, leading to cirrhosis and hepatocellular carcinoma (33). Factors that affect outcome include age, sex, and the immune status of the individual. Women, adults, and immune-competent individuals are more likely to have a self-limited infection. Neonates infected at birth have a 90% chance of chronicity. This decreases to approximately 10% if the person is infected in the teens. Healthy adult males with acute infection have an approximately 2% chance for chronic carriage.

The narrow host range of the virus (humans, gorillas, and chimpanzees) has necessitated studies with similar hepadnaviruses of other species, including the Eastern woodchuck, California ground squirrel, and Peking ducks (34). Recently, in vitro studies of HBV infection have been achieved with adult human hepatocytes (35), primary human fetal hepatocytes (36), and hepatoma cell lines (37) and by transfecting human hepatoma cell lines with multimers of the virus genome (38).

HBV is not exclusively hepatotropic. Viral DNA and antigens can be detected in such extrahepatic tissues as pancreas, kidney, skin (39), or cells of hematopoietic origin (40). Romet-Lemonne and colleagues determined that a small percentage of bone marrow cells from four HBV-infected patients contained HBsAg and HBcAg (41). They established an HBV-containing lymphoblastoid cell culture from the bone marrow of a patient (42). This culture also contained Epstein-Barr virus; whether the coinfection with Epstein-Barr virus promoted replication of HBV in this primary tissue culture is not known, but with long-term culture, the HBV-containing cells were no longer detectable. Others have identified HBV DNA sequences in the bone marrow of patients with leukemia (43) and in peripheral blood mononuclear cells (PBMC) of infected patients. HBV DNA (44,45), HBV RNA (46–48), and HBV-associated proteins (49–51) were detected in the PBMC. In a few cases, HBV DNA replicative intermediates were found; however, usually the HBV genome is primarily in a nonreplicative (46,49,52) or integrated form (44,53,54).

Viral infection of hematopoietic cells may have a primary or secondary role in the moderate bone marrow depression that occurs during acute disease and in the rare cases of aplastic anemia that follow. Our laboratory reported that HBV inhibited the differentiation and proliferation of human bone marrow progenitors (55). In vitro exposure of progenitor cells to HBV resulted in a dose-dependent inhibition of erythroid (CFU-E and BFU-E), myeloid (CFU-GM), and lymphoid (CFU-TL, T lymphocytes) hematopoietic stem cells (Figure 3). HBsAg was detected by immune electron microscopy in greater than 70% of immature hematopoietic cells, but HBcAg was observed in 5% of bone marrow cells (Fig. 4). Inhibition of progenitor colony formation did not occur after viral inactivation by physical (heat) or chemical (urea dialysis) means. The amount of inhibition was dependent on the ratio of the number of viruses per mononuclear cell and was blocked by antibody directed to epitopes on the viral surface (Fig. 5) (56). Monoclonal antibodies to HBcAg, HBeAg, interferon $\alpha$ and $\gamma$, and other nonviral proteins did not neutralize HBV-mediated cell growth inhibition. Thus, the inhibition of colony formation appeared to be direct. Purified Dane particles, but not viral DNA or proteins, inhibited colony formation. Tissue culture-derived virus also inhibited colony formation of highly purified bone marrow progenitor cells. In one experiment, one in five mononuclear cells formed colonies without exposure to HBV, but in these similarly purified progenitor cells incubated overnight with HBV colony formation was inhibited.

In an effort to extend these findings, we surveyed a number of cell lines of human origin to determine whether HBV would inhibit growth. Inhibition was tested in two ways: the growth of cells into colonies in semisolid suspensions, and the growth of cells in suspension or monolayer culture as measured

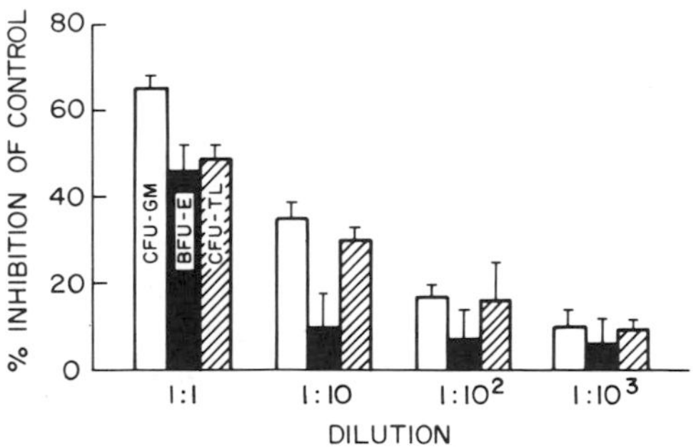


**Figure 3** Effect on hematopoietic colony formation of incubating MNC with serum containing HBV DNA. The data charted are the mean inhibitions and standard error of the mean of colony formation produced by exposure to a HBV DNA$^+$ serum compared to the number of colonies of a negative control serum. The serial logarithmic dilutions of sera were made in RPMI 1640 media. The number of colonies for the control serum for CFU-GM was 224 ± 8 (95% confidence interval, CI) per $10^5$ cells; for BFU-E, 230 ± 4; and for CFU-TL, 1228 ± 41. (From Ref. 55.)

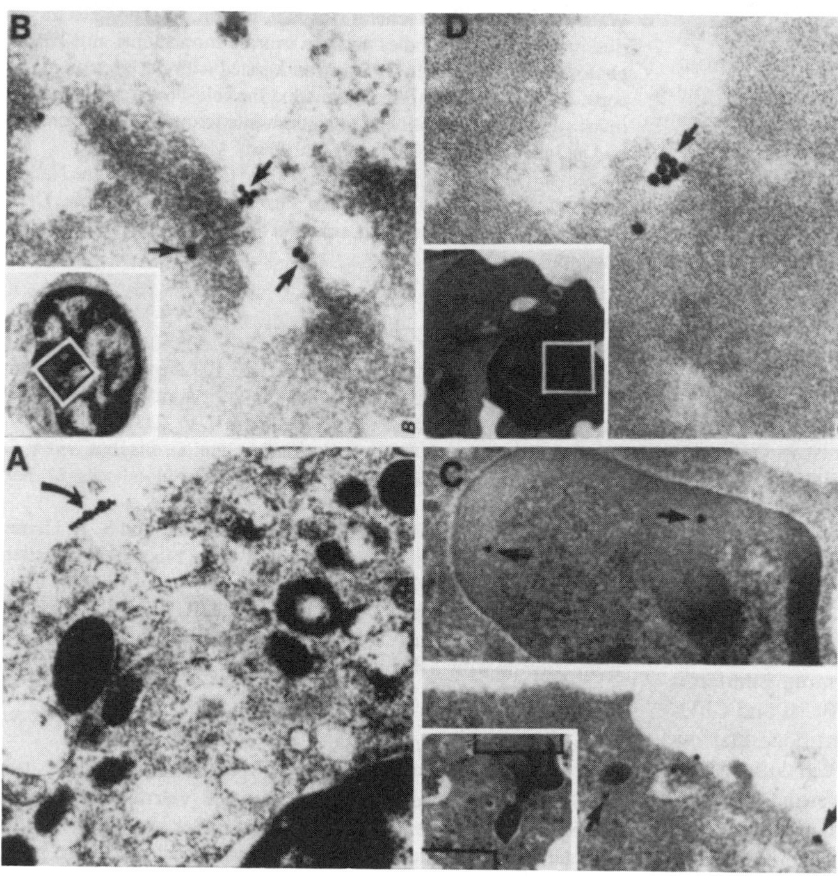


**Figure 4** Immune electron microscopy of bone marrow mononuclear cells incubated with HBV DNA$^+$ serum. (A) Myeloperoxidase-positive myelocyte with gold particles on the surface (× 4500); (B) myeloblast with nuclear labeling (× 14,000); (C) neutrophil with both cytoplasmic and nuclear labeling (× 4500); and (D) normoblast with nuclear labeling (× 20,000). Only MNC incubated with HBV and stained with murine monoclonal anti-HBs antibodies had clusters of two or more gold particles. MNC incubated with HBV and stained with nonspecific monoclonal antibody or MNC incubated with control sera and stained with monoclonal anti-HBs antibodies did not have clusters of gold particles. (From Ref. 55.)

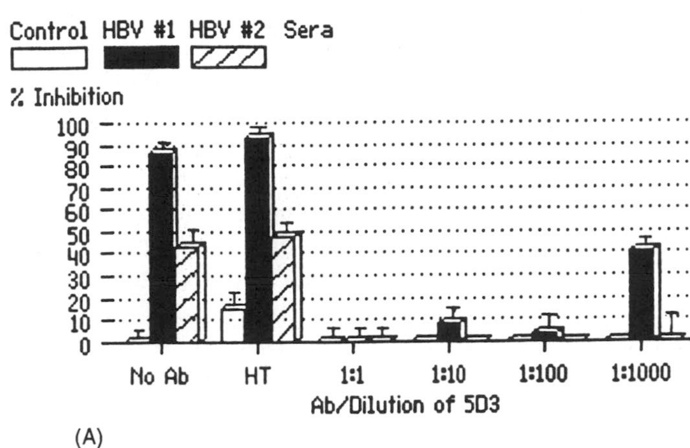


(A)

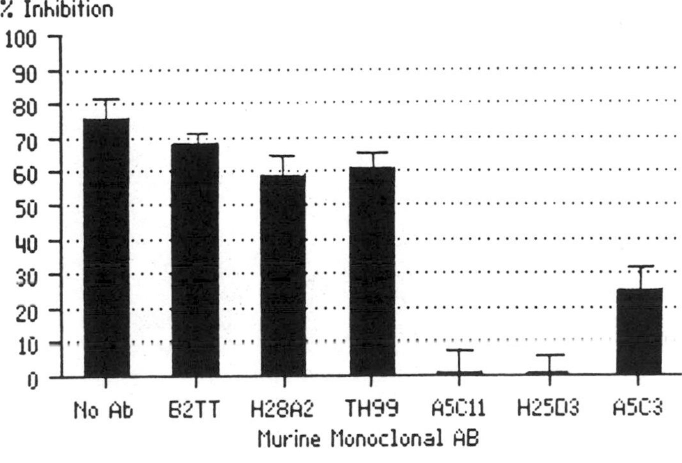


(B)

**Figure 5** (A) Anti-HBs antibodies reverse the HBV inhibition of CFU-E. Comparison of the effects of two HBV DNA-positive sera and two murine monoclonal antibodies on CFU-E. 5D3 is an IgM anti-HBs monoclonal antibody. The murine monoclonal antibody HT is an $IgG_{2a}$ that lacks anti-HBs specificity. The mean colony number and the 95% CI for the control were 94 ± 3 per $10^5$ cells. (B) Comparison of the effects of six murine monoclonal antibodies on HBV-mediated inhibition of CFU-E. B2TT ($IgG_1$), H25A2 (IgM), and TH99 ($IgG_{2a}$) lack anti-HBs specificity. A5C11 ($IgG_1$), H25D3 (IgM), and A5C3 ($IgG_{2a}$) were anti-HBs specific. Murine ascites were diluted 1:10. The mean colony number and the 95% CI for the control were 119 ± 14 per $10^5$ cells. (From Ref. 56.)

by MTT assay. MTT [3-(4,5-dimethylthiazol-2-yl)-2,5-diphenyltetrazolium bromide] is metabolized to form blue formazan crystals by labile cellular dehydrogenases that are found only in viable cells. The quantity of these labile cellular dehydrogenases are proportional to the number of viable cells in culture. After a period of time, the tissue culture cells are incubated with MTT for 6 h and the level of blue formazan is measured at an optical density of 510 nm (57). We determined that the growth of human hematopoietic cell lines of granulocyte, monocyte, and erythrocyte origin was inhibited by HBV, but the growth of nonhematopoietic cell lines derived from breast, colon, liver, and stomach were not (Fig. 6) (58). These data indicated that the HBV-mediated cell growth suppression is tissue specific. Intact virions were necessary for growth inhibition to occur (Fig. 7).

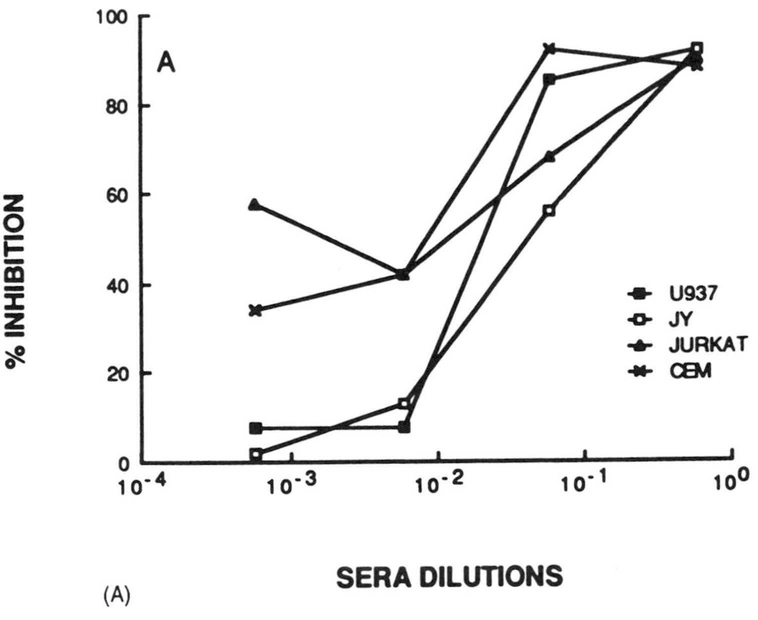


**Figure 6** Effect of HBV-positive sera on hematopoietic cell lines. (A) Effects on cell growth determined by MTT assay. The $OD_{490}$ (optical density, 490 nm) of the controls was 0.290 ± 0.006 for U937, 0.392 ± 0.006 for JY, 0.248 ± 0.0 for Jurkat, and 0.215 ± 0.004 for CEM. (B) Effects on colony formation. The control number of colonies was 57 ± 2 for K562, 34 ± 2 for U937, and 122 ± 3 for HL60. (C) Effect of HBV-positive serum on the growth of three nonhematopoietic cell lines by the MTT assay. The $OD_{490}$ of the controls was 0.220 ± 0.020 for T47D, 0.233 ± 0.010 for B5637, and 0.540 ± 0.010 for C247. (From Ref. 58.)

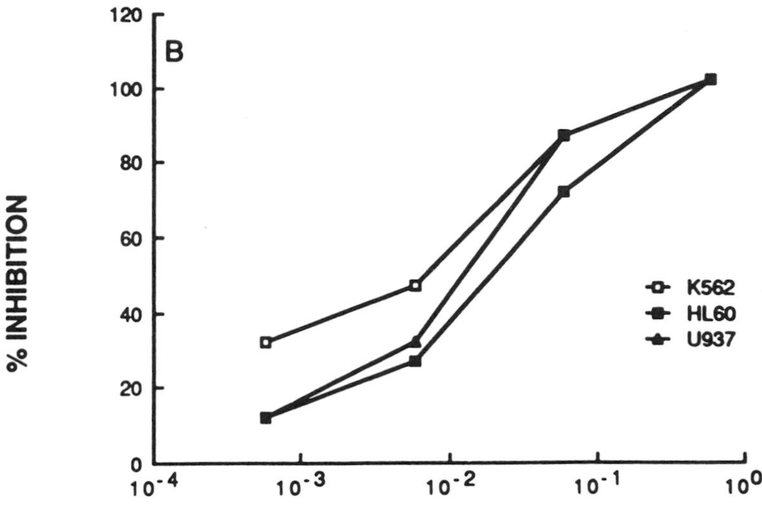
B
% INHIBITION
120
100
80
60
40
20
0
K562
HL60
U937
$10^{-4}$
$10^{-3}$
$10^{-2}$
$10^{-1}$
$10^{0}$
SERA DILUTIONS

(B)

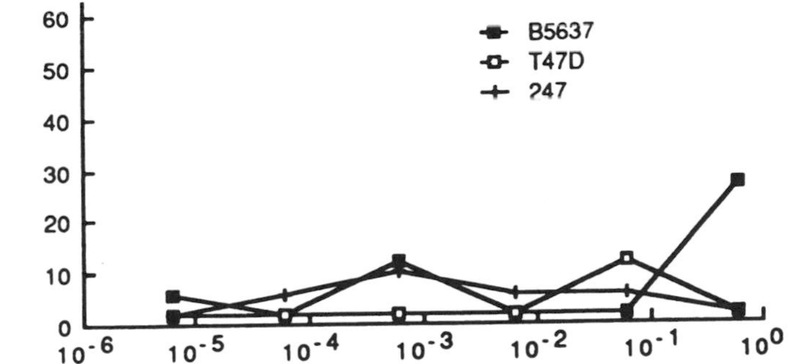
% INHIBITION
60
50
40
30
20
10
0
B5637
T47D
247
$10^{-6}$
$10^{-5}$
$10^{-4}$
$10^{-3}$
$10^{-2}$
$10^{-1}$
$10^{0}$
SERA DILUTIONS

(C)

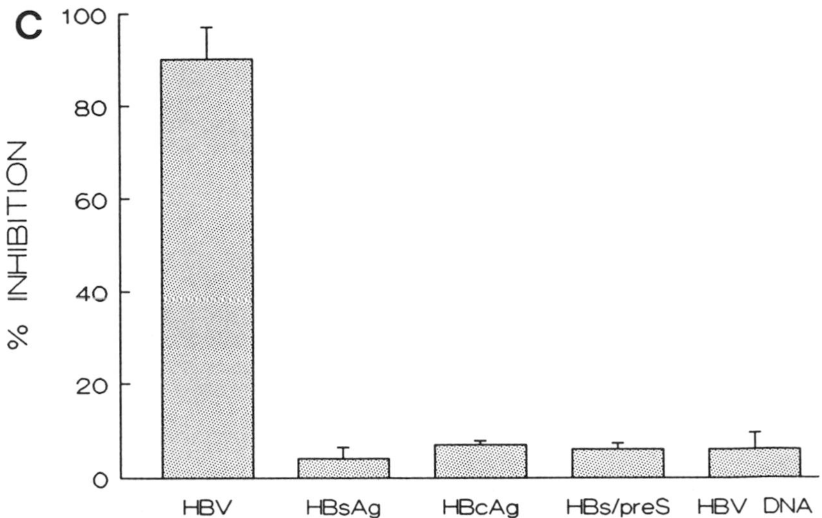


**Figure 7** Recombinant and purified HBV-related antigens do not inhibit K562 colony formation. HBV, serum containing HBV DNA so that the ratio of exposure (ROE) was $10^5$ virions per cell; HBsAg, recombinant small HBsAg at a concentration of 13 ng per cell; HBcAg, recombinant HBcAg; HBs/preS, large, middle, and small HBsAg purified from serum; HBV DNA, serum-derived HBV DNA after proteinase K digestion, phenol-chloroform extraction, ethanol precipitation, reconstitution in RPMI 1640, and exposure to K562 cells at an ROE of $3 \times 10^4$ DNA molecules per cell. (From Ref. 58.)

More recently, we surveyed a number of HBV-containing sera and the supernatants of cell lines that produce virus for their inhibitory effects on the growth of human hematopoietic cell lines. The sera and cell culture supernatants that inhibited cell line growth differed from the noninhibitory samples in only one aspect: when DNA and RNA were isolated from the exposed cells and tested for viral nucleic acid by polymerase chain reaction (PCR) and reverse transcriptase (RT) PCR, HBV DNA and RNA were detected only in cells exposed to the inhibitory samples. The cells in colonies and cells not in colonies that were present in methylcellulose culture were analyzed for viral DNA and mRNA by PCR and RT PCR. The cells from colonies did not contain viral nucleic acid; however, the viable cells (as judged by trypan blue exclusion) that failed to grow into colonies contained both HBV DNA and RNA. Thus, the growth inhibition was directly related to viral infection (Bouffard and Zeldis, manuscript submitted).

The mechanisms of suppression of cell proliferation and differentiation by HBV are not yet understood. HBV affects the functioning of a number of immunologically active cells. HBV inhibits interleukin-1 release from human mononuclear cells and the monocytelike cell line U937 (59–63). Furthermore, HBV exposure to T cells results in viral uptake, transcription, and a decline in the surface display of interleukin-2 receptors (Assounga, manuscript submitted), so that the T cells are more refractory to interleukin-2 stimulation. By analogy, the exposure and uptake of HBV by hematopoietic cells may cause growth inhibition by direct effects of the virus on cell functions or indirectly by making the cells less sensitive to growth factors. Alternatively, cells that are infected by virus may stop growing but display antigens on the surface that make them targets for cytotoxic T cells. These T cells may release cytokines that are inhibitory for hematopoiesis, or the T cells may destroy the microenvironment so that aplasia results.

Hepatitis D virus (HDV) is a defective RNA virus that depends on HBV for its release from infected cells (64). Its 1.7 kb circular RNA genome shares many properties with that of viroids and virusoids, including ribozymelike activity and a complicated secondary and tertiary structure. The viral genome is capable of replicating independently of HBV; however, the nascent HDV capsid particles require hepatitis B virus surface antigen for the viral envelope and secretion from cells. To date, no case of hepatitis-associated aplastic anemia has been reported in an HDV-infected individual. However, this lack of evidence for a role of HDV in severe bone marrow depression may reflect only that few if any investigators have analyzed the sera from cases of HBV-associated aplastic anemia for HDV RNA.

## NON-A, NON-B HEPATITIS VIRUSES AND BONE MARROW DISORDERS

Both aplastic anemia and agranulocytosis occur concurrently or shortly after acute non-A, non-B hepatitis disease (4,65–68). Before the discovery of hepatitis C and E viruses, the majority of cases of hepatitis-associated aplastic anemia were determined not to be due to HAV or HBV. For example, we determined that 13 of 16 cases of hepatitis-associated aplastic anemia who presented for therapy to the University of California–Los Angeles (UCLA) Center for the Health Sciences did not have evidence of either HAV or HBV infection (4). Immunologic defects reported in these patients included a reduction in the number of B and T cells, a decline in serum immunoglobulins, reduced T cell stimulation to mitogens, and a decline in cutaneous hypersensitivity. Nevertheless, it is unclear whether these immunologic disorders are the cause or the consequence of NANB hepatitis-associated aplastic anemia

(65). Studies of the role of putative non-A, non-B agents in causing hepatitis-associated aplastic anemia were limited until recently because of the unavailability of reagents that represented pedigreed viral strains and diagnostic tests that would allow the detection of virus-associated antigens, nucleic acids, and antibodies.

Before the isolation of hepatitis C virus, our laboratory determined that chimpanzee sera from the acute phase of hepatitis induced by parenteral non-A, non-B hepatitis inhibited the growth of human erythroid (CFU-E and BFU-E) and granulocyte-macrophage (CFU-GM) progenitor cells. Sera from the chimpanzees before inoculation with virus or after recovery from infection failed to inhibit stem cell growth (69). (The chimpanzees were inoculated from a chimpanzee-derived factor VIII made by Bradley of the Centers for Disease Control, Atlanta.) Plasma from chimpanzees inoculated with the same preparations were used to isolate HCV. We subsequently determined that the chimpanzees we studied had been infected with HCV.

Hepatitis C and E viruses are the major etiologies of parenterally transmitted and enterally transmitted non-A, non-B hepatitis, respectively. Hepatitis C virus causes more than 90% of posttransfusion NANB hepatitis. This flaviviruslike agent contains a positive-stranded RNA genome of approximately 9400 nucleotides, composed of at least three structural proteins and five nonstructural proteins (70,71). Acute HCV infection is usually mild, and fulminant hepatitis is rare (72). Chronicity results in greater than half of those infected. About 20% of patients with chronic hepatitis due to HCV develop chronic active hepatitis and cirrhosis 5–10 years after infection, but the determinants for the risk of developing progressive disease are unknown. Furthermore, a small percentage of patients with chronic hepatitis C eventually develop end-stage liver disease and hepatocarcinoma (73).

We and others are finding that approximately 10–15% of patients who present to transplantation centers with aplastic anemia have antibodies to HCV as detected by the relatively insensitive first-generation immunoassay (anti-C100) (51). The prevalence of anti-C100 antibodies in patients with hepatitis-associated aplastic anemia was only slightly higher than that for patients with aplastic anemia due to metabolic or idiopathic causes (51). When U.S. patients with hepatitis-associated aplastic anemia were analyzed for HCV RNA by RT PCR and for anti-HCV antibody by a relatively insensitive first-generation enzyme immunoassay, 12 of 24 patients were either antibody reactive or had serum HCV RNA. The presence of both virus and antibody correlated with the number of units of blood products received before testing. Those patients who received no blood products lacked markers for HCV infection (Young, personal communication). Furthermore, in Thailand, where the prevalence of serum HCV RNA in hospitalized patients without bone marrow depression is 5.1%, serum HCV RNA was found in 5.3% of untransfused patients with aplastic anemia. These unpublished data can be interpreted to mean that in both Thailand and the United States HCV may have a minor role as an etiologic agent for aplastic anemia and that other viral agents may be more involved in hepatitis-associated aplastic anemia. Despite this, we have identified individual cases of HCV-associated aplastic anemia and an effect of the virus on in vitro assays for hematopoietic progenitor cells (Zeldis and Bouffard, unpublished results).

We and others have found that HCV RNA is present in the PBMC and bone marrow of chronic carriers, and there is evidence that HCV capsid antigens are also detected in PBMC. HCV inhibits the growth of hematopoietic cells, including BFU-E, CFU-E, and CFU-GM. This inhibition is dependent upon the ratio of exposure of virus to mononuclear cells. Because HCV is much more labile than HBV, this had led to conflicting results among different investigators. UV exposure, freezing and thawing, and urea inactivate the HCV-mediated inhibition of stem cell growth and differentiation. The growth of not all human hematopoietic cell lines is affected by HCV as it is by HBV. The growth of the monocytelike cell line U937 is inhibited: cells cease growth but remain viable as measured by trypan blue exclusion. Preliminary studies reveal that viral antigens are present in these cells. Studies on viral uptake and antigen expression by these cells are ongoing. The HCV RNA is detected by polymerase chain reaction in all U937 cells after incubation with high titered HCV containing serum. Under certain culture conditions, the negative strand (replicative intermediate) is present. (Bouffard and Zeldis, unpublished data).

We are locating cases in which there are HLA identical bone marrow donors, to determine whether an immune mechanism is involved with HCV related aplastic anemia. The affected patient's lymphocytes are incubated with the donor's HLA-matched bone marrow and the cells are then placed into the various bone marrow progenitor cell assays. Prior to incubation the lymphocytes are exposed to irradiated monocytes with virus, UV inactivated virus, or recombinantly derived viral proteins. Also, prior to exposure to the lymphocytes, the donor bone marrow is exposed overnight to HCV. To date, the number of patients studied is to too small to derive meaningful conclusions about a possible role cellular immunity might have in causing severe bone marrow depression.

Hepatitis E virus (HEV), a Colissi-like agent, is primarily enterically transmitted (74). This has resulted in large water-borne epidemics in Asia, the Mediterranean, and Central America. Although cases of HEV hepatitis have been imported from endemic areas, no endogenously acquired clinical case of HEV hepatitis has yet been reported in the United States. Despite this, surveys of sera from Americans using newly developed HEV immunoassays have shown that 1–2% contain HEV-related antibodies. Whether HEV is a cause of clinically significant bone marrow depression is unknown and await the application of new immune assays and RT PCR tests for HEV RNA.

## CONCLUSIONS AND FUTURE DIRECTIONS

Our understanding of hepatitis-associated bone marrow inhibition is rudimentary. Hepatitis A, B, and C are definitely associated with mild transient bone marrow depression and aplastic anemia. Each virus inhibits in vitro assays of stem cell growth. No studies have yet assessed the effects of these viruses on stromal cell function or the responsiveness of the progenitor cells on growth factors vis-à-vis viral exposure. The effects of these viruses on protooncogene expression in hematopoietic progenitors and cell lines have not yet been determined. Also, little is known about the role cellular immunity may have in the induction of the bone marrow depression associated with viral hepatitis.

## REFERENCES

1. Smith D, Gribble TJ, Yeager AS, et al. Spontaneous resolution of severe aplastic anemia associated with hepatitis A in a 6 year old child. Am J Hematol 1978; 5: 247.
2. Casciato DA, Klein CA, Kapowitz N, Scott JL. Aplastic anemia associated with type B viral hepatitis. Arch Intern Med 1978; 138:1557.
3. Nakamura S, Sabo T, Maeda T, Sato Y. Viral hepatitis B and aplastic anemia. Tohoku J Exp Med 1975; 116:101-2.
4. Zeldis JB, Dienstag JL, Gale RP. Aplastic anemia and non-A non-B hepatitis. Am J Med 1984; 74:64–8.
5. Young NS, Mortimer PP. Viruses and bone marrow failure. Blood 1984; 63:729–37.
6. Bottinger LE, Westerholm B. Aplastic anemia I: incidence and etiology. Acta Med Scand 1972; 192:315.
7. Hagler L, Pastore R, Begin J. Aplastic anemia following viral hepatitis. Report of two fatal cases and literature review. Medicine (Baltimore) 1975; 54:139–64.
8. Young NS. Flaviviruses and bone marrow failure. JAMA 1990; 263:3065–8.
9. Piazza M, Piccinino F, Metano F. Haematological changes in viral (MHV-3) murine hepatitis. Nature 1965; 205:1034.
10. Jolicoeur P, Lamontagne L. Mouse hepatitis virus 3 pathogenicity expressed by a lytic infection in bone marrow 14.8$^+$ mu$^+$ B lymphocyte subpopulations. J Immunol 1989; 143:3722–30.
11. Lucchiari MA, Pereira CA. A major role of macrophage activation by interferon-gamma during mouse hepatitis virus type 3 infection. I. Genetically dependent resistance. Immunobiology 1989; 180:12–22.
12. Levy G, Abecassis M. Activation of the immune coagulation system by murine hepatitis virus strain 3. Rev Infect Dis 1989; 11 (Suppl 4):S712–21.
13. Blaine Hollinger F, Ticehurst J. Hepatitis A virus. In: Fields BN, Kniper DM, et al., eds. 2nd ed. Chap. 23, Vol. 1. New York: Raven Press, 1990; 631–67.
14. Lemon SM, Ping L-H, Day S, et al. Immunobiology of hepatitis A virus. In: Hollinger FB, Lemon SM, Margolis HS, eds. Viral hepatitis and liver disease, Baltimore: Williams & Wilkins, 1991; 20–4.

15. Najarian R, Caput D, Gee W. Primary structure and gene organization of human hepatitis A virus. Proc Natl Acad Sci U S A 1985; 82:2627–31.
16. Ticehurst JR, Racaniello VR, Baroudy BM, Baltimore D, Purcell RH, Feinstone SM. Molecular cloning and characterization of hepatitis A virus cDNA. Proc Natl Acad Sci U S A 1983; 80:5885–9.
17. Tratschin JD, Siegl G, Frosner GG, Dienhardt F. Characterization and classification of virus particles associated with hepatitis A. III. Structural proteins. J Virol 1981; 38:151–6.
18. Wheeler CM, Robertson BH, Van Nest G, Dina D, Bradley DW, Fields HA. Structure of the hepatitis A virion, peptide mapping of the capsid region. J Virol 1986; 58:307–13.
19. Maynard JE, Bradley DW, Gravelle CR, Ebert JW, Krushak DJ. Preliminary studies of hepatitis A in chimpanzees. J Infect Dis 1975; 131:194–6.
20. Leduc JW, Lemon SM, Keenan CM, Graham RR, Marchricki RH, Binn LN. Experimental infection of the new world owl monkey (*Aotus trivirgatus*) with hepatitis A virus. Infect Immun 1983; 40:766–72.
21. Provost PJ, Villajeros VM, Hilleman MR. Suitability of the rufiventer marmoset as a host animal for human hepatitis A virus. Proc Soc Exp Biol Med 1977; 155:283–6.
22. Bottinger LE, Westerholm B. Aplastic anemia. III. Aplastic anemia and infectious hepatitis. Acta Med Scand 1972; 192:323.
23. Aoyagi K, Ohhara N, Okamura S, et al. Aplastic anemia associated with type A viral hepatitis—possible role of T-lymphocytes. Jpn J Med 1987; 26:348–52.
24. Busch FW, de Vas S, Flehmig B, Hermann F, Sandler C, Vallbracht A. Inhibition of in vitro hematopoiesis by hepatitis A virus. Exp Hematol 1987; 15:978–82.
25. Stibbe W, Gerlich W. Structural relationship between minor and major proteins of hepatitis B surface antigen. J Virol 1983; 46:626–8.
26. Neurath AR, Kent SBH, Strich N, Taylor P, Stevens CDE. Hepatitis B virus contains pre S gene encoded domains. Nature 1985; 315:154–6.
27. Hoofnagle JH, Schafer DF. Serologic markers of hepatitis B virus infection. Semin Liver Dis 1986; 6:1–10.
28. Elfassi E, Haseltine WA, Dienstag JL. Detection of hepatitis B virus X product using an open reading frame *E. coli* expression vector. Proc Natl Acad Sci U S A 1980; 83:2219–22.
29. Mondelli M, Eddleston ALWF. Mechanisms of liver cell injury in acute and chronic hepatitis B. Semin Liver Dis 1984; 4:47–58.
30. Ferrari C, Penna A, Giuberti T, et al. Intrahepatic, nucleocapsid antigen-specific T cells in chronic active hepatitis B. J Immunol 1987; 139:2050–8.
31. Chisari FV. Analysis of hepadnavirus gene expression, biology, and pathogenesis in the transgenic mouse. Curr Top Microbiol Immunol 1991; 168:85–101.
32. Peters RL. Viral hepatitis: a pathologic spectrum. Am J Med Sci 1975; 270:17.
33. Beasley RP, Lin CC, Hwang LY, Chien CS. Hepatocellular carcinoma and hepatitis B virus: a prospective study of 22,707 men in Taiwan. Lancet 1981; 2:1129–33.
34. Barker LF, Chisari F, Ube Grath PP, Dalgard DW, Kirschstein R. Transmission of type B viral hepatitis to chimpanzees. J Infect Dis 1973; 127:648–62.

35. Gripon P, Diot C, Theze N, et al. Hepatitis B virus infection of adult human hepatocytes cultured in the presence of dimethyl sulfonide. J Virol 1988; 62: 4136–43.
36. Ochya T, Tsurumoto T, Ueda K, Okubo K, Shiozawa M, Matsubara K. An in vitro system for infection with hepatitis B virus that uses primary human fetal hepatocytes. Proc Natl Acad Sci U S A 1989; 86:1875–9.
37. Bchini R, Capel F, Dauguet C, Dubanchet S, Petit MA. In vitro infection of human hepatoma (Hep G2) cells with hepatitis B virus. J Virol 1990; 64:3025–32.
38. Sells MA, Chen ML, Acs G. Production of hepatitis B virus particles in Hep G2 cells transfected with cloned hepatitis B virus DNA. Proc Natl Acad Sci U S A 1987; 84:1005–9.
39. Dejean A, Lugassy C, Zafrani S, Tiollais P, Brechot C. Detection of hepatitis B virus DNA in pancreas, kidney and skin of two human carriers of the virus. J Gen Virol 1984; 65:651–5.
40. Lamelin JP, Trepo C. The hepatitis B virus and the peripheral blood mononuclear cells: a brief review. J Hepatol 1990; 10:120–4.
41. Romet-Lemone JL, McLane MF, Elfassi E, Haseltine WA, Azocar J, Essex M. Hepatitis B virus infection in cultured human lymphoblastoid cells. Science 1983; 221:667–9.
42. Effassi E, Romet-Lemonne JL, Essex M, MacLane MF, Haseltine WA. Evidence of extrachromasomal forms of hepatitis B viral DNA in a bone marrow culture obtained from a patient recently infected with hepatitis B Virus. Proc Natl Acad Sci U S A 1984; 81:3526–8.
43. Pontisso P, Locasciutti A, Sohiavon E, et al. Detection of hepatitis B virus DNA sequences in bone marrow of children with leukemia. Cancer 1987; 59:292–6.
44. Pontisso P, Poon MC, Tiollais P, Brechot C. Detection of HBV DNA in mononuclear blood cells. Br Med J 1984; 288:1563–6.
45. Sugai Y, Okamoto H. State of hepatitis B virus DNA in peripheral blood mononuclear cells from persistently infected individuals: correlation with e antigen and viral DNA in the serum as well as with the activity of liver disease. Tohoku J Exp Med 1989; 158:73–84.
46. Hadchouel M, Pasquinelli C, Fournier JG, et al. Detection of mononuclear cells expressing hepatitis B virus in peripheral blood from HBsAg positive and negative patients by in situ hybridization. J Med Virol 1988; 24:27–32.
47. Baginski I, Chemin I, Bouffard P, Hantz O, Trepo C. Detection of polyadenylated RNA in hepatitis B virus infected peripheral blood mononuclear cells by polymerase chain reaction. J Infect Dis 1990; 163:996–1000.
48. Lobbiani A, Lalatta F, Lugo F, Colucci C. Hepatitis B virus transcripts and surface antigen in human peripheral blood lymphocytes. J Med Virol 1990; 31: 190–4.
49. Bouffard P, Lamelin JP, Zoulin F, Pichoud C, Trepo C. Different forms of hepatitis B virus DNA and expression of HBV antigens in peripheral blood mononuclear cells in chronic hepatitis B. J Med Virol 1990; 31:312–7.
50. Zoulim F, Vitvitski L, Bouffard P, et al. Detection of pre $S_1$ proteins in peripheral blood mononuclear cells from patients with HBV infection. J Hepatol 1991; 12:150–6.

51. Parvaz P, Lamelin JP, Vitvitski L, et al. Prevalence and significance of hepatitis B virus antigens: expression in peripheral blood mononuclear cells in chronic active hepatitis. Clin Immunol Immunopathol 1987; 43:1–8.
52. Davison F, Alexander GJM, Anastassakos C, Fagan EA, William R. Leucocyte hepatitis B virus DNA in acute and chronic hepatitis B virus infection. J Med Virol 1987; 22:379–85.
53. Gu JR, Chen YC, Jiang HO, et al. State of hepatitis B virus DNA in leucocytes of hepatitis B patients. J Med Virol 1985; 17:73–81.
54. Laure F, Zagury D, Saunot AG, Gallo RC, Hahn BH, Brechot C. Hepatitis B virus DNA sequences in lymphoid cells from patients with AIDS and AIDS related complex. Science 1985; 229:561–3.
55. Zeldis JB, Mugishima H, Steinberg HN, Nir E, Gale RP. In vitro hepatitis B virus infection of human bone marrow cells. J Clin Invest 1986; 78:411–7.
56. Zeldis JB, Farraye FA, Steinberg H. In vitro hepatitis B virus suppression of erythropoiesis is dependent on the multiplicity of infection and is reversible with anti-HBs antibodies. Hepatology 1988; 8:755–9.
57. Carmichael J, De Graff WG, Gazdar AF, Minna JB, Mitchell JB. Evaluation of tetrazolium-based semi-automatic assay. Cancer Res 1987; 47:936–46.
58. Steinberg H, Bouffard P, Trepo C, Zeldis JB. In vitro inhibition of hemopoietic cell line growth by hepatitis B virus. J Virol 1990; 64:2577–81.
59. Jochum C, Voth R, Rossol S, et al. Immunosuppressive function of hepatitis B antigens in vitro: role of endoribonuclease V is one potential trans-inactivation for cytokines in macrophages and human hepatoma cells. J Virol 1990; 64:1956–63.
60. Knudsen PJ, Strom TB, Vogel H, Zeldis JB. Interaction of hepatitis B virus with U937 cells causes a block in the induction of interleukin-1 release. In: Zuckerman AJ, ed. Viral hepatitis and liver disease. New York: Alan R. Liss, 1988; 691–3.
61. Tru JS, Lee CH, Lin PM, Schloemer RH. Hepatitis B virus suppresses expression of human beta-interferon. Proc Natl Acad Sci U S A 1988; 85:252–6.
62. Tru JS, Scholoemer RH. Transcription of the human beta-interferon gene is inhibited by hepatitis B virus. J Virol 1989; 63:3065–71.
63. Whitten TM, Quets AT, Schloemer RH. Identification of the hepatitis B virus factor that inhibits expression of the beta-interferon gene. J Virol 1991; 65:4699–704.
64. Taylor JM, Chao M, Hsieh SY, Luo G, Ryo WS. Structure and replication of hepatitis delta virus. In: Hollinger FB, Lemon SM, Margolis HS, eds. Viral hepatitis and liver disease. Baltimore: Williams & Wilkins, 1991; 460–3.
65. Foon KA, Mitsuyasu RT, Schroff RW, McIntyre RE, Champlin R, Gale RP. Immunologic defects in young male patients with hepatitis-associated aplastic anemia. Ann Intern Med 1984; 100:657–62.
66. Stook PG, Stiner ME, Freese D, Sharp H, Ascher NL. Hepatitis-associated aplastic anemia after liver transplantation. Transplantation 1987; 43:595–7.
67. Kojima S, Matsuyama K, Kodera Y. Bone marrow transplantation for hepatitis-associated aplastic anemia. Acta Haematol (Basel) 1988; 789:7–11.

68. Pol S, Driss F, Devergie A, Brechot C, Berthelot P, Gluckman E. Is hepatitis C virus involved in hepatitis-associated aplastic anemia? Ann Intern Med 1990; 113:435–7.
69. Zeldis JB, Boender PJ, Hellings JA, Steinberg H. Inhibition of human hematopoiesis by non-A, non-B hepatitis virus. J Med Virol 1989; 27:34–8.
70. Choo Q-L, Kuo G, Weiner AJ, Overby LR, Bradley DW, Houghton M. Isolation of a cDNA derived from a blood-borne non-A, non-B viral hepatitis genome. Science 1989; 244:359–62.
71. Choo Q-L, Richman KH, Han JH, et al. Genetic organization and diversity of the hepatitis C virus. Proc Natl Acad Sci U S A 1991; 88:2451–5.
72. Dienstag JL, Alter JH. Non-A, non-B hepatitis: evolving epidemiologic and clinical perspective. Semin Liver Dis 1986; 6:67–81.
73. Nalpas B, Driss F, Pol S, et al. Association between HCV and HBV infection in hepatocellular carcinoma and alcoholic liver disease. J Hepatol 1991; 12:70–4.

# V

# RETROVIRUSES

# 9

# Human Immunodeficiency Virus and the Bone Marrow

**Jerry L. Spivak**

*Johns Hopkins University School of Medicine*
*Baltimore, Maryland*

**Barbara Potts**

*Repligen Corporation*
*Cambridge, Massachusetts*

## INTRODUCTION

In July 1982, a 37-year-old homosexual man was admitted to the Johns Hopkins Hospital for evaluation of anorexia, weight loss, intractable diarrhea, and fever (1). Apart from wasting and thrush, the physical examination was normal, but gastrointestinal evaluation revealed esophagitis due to cytomegalovirus and *Candida albicans*, jejunal giardiasis, and *Entamoeba coli* trophozoites in the stool. Cytomegalovirus was also present in the urine, and serologic studies indicated previous infection with hepatitis B, herpes simplex, and *Treponema pallidum*. There was cutaneous anergy, an absolute lymphopenia with less than 400 T cells $mm^{-3}$, and a $CD4^{+}/CD8^{+}$ ratio of 0.3 (normal 1.2).

The patient's illness fit all the clinical criteria for what had been newly appreciated a year previously as an acquired immune deficiency syndrome of unknown cause occurring mainly in homosexuals, intravenous drug users, recipients of blood products, and the children or consorts of afflicted individuals (2–5). Since no etiology had been established, the diagnosis of this acquired immunodeficiency syndrome, or AIDS as it quickly came to be known, was solely based on clinical criteria. The principal target organs for the disorder were considered the lymphatic system, the gastrointestinal tract, the lungs, and the central nervous system.

This patient clearly had AIDS, but his illness was noteworthy for the additional reason that striking abnormalities of the blood and marrow were also present. Thus, early in the initial hospitalization, pancytopenia developed with an hematocrit of 35%, a leukocyte count of 2960 $mm^{-3}$ with 18% band forms, 42% segmented neutrophils, 26% lymphocytes, 8% monocytes, 5% eosinophils, and 1% basophils, and a platelet count of 87,000 $mm^{-3}$. The peripheral blood smear was noteworthy for the presence of atypical vacuolated monocytes, and a bone marrow aspirate contained many histiocytes, some of which had ingested myeloid and erythroid cells and platelets. Plasma cells were increased in number, and there was a shift left in the myeloid series. Marrow cellularity was quantitatively reduced, with an increase in reticulin.

Although the initial clinical reports of this newly described acquired immunodeficiency syndrome suggested that anemia and leukopenia were not uncommon, there was no indication in any previous study that the bone marrow was a target organ in AIDS, nor were there any descriptions of blood and marrow abnormalities similar to those observed in our patient. The hematologic abnormalities, however, resembled those in patients receiving immunosuppressive drugs who were infected with cytomegalovirus (CMV), Epstein-Barr virus (EBV), herpes simplex, or adenovirus, and these abnormalities had been given the designation of the virus-associated hematophagocytic syndrome (6). Since at that time no other AIDS patients were available to us for comparative studies, we assumed that out patient's hematologic abnormalities reflected the presence of an infection with an organism like CMV in an immunodeficient host and could therefore not only serve as a marker for an immunodeficient state but might also be expected to occur in other AIDS patients as well, a prediction that proved to be true (7).

There the matter would have rested had it not been for several outbreaks of an unusual immune deficiency syndrome associated with weight loss, fever, diarrhea, anemia, neurologic abnormalities, and lymphomas occurring in primate colonies in both California and New England (8,9). This simian immune deficiency syndrome (SAIDS) was considered clinically similar but not identical to human AIDS (10). The most obvious difference frequently cited was the presence in the monkeys of a bizarre early monocyte in the peripheral blood and marrow.

The published illustration of these "bizarre" monocytes was indistinct (8), but they appeared to resemble the unusual circulating monocytes we observed in our AIDS patient (1). Accordingly, we exchanged blood smears and slides with Letvin at the New England Regional Primate Center, and it was immediately evident that the atypical circulating monocytes associated with AIDS and SAIDS were identical in appearance. This observation led us to examine the hematologic status of other AIDS patients as the epidemic unfolded, and it soon became apparent that the bone marrow was unequivocally a target organ in this disorder (7).

Subsequently, it was discovered that AIDS was due to a specific retrovirus, now called the human immunodeficiency virus (HIV), and SAIDS to a closely related retrovirus. Thus, it became possible to examine the natural history of the hematologic abnormalities occurring during the course of infection with these retroviruses and the mechanisms for them. In this chapter, we review the blood and bone marrow abnormalities associated with HIV infection and their pathophysiology.

## THE HUMAN IMMUNODEFICIENCY VIRUS

The human immunodeficiency viruses, HIV-1 and HIV-2, members of the lentivirus subfamily of retroviruses, are different from the previously identified human retroviruses, human T cell leukemia virus types I and II (HTLV-I and II), which are members of the oncornaviruses subfamily, in that the lentiviruses do not produce tumors or myelopathic disorders (11,12).

Other members of the lentiviruses subfamily include the primate lentiviruses, simian immunodeficiency virus (SIV) in African green monkeys (SIV/AGM) (13) and SIV in macaques (SIV/MAC) (10), and four nonprimate lentiviruses, including equine infectious anemia virus (EIAV) in horses (14,15), visna in sheep (16), caprine arthritis encephalitis virus (CAEV) in goats (17), and feline immunodeficiency virus (FIV) in cats (18). Although these viruses are quite diverse, there is considerable genetic relatedness between isolates in their reverse transcriptase enzyme (17,19). A schematic of this relationship is shown in Figure 1.

The lentiviruses share a distinctive morphology: the virion buds without the appearance of preformed nucleoids (Fig. 2). They also have a similar pathogenesis, which includes a persistent viremia with moderate neutralizating antibody responses, a prolonged incubation period, neuropathology, viral infection of select blood cell populations, including macrophage tropism, abnormalities in hematopoiesis, and a marked antigenic variation of the envelope (14,16).

The complexity of the HIV-1 genome has been unraveled at a fast pace, especially the function of the proteins encoded by the viral regulatory genes (Fig. 3) (20). A more detailed review of these gene products may be found in recent reviews (21,22). The importance of regions of the envelope for specific tropism has been proposed, with a focus on monocyte tropism (23–26); however, no detailed studies have been made concerning HIV in bone marrow cultures. Our recent work attempted to solve this problem by examining the effect of several different HIV-1 isolates and one HIV-2 isolate on in vitro

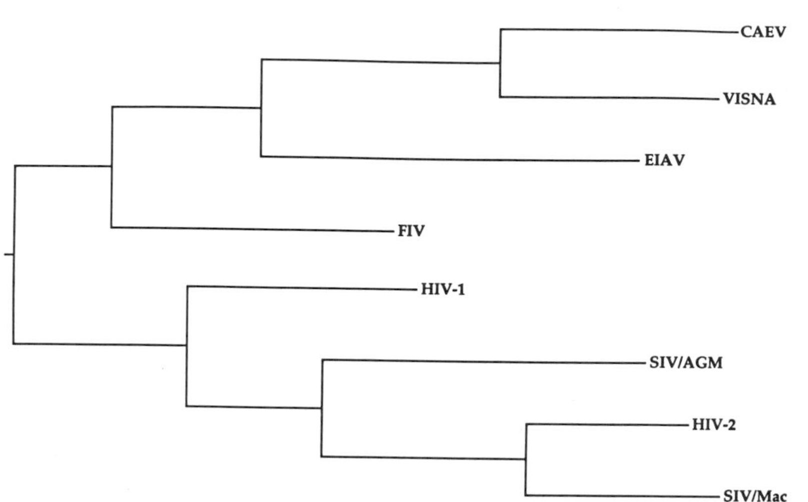


**Figure 1** Phylogenetic tree of lentivirus reverse transcriptase.

colony formation by erythroid progenitor cells (burst-forming units-erythroid, BFU-E) and granulocyte-macrophage progenitor cell (colony-forming units–granulocytes-macrophages, CFU-GM) from normal human marrow (27). Marrow cells plated in methylcellulose in the presence of saturating concentrations of erythropoietin and leukocyte-conditioned medium were inoculated after 7 days of culture with various virus isolates that had been passaged only in peripheral blood lymphocytes (PBL) or monocytes (28). Viral replication was monitored by reverse transcriptase (RT), indirect immunofluorescence (FA), electron microscopy (EM), and in situ hybridization. The effect of viral replication on colony fromation was determined by counting BFU-E and CFU-GM. These studies demonstrated HIV isolate-specific and lineage-restricted lysis of committed human marrow erythroid and myeloid cells by what is presumably a factor produced as a result of HIV replication in monocytes. These studies correlate well with in vivo studies that demonstrate global hematopoietic dysfunction in AIDS patients, although little virus is detectable (29).

A key issue in studies of HIV in primary culture systems is the passage history of the virus. If a laboratory strain passaged in transformed T cell lines is studied, then multiple passages in a new host system may be required before optimal replication can be reached. This has been noted with a transformed T cell adapted isolate, MN (30). This HIV isolate required two passages in peripheral blood lymphocytes before a significant infectious virus was noted. In our bone marrow studies, all viral isolates came from primary

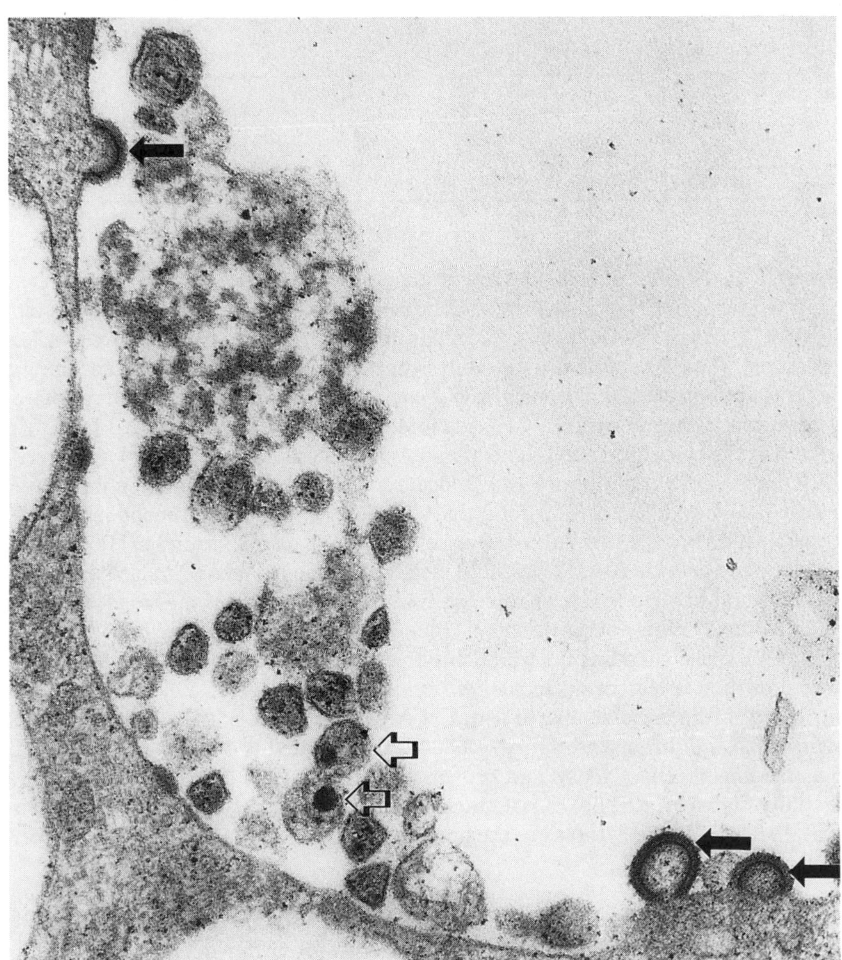

**Figure 2** Electron micrograph of an HIV-1 (AD-87 M-P)-infected bone marrow promonocyte. Immature particles without the appearance of preformed nucleoids are seen budding into a vacuole within the cytoplasm (closed arrows). The vacuole also contains mature virion particles with formed nucleoids (open arrows). Magnification × 94,000.

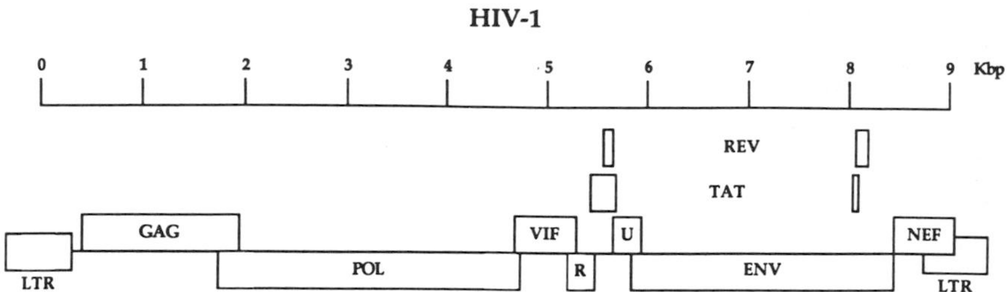


**Figure 3** HIV genome structure and protein processing. GAG: gene encoding the group-specific antigens or core proteins, the myristoylated precursor of which is typically 55 kD; fragments from the C terminus of the *gag* precursor have special roles; for example, the p7 peptide is a zinc-finger binding protein. POL: gene encoding a polymerase polyprotein that upon cleavage yields a protease, a reverse transcriptase, and an endonuclease-integrase. VIF: viral infectivity factor, typically a 23 kD protein (localized in the cytoplasm and cell membrane) that determines the rate of viral spread. VPR(R): gene product of about 15 kD localized in the nucleus; function unknown; found in HIV-1 and HIV-2/SIV but not SIV/AGM. VPU(U): gene encoding a 15–20 kD cytoplasmic protein that functions to release viral particles; found in HIV-1 only. REV: gene product of 20 kD (typically) localized in the nucleus or nucleolus; facilitates structural protein synthesis through transport of unspliced messages; interacts with RRE, the "*rev*-responsive element" found in the envelope coding region of transcripts. TAT: gene encoding the transactivating regulatory protein of typically 14 kD, localized in the nucleus or nucleolus; *tat*$^-$ mutants do not replicate; tat protein has been found in the extracellular milieu. ENV: gene product is the envelope or coat protein consisting of at least an extracellular glycosylated protein of about 120 kD and a transmembrane glycosylated protein of about 41 kD. NEF: gene encoding a potentially myristoylated protein of about 27 kD, the functions of which are controversial; localized in the cytoplasm, the protein is the most immunogenic of the accessory proteins.

PBL or macrophage cultures (27,28). Attempts by other investigators to replicate HIV in bone marrow cultures have been either negative (31) or inefficient (32), probably because of their choice of viral isolates and the passage history of these isolates. In addition, some isolates may lack the ability to replicate in a host system as a result of a major genetic change. This is apparent with PBL isolates, which do not adapt to optimal growth in primary human monocyte-macrophage cultures. We found that Z3, a PBL isolate, and LAV, the prototype laboratory strain, could not be adapted to grow well in monocytes, even after multiple passages (Fig. 4B) (28). A comparison of the replication of various HIV isolates in macrophages, PBL, and bone marrow cultures is shown in Figure 4. The variable replication of different isolates in different culture systems may reflect the variability of HIV replication in vivo. What should be kept in mind, though, is that suboptimal rep-

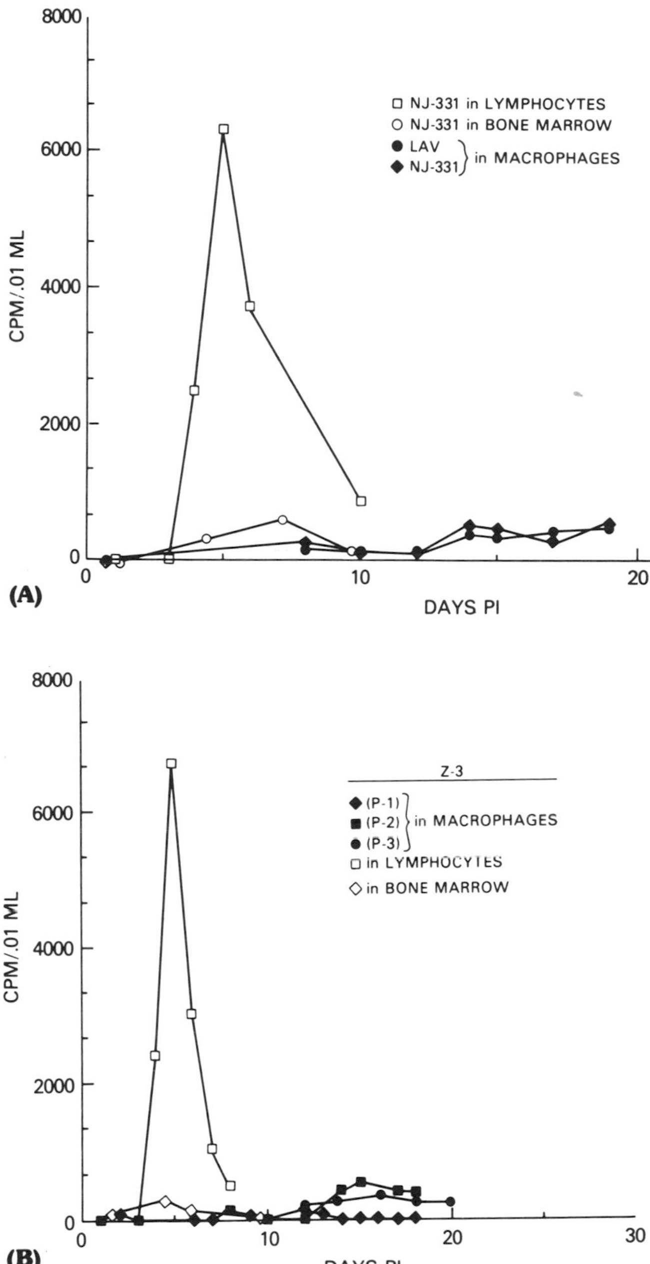


**Figure 4** Growth curves of T cell tropic (A, B, and C) and monocyte tropic (D) HIV isolates in human peripheral blood lymphocytes, bone marrow, and macrophage cultures. At indicated times, 10 $\mu$l aliquots of the cell-free supernatants were removed and the virion-associated reverse transcriptase (RT) activity was measured. Values expressed are net counts from which mock-infected samples (50–100 cpm per 0.01 ml) have been substracted.

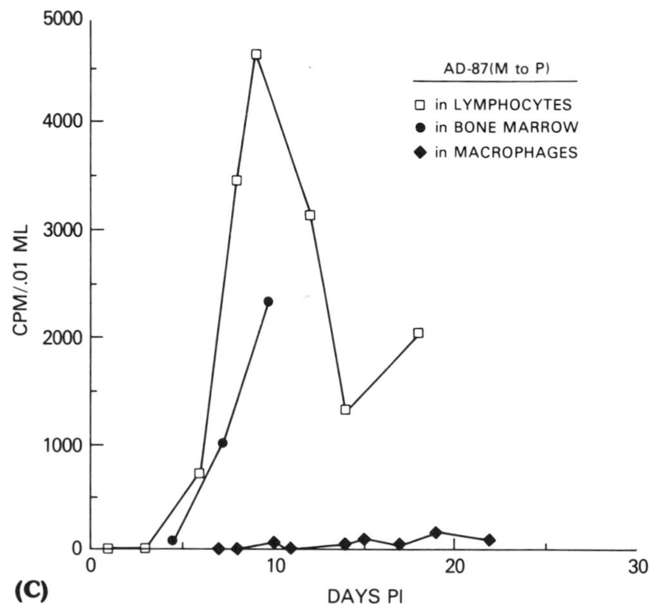


(C)

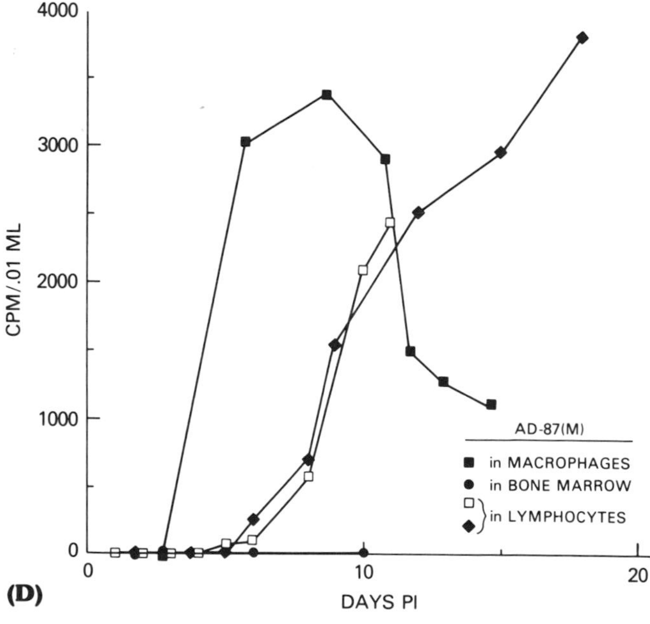


(D)

**Figure 4** (continued)

lication of a virus in vitro, such as Z3 in macrophages, results in only 10–100 infectious units/ml—not useful for in vitro studies but a significant load of virus in vivo.

Many lentiviruses of both primates and nonprimates show bone marrow involvement (33–36), documented in both in vivo and in vitro studies. These animal models may serve as valuable tools to determine the mechanism of HIV destruction of bone marrow (33). Studies of SIV/MAC have demonstrated both in vivo and in vitro that bone marrow harbored SIV in macrophages, not T lymphocytes, and that the SIV infection resulted in inhibition of colony formation. These data, like ours (27), suggest that suppression of colony growth may be mediated by a factor produced as a result of SIV infection of macrophages. This animal model is very important for evaluating drug effects on lentivirus load and hematopoietic functions.

The factor produced as a result of HIV infection of bone marrow macrophages, which are responsible for the lysis of committed human marrow cells, may be a cytokine (37–40), a toxin (41), or possibly a viral product, such as TAT. Studies have shown a specific glycoprotein associated with defective in vitro hematopoietic colony formation (39), and a toxin has been proposed as the cause of neuron destruction in the central nervous system (CNS) (41). This toxin is produced by HIV-1-infected CNS microglia and macrophages. The pathogenesis of AIDS encephalopathy clearly parallels that seen in the bone marrow, namely, marked dysfunction over time despite subtle or minimal neuropathic changes or detectable virus (42), suggesting a similar underlying pathophysiology.

## EARLY HEMATOLOGIC ABNORMALITIES ASSOCIATED WITH HIV INFECTION

In contrast to the global impairment of hematopoiesis that is usually evident in the later stages of HIV-1 infection (7), hematologic abnormalities occurring early during the course of the infection are either transient or restricted in their extent. Latency and a long incubation period are characteristic features of a lentivirus infection, and progression from the asymptomatic HIV carrier state to clinical manifestations occurs at a rate of approximately 5–8%/year. Exceptions include the acute viral or glandular syndrome and the acute thrombocytopenia associated with early HIV infection.

### Acute Viral Syndrome

First described anecdotally in 1984 (43), the acute viral syndrome is the earliest clinical manifestation of HIV infection and represents a host reaction to tissue invasion by the virus. Based on the probable time of exposure, the incubation period may be as brief as 6–14 days, which is much shorter than the incubation period for the acute viral syndrome caused by Epstein-Barr virus (44,45). The acute viral syndrome associated with HIV infection is associated variously with fever, night sweats, chills, pharyngitis, myalgia, arthralgia, rash (maculopapular or urticarial), headache, lymphadenopathy, neuritis, meningitis, splenomegaly, and diarrhea, with fever, night sweats, and headache the most characteristic complaints (44–49). The total leukocyte count is usually normal, but leukopenia or leukocytosis may occur, most often due to changes in the number of circulating lymphocytes. The proportion of circulating atypical lymphocytes is increased, and these cells are indistinguishable from those seen with an EBV or CMV infection (47). A reversal of the $CD4^+/CD8^+$ lymphocyte ratio also occurs and is usually due to proliferation of $CD8^+$ lymphocytes, but a reduction in circulating $CD4^+$ cells may be seen (44,48). Cutaneous anergy is also present (45,47). Following clinical recovery, the $CD4^+/CD8^+$ ratio may eventually return to normal. Anemia rarely occurs and is usually of a mild degree. Thrombocytopenia, also usually mild, may develop and neutropenia has also been documented. Elevations of the serum transaminases and alkaline phosphatase have been observed. The onset of the illness is usually sudden, but as is the case with EBV infection, signs and symptoms may evolve over a period of weeks. The duration of symptoms may be as short as 3 days but 2 weeks is the norm, and in some patients 4–8 weeks may be required for complete recovery. Seroconversion with antibodies to HIV has been documented from 15 to 99 days after onset of symptoms; antibodies to the viral proteins gp160, gp120, and p24 appear before antibodies to p41 (46).

As evident from its description, the acute viral syndrome following exposure to HIV is clinically indistinguishable from the infectious mononucleosis syndrome associated with EBV or CMV infection (50–52), but careful serologic studies in a number of patients have documented the absence of these or other infectious agents, such as the hepatitis viruses, toxoplasma, or *T. pallidum*, which are frequently acquired by sexual contact or transfusion and cause similar symptoms. Although anti-i cold agglutinins are produced with EBV infection, anti-I cold agglutinins are produced in the HIV-related acute viral syndrome (47). Of course, HIV-infected patients may fail to have an appropriate immune response, and the absence of positive serologic tests does not exclude another organism as the cause of symptoms (53). When studied, HIV could be isolated from the blood and, in one patient with aseptic meningitis, from the spinal fluid, within a week of the onset of clinical symptoms, proving conclusively that HIV per se can cause an infectious mononucleosis-like syndrome (46).

The frequency of an acute viral syndrome following acquisition of HIV is unknown since most reports are anecdotal or retrospective. In a group of

12 seroconverters, however, 11 were documented to have a clinically apparent acute viral syndrome associated with seroconversion (44). In another well-controlled prospective study, symptoms compatible with an acute viral syndrome occurred in 55% of a group of seroconverters (49). Subclinical infection with HIV is probably common, similar to infection with EBV or CMV. It is also important to note that the symptoms associated with acquisition of HIV are sufficiently nonspecific and often sufficiently mild enough to be overlooked (49). The presence of circulating atypical lymphocytes is a helpful clue to pursue the appropriate serologic studies.

HIV-infected individuals may also develop generalized lymphadenopathy. In a series of 90 such patients, lymphadenopathy was preceded in 23 by pharyngitis, fever, and myalgia (54). In 1 patient, HIV was present in the spinal fluid 2 weeks before the development of generalized adenopathy (46). Generalized persistent lymphadenopathy in HIV-infected patients has been classified as a distinct stage in the disease process, but in some patients it appears that it may develop directly from the acute viral syndrome without an intervening, asymptomatic interval (47).

## HIV-Associated Thrombocytopenia

Apart from lymphopenia, especially a reduction in circulating $CD4^+$ lymphocytes, thrombocytopenia is the earliest quantitative abnormality occurring as a consequence of HIV infection. Generally, isolated thrombocytopenia, so called "ITP," in the absence of concomitant drug or ethanol ingestion, overt infection, splenomegaly, or bone marrow damage, occurs most often in women (male-female ratio of 1:3) in the reproductive age range. Beginning in 1982, however, shortly after the acquired immunodeficiency syndrome was recognized, an unusual frequency of isolated thrombocytopenia in men was reported in three groups at high risk of HIV infection, homosexuals (55), hemophiliacs (56), and intravenous drug abusers (57). Clinically, most of these patients fulfilled all the criteria for ITP, although in some mild anemia and neutropenia alone or together were also present. In others splenomegaly (mild and not of the degree associated with significant platelet sequestration) was also observed, and many had generalized lymphadenopathy. As expected for these high-risk groups, when tested the thrombocytopenic patients uniformly expressed antibodies to HIV-related proteins; many subsequently progressed clinically to AIDS. Further proof of the relationship between HIV infection and isolated thrombocytopenia was provided by the observation of acute thrombocytopenia developing in association with HIV seropositivity in men or women following heterosexual contact with consorts from a group at high risk for HIV infection (58).

Although the frequency of severe thrombocytopenia (platelet count less than 20,000 $mm^{-3}$) associated with HIV infection before the development of AIDS is unknown, the overall incidence of thrombocytopenia in one series was 3% of a group of 359 homosexuals and 9% of 321 intravenous drug abusers (59). In a large prospective study of HIV-positive homosexual men, the incidence of thrombocytopenia was 6.7% over a 12 month interval compared to 1.5% in an HIV-negative control group, and there was no difference in the incidence when the thrombocytopenia was associated with generalized lymphadenopathy (60). In a retrospective study of 102 HIV-positive individuals, 12% of both asymptomatic individuals and those with AIDS-related complex were thrombocytopenic compared to 24% of patients with Kaposi's sarcoma and 43% of patients with AIDS (61). A correlation of thrombocytopenia with the $CD_{4+}$ lymphocyte count has also been observed, in keeping with the increased frequency of thrombocytopenia in HIV-infected patients who progress to AIDS (60).

The degree of thrombocytopenia in HIV-positive patients varies from severe to mild, and in many patients the platelet count fluctuates in the absence of treatment or clinically evident signs of disease progression. In one series, HIV-positive intravenous drug abusers had more profound thrombocytopenia as a group than HIV-positive homosexuals (59). Because the development of isolated thrombocytopenia is unusual in men and because of the multiple possibilities for this in addition to autoimmune mechanisms, HIV-associated thrombocytopenia has been carefully studied (62).

The presence of adequate numbers of megakaryocytes is one criterion for ITP, and this has usually been the case in HIV-associated thrombocytopenia. Although it has been stated that a compensatory increase in marrow megakaryocytes is lacking in some patients, this is certainly not the case in others. Most of these patients lack the characteristic bone marrow abnormalities seen in AIDS patients, nor is there any evidence of opportunistic infection involving the marrow. Several groups have described morphologic abnormalities of the megakaryocytes in thrombocytopenic AIDS patients, particularly at the ultrastructural level (63–66), and as discussed in more detail later, in situ hybridization studies have revealed the expression of HIV RNA by megakaryocytes of thrombocytopenic AIDS patients (63).

Serologically, patients with HIV-associated thrombocytopenia were found by one group to have elevated platelet-associated IgG and complement, circulating immune complexes, and negative antinuclear antibody titers (67). Serum antiplatelet antibodies were also identified, and the serologic findings were not different in patients with AIDS than in those patients who had not yet progressed to AIDS (66). HIV-positive thrombocytopenic intravenous drug abusers studied by the same investigators had elevated platelet-associated IgG, IgM, and complement. Circulating immune complexes and serum antiplatelet antibodies were also present (57). Similar findings were observed in a group of HIV-positive hemophiliacs (68). In general, the quantity of platelet-associated IgG or IgM, complement and immune complexes exceeded that found in patients with non–HIV-associated autoimmune thrombocytopenia (68). Thrombocytopenic HIV-infected homosexuals appeared to differ from some of the intravenous drug abusers, hemophiliacs, and patients with classic autoimmune thrombocytopenia because neither the eluted platelet-associated IgG nor serum IgG usually bound to platelets (57, 67,68). Based on these observations, it was concluded that the mechanism for acute thrombocytopenia in HIV-positive homosexuals was most likely related to the deposition of immune complexes on platelets.

In contrast to these observations, other laboratories have identified classic specific antiplatelet antibodies on the platelets of HIV-positive homosexuals and in their serum (69–71). These antibodies were either IgG or IgM; no platelet-associated complement was identified, and there was no correlation between platelet-associated antibody and circulating immune complexes (71). In HIV-positive thrombocytopenic hemophiliacs, all major classes of immunoglobulin were found on platelets, in contrast to patients with classic autoimmune thrombocytopenia in whom only IgG and IgM were identified. Interestingly, in this study, as noted previously for homosexual patients but not for hemophiliac patients, platelet immunoglobulin eluates did not have platelet reactivity (72).

The nature of the circulating immune complexes in HIV infection has been investigated by a number of groups, and both virus and viral antigens have been identified in these immune complexes (74,75). In one laboratory, however, neither HIV nor its viral antigens were identified in either circulating or platelet-associated immune complexes in thrombocytopenic homosexuals and narcotic addicts; instead, IgG antibodies directed against HIV antibodies were identified (76). Antibodies against other viruses were also not present in the immune complexes.

The complexity of the serologic observations in HIV-infected thrombocytopenic patients is not unique and resembles results in classic autoimmune thrombocytopenia. Thus, although most patients with autoimmune thrombocytopenia have IgG-mediated platelet destruction, some have complement-mediated platelet destruction (77), and as in HIV infection (67), an apparent lack of correlation between platelet-associated IgG and platelet count has also been observed (78). This latter observation can be reconciled with the observations that in some patients with autoimmune thrombocytopenia, platelet life span is not markedly reduced, implicating a defect in platelet production (79), in others thrombocytopenia is due to increased platelet destruction, and in some patients with elevated platelet-associated IgG and a normal platelet count, impaired reticuloendothelial function has been documented (78).

Viewed in this context, the thrombocytopenia associated with HIV infection appears similar to autoimmune thrombocytopenia. First, a shortened platelet life span has been observed in some HIV-infected patients (80). Second, elevated levels of platelet-associated IgG in other patients with a low or even normal platelet count may merely reflect the nonspecific elevation of circulating immunoglobulin that occurs in this disorder (81). Alternatively, intrinsic marrow damage due to HIV infection may account for thrombocytopenia in certain patients. HIV-infected thrombocytopenic patients, like some patients with autoimmune thrombocytopenia, may demonstrate impaired reticuloendothelial function with respect to Fc receptor-mediated clearance of antibody-coated cells (82). In HIV-infected patients, the clearance abnormality appeared to correlate with the severity of the thrombocytopenia, not with the presence of platelet-associated IgG or circulating immune complexes (71). No abnormality of Fc receptor-mediated clearance has been observed in nonthrombocytopenic HIV-positive homosexuals (82).

Thus, the differences between HIV-associated thrombocytopenia and autoimmune thrombocytopenia are more apparent than real. Serologic disparities may indicate multiple mechanisms or reflect differences in laboratory techniques. Certainly HIV-associated thrombocytopenia responds to the same treatments employed for autoimmune thrombocytopenia. Many patients respond to corticosteroid therapy, although the response is not always durable (59,83–87). Splenectomy has also been effective in alleviating thrombocytopenia refractory to corticosteroids (80,83,84,86,87). The response to intravenous immunoglobulin appears to be even better than in adults with autoimmune thrombocytopenia (86,88,89). It is thus not surprising that other forms of therapy that have been anecdotally reported to be successful in autoimmune thrombocytopenia have been anecdotally beneficial in HIV-associated thrombocytopenia, including danazol (90), anti-Rh antibody (91), interferon-$\alpha$ (92,93), and vincristine (94). Additionally, zidovudine (azidothymidine, AZT) alleviates HIV-associated thrombocytopenia (95–98). This is of substantial interest with regard to mechanism, since as mentioned earlier, HIV-related RNA has been identified in the megakaryocytes of AIDS patients (63) and because zidovudine has proved otherwise toxic for erythroid and myeloid progenitor cells (98).

Concern has been expressed that treatment of HIV-associated thrombocytopenia with corticosteroids or splenectomy would place these patients at risk of disease progression or increase the incidence of opportunistic infection (99). These adverse effects have not been demonstrated clinically, and indeed, in vitro data indicate that corticosteroids do not enhance HIV activation or replication (100). At present, until more is known about the use of zidovudine in this situation, patients with HIV-associated thrombocytopenia should be treated like patients with classic autoimmune thrombocytopenia, remembering that in contrast to those with autoimmune thrombocytopenia, many of these patients improve spontaneously (83,85).

### Thrombotic Thrombocytopenic Purpura and Other Abnormalities of the Coagulation System

Thrombotic thrombocytopenic purpura (TTP) is an illness of unknown etiology that is defined clinically by the pentad of thrombocytopenia, microangiopathic hemolytic anemia, neurologic abnormalities, renal dysfunction, and fever. Recently, several reports have described this syndrome in HIV-infected patients (101,102); an additional report documented a variant of TTP, the hemolytic uremic syndrome, in an additional patient (103). How these disorders are linked to HIV infection is unclear, but symptomatic HIV infection or AIDS is not a prerequisite for their occurrence.

Coagulation inhibitors of the lupus type have also been described in a significant number of HIV-infected individuals (104,105). In some patients, the inhibitor developed in the setting of an infection and disappeared with resolution of the infection. Anticardiolipin antibodies have also been identified in HIV-positive subjects (106). Neither bleeding nor thrombosis has been associated with these serologic nor in vitro coagulation abnormalities.

## HEMATOLOGIC ABNORMALITIES ASSOCIATED WITH PROGRESSIVE HIV INFECTION

Although not all HIV-infected patients develop acute thrombocytopenia or the stigmata of the acute viral syndrome early in the course of the infection, they invariably manifest distinctive hematologic abnormalities as the infection progresses. No systematic prospective study of abnormal blood counts in a large cohort of patients has been performed, but on the basis of a variety of small studies (Table 1) a reasonably estimate of the incidence of anemia, leukopenia, and thrombocytopenia can be derived. Anemia and leukopenia, particularly lymphopenia, are the most common quantitative abnormalities, and they are more common with AIDS than in the less advanced stages of HIV infection. With respect to homosexuals, when a simultaneous control group, seronegative for HIV, was studied, similar blood count abnormalities were not observed. This was not true, however, of HIV-positive and HIV-negative hemophiliacs: in one study, 57% of HIV-positive patients were anemic, 60% leukopenic, and 70% thrombocytopenic compared with incidences of 16, 50, and 16%, respectively, for the HIV-negative group (64). The high incidence of abnormal blood counts in both groups of hemophiliacs probably reflects their common and chronic exposure to blood products that can cause hematologic abnormalities in the absence of HIV transmission.

**Table 1** Incidence of Hematologic Abnormalities (%) in HIV Infection

| | $HIV^+$ | ARC | AIDS |
|---|---|---|---|
| Anemia | 12 | 14 | 79 |
| Leukopenia | 4 | 10 | 58 |
| Lymphopenia | 15 | 25 | 77 |
| Neutropenia | 15 | 22 | 50 |
| Monocytopenia | ND[a] | ND | 50 |
| Thrombocytopenia | 8 | 17 | 38 |

[a]Not determined because of insufficient data.
*Source*: Data compiled from References 7, 61, 69, 70, 118, 120, and 124.

With the exception of lymphopenia, which occurs primarily as a result of HIV infection alone, there are a variety of potential causes for the other blood abnormalities in HIV-infected patients.

## Anemia

The anemia associated with HIV infection is usually mild at inception, with a hemoglobin deficit of less than 2.0 g per 100 g, but may become profound during the advanced stages of the illness. Morphologically, the anemia is normochromic and normocytic. As a consequence of the polyclonal hyperglobulinemia associated with HIV infection, rouleau formation may obscure red cell morphology. There are many possible causes for anemia in HIV infection, as listed in Table 2. The frequency varies, and often more than one cause is present in a given patient. Most commonly the anemia associated with HIV infection represents a fundamental reaction of the bone marrow to systemic infection and inflammation, not to a more specific anatomic lesion or immunologic or infectious insult. This nonspecific reaction, the anemia of chronic disease, is characterized by normochromic, normocytic, or occasionally microcytic red cells, a low reticulocyte count, morphologically normal erythroid progenitor cells, adequate to increased marrow iron stores with a low serum iron and iron binding capacity, and a low transferrin saturation and elevated serum ferritin level, all in the setting of a systemic illness. There is usually only a modest reduction in red cell life span. Invariably, impaired red cell iron reutilization leads to these abnormalities in iron metabolism. By definition correction or amelioration of the underlying disorder should alleviate the anemia, but because HIV-infection is inexorable, the anemia is usually progressive despite therapy (107). HIV infection also

**Table 2** Etiology of Anemia Associated with HIV Infection

| |
|---|
| Infection |
| Viral, fungal, myobacterial, parasitic |
| Drugs |
| Zidovudine, trimethoprim-sulfamethoxazole, gancyclovir |
| Inflammation |
| Inanition and malabsorption |
| Erythropoietin lack |
| Neoplasia |
| Lymphoma, Kaposi's sarcoma |
| Hematophagic histiocytosis |
| Autoantibodies |
| Myelofibrosis |
| Marrow necrosis |

imposes additional burdens on the host not usually seen in most other chronic disorders causing anemia: inanition, profound wasting, and often intractable diarrhea due to gastrointestinal involvement by the virus or infection with a variety of opportunistic organisms.

An adequate supply of erythropoietin is central to maintaining erythropoiesis. In simple uncomplicated anemias, such as those due to blood loss, iron deficiency, or hemolysis, there is a substantial increase in erythropoietin production as the hemoglobin level falls (108). With HIV infection, there is a disturbance of the normal feedback mechanism between tissue hypoxia and erythropoietin production. In a large series of anemic AIDS-related complex (ARC) and AIDS patients with normal renal function, serum immunoreactive erythropoietin levels were inappropriately low for the degree of anemia, and the expected inverse correlation between hemoglobin and serum erythropoietin was profoundly blunted compared to that in anemic patients with uncomplicated iron deficiency (109). No correlation was found in these anemic ARC and AIDS patients between serum erythropoietin levels, serum albumin, liver function tests, the presence of opportunistic infections, or Kaposi's sarcoma. The administration of zidovudine was associated with a marked increase in serym erythropoietin in many patients (109). The increase was such that, for any given degree of anemia, serum immunoreactive erythropoietin was higher than in iron-deficient controls with comparable degrees of anemia. The increase in erythropoietin levels was not associated with changes in p24 antigen, HIV positivity, or $CD_{4+}$ cell number. These observations suggest that HIV infection suppresses erythropoietin production so that the capacity for erythropoietin synthesis is enhanced but net production of the hormone is blunted. There are no data concerning erythropoietin metabolism in HIV infection, but it is sufficiently invariant in other situations that an abnormality in production is much more likely.

## Red Cell Autoantibodies

Although there is a high incidence of red cell autoantibodies in HIV-infected patients, overt antibody-mediated hemolysis is uncommon (73). In one study, 43% of the patients studied had a positive direct antiglobulin test (110); in two others, the incidence was 18 and 21% (61,111), and in a fourth, the incidence was 85% of AIDS patients, 68% of ARC patients, and 43% of asymptomatic HIV-infected patients (112). Anti-i and anti-U antibodies have been identified in a number of patients. Most of the patients expressing anti-i had positive cultures for either EBV or CMV. In some patients, the anti-i antibody had a high thermal amplitude, and most anti-i and anti-U patients had hemoglobin levels lower than patients not expressing these antibodies (110). As mentioned earlier, during the acute viral syndrome that frequently heralds the acquisition of HIV, anti-I cold agglutinins can be present (47).

HIV-positive patients with a positive direct antiglobulin test can have IgA, IgG, and complement or complement alone on their red cells. In general, the IgG eluted from the red cells is usually not reactive with erythrocytes, suggesting that the positive antiglobulin test is a nonspecific consequence of the polyclonal hyperglobulinemia of AIDS (111). Alternatively, it may reflect the binding of immune complexes to red cell complement receptors, a process that appears to increase with the progression to AIDS (112). The cold agglutinin anti-Pi was found in several nontransfused AIDS patients, and care should be taken in selecting blood for these patients (110). Platelets also express the i antigen and neutrophils express U; perhaps the antibodies to these antigens could be involved in the thrombocytopenia and neutropenia seen with HIV infection (110).

## Neutropenia

Mild to severe neutropenia is common in HIV-infected patients and, like anemia, is progressive during the course of the illness (Table 1). Neutropenia, because of the underlying infections and inflammatory process, is characterized by an increase in the proportion of band forms and the presence of toxic granulation, Dohle bodies, and occasionally vacuoles (7). Giant neutrophils (or "macropolys"), neutrophils that have failed to separate after mitosis, are seen in the blood of AIDS patients (113). These unusual cells are a nonspecific finding: they are also seen in patients without HIV. On occasion, circulating neutrophils or monocytes in AIDS patients may provide the first clue to an underlying infection by the presence of ingested organisms, such as histoplasma or *Myobacterium avium-intracellularis* (114–116).

Neutropenia associated with granulocyte antibodies has been described in non–HIV-positive homosexuals (117), and antibodies have been identified on the neutrophils of HIV-infected patients as well (69,70). In some instances, the eluted antibodies were reactive with other neutrophils, suggesting that they were autoantibodies (70). In other instances, the eluates were nonreactive and possibly represented immune complexes. No correlation was found, however, between circulating immune complexes and neutrophil antibodies, nor was there any correlation between the presence of neutrophil antibodies and the neutrophil count (70). As might be expected from the high incidence of anemia and neutropenia in AIDS patients, these abnormalities frequently coexist; their association with thrombocytopenia is less frequent and the incidence of pancytopenia in AIDS patients is approximately 40%.

Although less well studied, monocytopeniaa occurs in HIV-infected patients (118). Frequently the monocytes are morphologically atypical, with spreading cytoplasm, vacuoles, and phagocytic inclusions (1,118).

## HISTOLOGIC CHANGES IN THE BONE MARROW

Histologic abnormalities of the bone marrow are common with HIV infection (Table 3) (7,61,64,118–124). First described in 1983, these abnormalities involve changes in cell number, cell morphology, cell populations, and bone marrow architecture (1). The abnormalities do not correlate with either the clinical stage of the infection or the route of HIV acquisition (7), but they are more frequent in patients who have advanced to the stage of AIDS. Hypercellularity and myelofibrosis can be seen early in the course of the infection; serous fat atrophy, which reflects inanition and wasting, and bone marrow necrosis are generally late complications. Characteristically, there is a shift left in the myeloid series and an increase in normal-appearing plasma cells; eosinophilia is also common. In some patients, megaloblastoid or megaloblastic erythroid and granulocytic maturation occur, unassociated with folic acid or vitamin $B_{12}$ deficiency.

Some authors have applied the term "myelodysplasia" to the morphologic abnormalities of erythroid and myeloid precursor cells associated with HIV infection (125). Although phenotypically correct, *myelodysplasia* is usually employed to describe the panmyelopathy involving hematopoietic cells as a consequence of neoplastic transformation. Although a true "myelodysplastic syndrome" has been described in an HIV-infected individual (126), there is no evidence that this is the cause of the bone marrow morphologic abnormalities in the majority of HIV-infected patients, and it is also

**Table 3** Histologic Bone Marrow Abnormalities Associated with HIV Infection

| Histologic feature | % |
|---|---|
| Cellularity | |
| Increased | 36 |
| Normal | 46 |
| Reduced | 18 |
| Dyspoiesis | |
| Myeloid | 35 |
| Erythroid | 76 |
| Megakaryocytes | |
| Increased | 47 |
| Normal | 43 |
| Decreased | 10 |
| Plasmacytosis | 59 |
| Lymphoid aggregates | 42 |
| Increased reticulin | 55 |
| Eosinophilia | 45 |
| Phagocytic histocytes | 20 |
| Serous fat atrophy | 34 |
| Granulomas | 17 |

*Source*: Data compiled from References 7, 61, 118, and 120–125.

worth remembering that phenotypic abnormalities frequently have no relationship to genotypic abnormalities (127). Thus, it seems reasonable not to apply the term "myelodysplastic" to the morphologic changes observed in the marrow as a consequence of HIV infection.

Atypical collections or aggregates of lymphocytes usually not in a paratrabecular location or a diffuse increase in small lymphocytes are other features of the bone marrow in HIV infection. Bone marrow lymphoid aggregates are usually noticed in an older age group than the population affected with HIV. The etiology of these lymphoid aggregates or the marrow lymphocytosis associated with HIV infection is unknown; their presence does not correlate with the later development of a lymphoma and probably relates to the polyclonal B cell inactivation that occurs with HIV infection (81).

Granulomas may also be observed in the bone marrow of HIV-infected patients. They are usually noncaseating, often small, lacking giant cells, and not always associated with an identifiable infectious organism by stain or culture. On the other hand, because of immunosuppression, many HIV-infected patients fail to develop granulomas in association with mycobacterial or fungal infections.

Increased marrow reticulum and phagocytic histiocytosis are two frequently observed abnormalities in HIV-infected patients. Of unclear pathogenesis, these abnormalities are not specific to HIV. For example, an increase in marrow reticulum is seen with other viral infections and autoimmune disorders in which there is immunosuppression (6,128). Any type of infection can give rise to hematophagic histiocytosis, and this abnormality is especially frequent in immunosuppressed patients (6,129). The depression of peripheral blood counts that is characteristic of HIV infection is in some patients likely in part caused by hematophagocytosis.

An increase in marrow reticulum is not the only reason for a "dry tap" in HIV-infected patients. We have documented the presence of Kaposi's sarcoma antemortem in an AIDS patient on more than one occasion (130). Characteristically, there is dense marrow fibrosis with the presence of slit-like spaces and endothelial cell-lined channels. Factor VIII staining or electron microscopy can be used to confirm the diagnosis.

The presence or absence of an opportunistic infection or drug therapy does not appear to influence markedly bone marrow morphology, except perhaps for the presence of hypocellularity. However, although not diagnostic for HIV infection or necessarily diagnostic of the etiology of depressed blood counts, a bone marrow aspiration and biopsy should be performed on every patient who is febrile or who manifests a change in peripheral blood counts. Bone marrow aspiration and biopsy are simple and excellent techniques for identifying the presence of opportunistic organisms. Overwhelming invasion of the marrow by mycobacteria or fungi is often observed, and consequently, a diagnosis can often be made well in advance of culture studies (116). Infectious organisms documented by histologic examination of marrow include tuberculosis (64,123,131), histoplasmosis (114–132,133), leishmaniasis (134), and *Pneumocystis carinii* (135). Even with a dry tap, careful scrutiny of macrophages on the touch preparation may reveal intracellular organisms. A substantial number of mycobacteria can be present in the absence of granulomas, although histiocytes laden with these organisms are often present.

Normal or even increased cellularity of the marrow in the presence of reduced peripheral blood counts is a feature of HIV infection. Even if marrow cellularity is reduced, megakaryocytes are usually preserved. A similar discordance is also observed in patients infected with CMV (129). The disparity between marrow cellularity and peripheral blood counts suggests increased destruction of the circulating blood cells but does not exclude ineffective hematopoiesis. However, anemia was found to be more frequently associated with marrow hypercellularity than normocellularity, suggesting some degree of attempted marrow compensation. No such correlations have been observed for either granulocytes or platelets (61).

Red cell aplasia and total marrow hypoplasia occur with HIV infection, but their frequency is low. Infection, drugs, or malignancy is most often responsible for these abnormalities. One agent recently documented as a cause of red cell aplasia in HIV-infected patients is parvovirus B19 (see Chap. 3) (136). Parvovirus B19 infects erythroid progenitor cells, but the hematologic consequences are usually insignificant unless hemolysis is present or there is marked immunosuppression preventing the development of viral immunity. HIV-infected patients fall into the latter category and benefit from the passive immunization provided by intravenous administration of gammaglobulin (136).

## DRUG-INDUCED MARROW DYSFUNCTION

HIV-infected patients are frequently treated with drugs that are myelotoxic. These include zidovudine (AZT), pentamidine, trimethoprim-sulfamethoxazole, pyrimethamine, and gancyclovir. The myelotoxicity of trimethoprim-sulfamethoxazole was recognized early in the course of the HIV epidemic, when several patients treated with this drug for pneumocystis pneumonia developed profound leukopenia and neutropenia 9–31 days after beginning therapy. The white cell promptly rebounded when the drug combination was discontinued (137,138). Bone marrow aspiration did not eveal megaloblastic changes, and folinic acid did not reverse the neutropenia due to trimethoprim-sulfamethoxazole. Other toxicities due to trimethoprim-sulfamethoxazole include fever, rash, thrombocytopenia, and transaminase elevations. Similar toxic reactions but at a lower frequency are seen with pentamidine, which also causes azotemia and hypoglycemia. Toxic reactions also appeared to be more common in AIDS patients treated with trimethoprim-sulfamethoxazole than in patients receiving the drug who were not infected with HIV (138). Similar drug hypersensitivity is seen with other virus infections, such as EBV or CMV, presumably through a loss of immune control.

The most common myelotoxic drug used to treat HIV-infected patients is zidovudine. In a large clinical trial anemia developed in 24% of patients taking zidovudine, and 31% required transfusions. Neutropenia developed in 16%; suppression of the platelet count was infrequent and mild, and in some patients an increase in platelet number was observed (98). Progressive macrocytosis unassociated with low serum vitamin $B_{12}$ or folate levels is a common consequence of zidovudine therapy (98,139). The patients most susceptible to zidovudine-associated myelotoxicity include those with AIDS, those already anemic or neutropenic, and those with a low $CD_4$ count and a low serum vitamin $B_{12}$ level (98). In general, anemia or neutropenia developed within 6 weeks, and concomitant administration of acetaminophen appeared to increase the frequency of myelotoxicity. A recent study suggests that serum thymidine kinase activity may be a marker for impending marrow suppression, since a high serum thymidine kinase level after 4 weeks of zidovudine therapy correlated with the development of marrow failure (140). A low serum vitamin $B_{12}$ level in the absence of vitamin $B_{12}$ malabsorption is not uncommon in AIDS patients (141).

Morphologically, erythroid hypoplasia and pure red cell aplasia have been observed in anemic patients taking zidovudine (139), and in some patients marked marrow hypocellularity in conjunction with pancytopenia has been described (142). Marrow recovery usually occurs when the zidovudine is stopped, but with pancytopenia recovery can be very slow and in sometimes marrow hypoplasia is persistant (142). Generally, those patients who developed pancytopenia with marrow hypoplasia had been taking the drug for more than 3 months.

The mechanism for zidovudine-induced marrow suppression appears to be largely a direct effect of the drug on hematopoietic cells. With respect to anemia, a deficiency of erythropoietin cannot be evoked since zidovudine did not inhibit erythropoietin production in anemic mice (143) and serum immunoreactive erythropoietin levels in patients taking zidovudine are much higher than the pretreatment value for any degree of anemia (109). Indeed, for unknown reasons, erythropoietin levels are higher in some anemic patients taking zidovudine than in iron-deficient patients with the same degree of anemia (109). Nevertheless, anemic AIDS patients taking zidovudine respond to erythropoietin, especially if the erythropoietin level is less than 500 mU/ml (144,145). It is likely that those patients with very high serum erythropoietin levels ($>$500 mU/ml) have either a reduced population of erythroid progenitor cells or are more sensitive to the suppressive effects of zidovudine, or both.

Several studies have addressed the role of zidovudine cellular toxicity using in vitro clonal assays for hematopoietic progenitor cells (146–150). There were some differences in the near effective dose ($ED_{50}$) and target cell sensitivity among these studies, which may reflect technical differences. Nevertheless, zidovudine suppressed hematopoietic cell proliferation in vitro in a dose- and time-dependent fashion, and its effects were reversible by deoxythymidine (148). Both myeloid and erythroid progenitor cells were sensitive to suppression by zidovudine, and the in vitro suppressive concentrations of zidovudine were compatible with those achieved in vivo. Marrow progenitors from AIDS patients appeared to be more susceptible to zidovudine-induced growth inhibition than those from normal individuals (147). Other myelotoxic drugs employed in HIV-infected patients, such as gancyclovir and DDC, inhibited marrow hematopoietic progenitor cell proliferation as well, but acyclovir, which is not myelotoxic, did not (148). The combination of zidovudine and gancyclovir is extremely myelotoxic in patients (151).

These in vitro studies may not truly reflect in vivo behavior, however. For example, in a recent study using oral zidovudine-treated, virally immunosuppressed mice, the number of BFU-E was increased, as was their sensitivity to erythropoietin with respect to colony formation (143). Furthermore, hemin can antagonize the in vitro inhibitory effect of zidovudine on colony formation by BFU-E, suggesting that the drug may exert its effect on terminal erythroid differentiation, not earlier in erythropoiesis (143,152). However, intraperitoneal administration of zidovudine in mice caused a rapid but reversible suppression of both hematopoietic progenitor cell numbers and total marrow cellularity, suggesting that zidovudine can act on hematopoietic cells at different stages of development (153).

## HEMATOPOIETIC PROGENTIOR CELLS IN HIV INFECTION

A number of studies have addressed the in vitro behavior of hematopoietic progenitor cells following HIV infection and whether these cells are infected by the virus. In one study, there was impaired colony formation by granulocyte-macrophage progenitor cells (CFU-GM) in 70 of 78 patients with AIDS or ARC (erythroid progenitor cells were not evaluated) (39). Impaired colony formation by CFU-GM was thought to be due to the inhibitory effect of an 84,000 molecular weight (kD) protein that could be isolated from medium conditioned by bone marrow cells of AIDS patients. This protein, but not serum from HIV-infected patients, inhibited colony formation by CFU-GM from normal donors. Colony formation by early (BFU-E) or late (CFU-E) erythroid progenitor cells was not inhibited by the 84 kD protein. The nature of this protein and its origin remain unknown because it was not reactive with antibodies against known HIV antigens (39).

In a more extensive study of bone marrow hematopoietic progenitor cell proliferation from patients with AIDS or ARC, significant impairment of colony formation compared with normal control subjects was observed not only for CFU-GM but also for multipotential hematopoietic progenitor cells (CFU-GEM), megakaryocytic progenitor cells (CFU-MK), and early erythroid progenitor cells (BFU-E), indicating a global defect in marrow progenitor cell behavior (154). T lymphocyte depletion enhanced colony formation by hematopoietic progenitor cells from AIDS or ARC patients but not normal individuals, but addition of autologous T cells suppressed colony formation by progenitor cells from the AIDS or ARC patients. The inhibitory effect of the added T cells was inversely proportional to the $T_4$ (helper) $T_8$ (suppressor) lymphocyte ratio, and no differences were observed between peripheral blood and marrow T lymphocytes. Macrophages did not seem to be involved since their removal did not enhance colony formation, nor were soluble factors released by AIDS or ARC marrow cells able to suppress colony formation by normal bone marrow progenitor cells (154). In contrast, in another study of peripheral blood hematopoietic progenitor cells during early HIV infection, a reduction in the number of CFU-GM, BFU-E, and CFU-MK was observed even in T cell-depleted cultures. No such deficit was observed with marrow progenitors, and there was no correlation with CD4$^+$ cell number (155).

In contrast to these observations, normal colony-forming behavior by hematopoietic progenitor cells from AIDS or ARC patients has also been described (31,156). In one particular study, hematopoietic progenitor cells responded normally in vitro to recombinant erythropoietin and granulocyte-macrophage colony-stimulating factor. However, when sera from AIDS or ARC patients were added to the marrow cultures, colony formation by BFU-E and CFU-GM was suppressed; no such inhibitory effect was seen with normal marrow cells. The inhibitory component of the serum, appeared to be an antibody against the major envelope protein of HIV, gp120. However, a subsequent study from the same laboratory, although affirming normally responsive marrow hematopoietic progenitor cells from AIDS patients, failed to detect HIV expression by these cells (31). Studies of in vitro colony formation by CFU-GM from hemophiliacs with AIDS have also failed to demonstrate abnormalities (157).

The conflicting results concerning the proliferative behavior of marrow hematopoietic progenitor cells in HIV infection may be the consequence of differing patient populations or technical differences with respect to the particular marrow cell populations studied—that is, lymphocyte depleted, macrophage depleted, or not depleted at all—or the type of culture system employed. Recent studies in monkeys as well as humans have shed sufficient light on the behavior of hematopoietic progenitor cells following HIV infection to partially resolve this issue.

As mentioned earlier, monkeys infected with a simian lentivirus (SIV) related to HIV develop qualitative and quantitative abnormalities that are quite similar to those in HIV-infected humans (7,8). In these monkeys, colony formation by CFU-GM and BFU-E is depressed (33). In vitro culture of monkey marrow cells with an SIV strain isolated from marrow macrophages resulted in productive infection within 2 weeks, and although the marrow cells remained viable, colony formation by CFU-GM and BFU-E was reduced (33). Depletion of T lymphocytes was without effect, but inhibition of macrophage replication restored colony formation by CFU-GM. Depression of colony formation was also correlated strongly with the SIV content of the marrow. The virus was identified only in CD4$^+$ macrophages immunologically and by electron microscopy, a not surprising result, since this SIV strain was trophic for macrophages. Lymphocyte-mediated marrow cell dysfunction in HIV-infected patients is not excluded by these observations, but importantly, macrophage-mediated suppression of progenitor cell proliferation was established. In vivo administration of recombinant soluble CD4 ameliorated depression of hematopoietic progenitor cell proliferation (158).

Although it is well accepted that CD4$^+$ lymphocytes (159,160) and monocytes (27,161–163) can be infected by HIV, there has been controversy over whether other hematopoietic cells can be infected by the virus. Our studies failed to identify HIV in either myeloid or erythroid cells (27), nor was the virus present in these cells in SIV-infected marrow (33). Using in situ hybridization of marrow specimens from HIV-infected patients, however, one group has claimed on morphologic grounds to identify HIV in myeloid and erythroid cells but not megakaryocytes (124); others, also using in situ hybridization, identified expression of HIV RNA in megakaryocytes of AIDS patients (63) as well as internalization of the virus by both megakaryocytes and platelets (164), and recently productive infection of a $CD4^+$ megakaryocyte cell line was established (165). Infection was more easily achieved with HIV-2 than HIV-1. The possibility that HIV could infect primitive hematopoietic progenitor cells was supported by experiments in which purified $CD34^+$ (My-$10^+$) cadaver marrow cells were infected with HIV (166). After 30 days, reverse transcriptase activity was identified, and the harvested cells were found to be $CD34^-$ but $CD4^+$ and positive for nonspecific esterase (166). The cells had the features of monocytes, and virus was present in vacuoles. It is possible that in these experiments the virus infected a primitive hematopoietic progenitor cell, but it is equally likely that the virus infected the monocytes that survived under the culture conditions employed (167). In this regard, it is important to remember that in vitro infection with HIV may not faithfully recapitulate the in vivo behavior of the virus or the pathways by which natural infection occurs (168). Furthermore, tissue culture variants of the virus may not behave in the same fashion as freshly explanted wild-type virus (27).

That HIV probably does not invade hematopoietic progenitor cells is suggested by other studies. In a study of hematopoietic cells, including the $CD34^+$ population, isolated from HIV-infected patients using the polymerase chain reaction (PCR), HIV was identified in $CD4^+$ cells and some B lymphocytes in all patients but only once in $CD34^+$ cells. No proviral DNA was found in granulocytes, nor was there depletion of $CD34^+$ cells (169). In another study using PCR, no HIV DNA was detected in myeloid or erythroid colonies from HIV-positive patients, nor was any detected in colonies grown from marrow infected in vitro with the virus (31).

Although detectable HIV infection of hematopoietic progenitor cells has been difficult to substantiate, the virus can infect marrow stroma fibroblasts (170), which may, in addition to $CD4^+$ lymphocytes and monocytes, serve as a reservoir for the virus. These data support the contention that inhibition of hematopoietic progenitor cell proliferation is an indirect effect of HIV infection and that the marrow hematopoietic progenitor cell number is not necessarily depleted in this situation. Further support comes from the observations that administration of recombinant GM-CSF, G-CSF, or erythropoietin enhances marrow cell proliferation and increases the number of circulating BFU-E in HIV-infected patients (171) and lithium carbonate can increase the granulocyte count in those patients receiving zidovudine (172).

The extent to which monocytes and macrophages are affected in HIV-positive patients has been a matter of controversy. Some studies suggest that the monocyte population is not a very significant reservoir of HIV (173, 174). Certainly, only a subpopulation of monocytes that are $CD4^+$ is susceptible to infection, and in several studies lymphocytes were more readily infected than monocytes in vitro. However, HIF is not cytopathic to monocytes; the virus accumulates in cytoplasmic vacuoles of monocytes (27), suggesting that monocytes may serve as protective reservoirs for the virus. In the bone marrow, where $CD4^+$ lymphocytes are depleted, monocytes could be a major reservoir of virus and also provide a source of cells to contaminate the central nervous system. Eosinophils are also $CD4^+$, but to date no studies have shown them to contain HIV (175).

Although HIV is not cytopathic to monocytes, infection with the virus causes impairment of intracellular killing (176) and chemotaxis (177,178). Granulocyte phagocytosis may be impaired in HIV infection (179), and since these cells do not carry the virus, mechanisms other than direct infection may also be involved in monocyte dysfunction as well. Because monocytes harbor HIV, stimulation by agents directed at improving leukocyte production and function, like GM-CSF, could potentially enhance HIV replication in these cells. Monocytic and myeloid cell lines could be productively infected by HIV in vitro, but only after induction of differentiation (28,167,180,181). In freshly explanted human peripheral blood monocytes, GM-CSF enhanced the replication of both monocytotropic and lymphocytotropic HIV strains; a similar effect was not observed with lymphocytes (182) or G-CSF (167). Interleukin-3 (IL-3), CSF-1, and GM-CSF had similar actions in freshly explanted HIV-infected monocytes (183). These observations suggest that factors associated with cell differentiation may be required for optimal viral replication, but in another study, GM-CSF inhibited HIV proliferation in a monocytic cell line (184). GM-CSF also enhanced the antiviral activity of zidovudine in HIV-infected cells (182) and enhanced in vitro colony formation by CFU-GM in the presence of zidovudine (150). GM-CSF also potentiated the effect of zidovudine on HIV-infected alveolar macrophages but did not enhance HIV replication in these cells (185). IL-3, while enhancing HIV replication in peripheral blood monocytes, did not impair the antiviral effect of zidovudine (186), suggesting that IL-3 as well as GM-CSF can be used safely in HIV-infected patients treated with zidovudine. It is also noteworthy that GM-CSF can correct occasionally observed neutrophil functional defects in AIDS (179).

## HIV-RELATED LYMPHOMAS

Abnormalities of the lymphoid system are a primary feature of HIV infection and extend from lymphopenia and suppression of the circulating $CD4^+$

lymphocyte count to aggressive non-Hodgkin's lymphomas. In between are the consistent findings of polyclonal hypergammaglobulinemia due to unregulated B cell function (81) and the frequent occurrence of persistent generalized lymphadenopathy, often an early manifestation of HIV infection (47,54). Although multiple myeloma is not causally associated with HIV infection, there is a low frequency of paraproteins, either IgG or IgM, usually with $\kappa$ light chains, (187). A careful study of one patient showed that the paraprotein was not truly monoclonal and had anti-HIV specificity. Since some of the paraproteins occurred in the setting of polyclonal hypergammaglobulinemia, without other features of a plasma cell dyscrasia, they are probably another manifestation of HIV infection. Angioimmunoblastic lymphadenopathy with dysproteinemia (AILD) has also been described in patients with a potential AIDS-defining illness (188); both AIDS and AILD share a number of clinical features, including the development of Kaposi's sarcoma (189).

The syndrome of generalized persistent lymphadenopathy associated with HIV infection is of interest since the associated hematologic abnormalities span the full spectrum observed in HIV-infected patients (54). Generalized lymphadenopathy is classified as a distinct stage of HIV infection and can be seen with the acute viral syndrome and in the setting of isolated acute thrombocytopenia, both generally early manifestations of infection with HIV. Although the adenopathy regresses in some patients, opportunistic infections, Kaposi's sarcoma, or lymphomas, all AIDS-defining illnesses, have developed in others. Leukopenia, lymphopenia, neutropenia, thrombocytopenia, bone marrow hypercellularity with lymphocytosis, and occasionally marrow hypoplasia have been observed in patients with generalized lymphadenopathy, suggesting that the lymphadenopathy itself may not define the prognosis (54,190,191).

The incidence of non-Hodgkin's lymphoma is increased in HIV-infected patients (192). Although a full discussion of these lymphomas is beyond the scope of this review, they are noteworthy not only because the bone marrow is frequently involved but also because with the increased longevity of HIV-infected patients, these lymphomas are becoming more prevalent (193). Histologically, the lymphomas commonly seen in HIV-infected patients are either high grade (small noncleaved or large cell immunoblastic) or intermediate grade (diffuse large cell). Many immunoblastic lymphomas, the most common subtype, are polyclonal, but expression of EBV DNA is uncommon (194). These tumors are characterized by presentation of an advanced stage and a high frequency of extranodal disease, particularly in the central nervous system, gastrointestinal tract, and liver. In one series, bone marrow involvement occurred in approximately 40% of patients with small noncleaved cell tumors and 16% of large cell immunoblastic lymphomas (195). Occasionally

T cell leukemias (196) or lymphomas (197) have been observed. Although Hodgkin's disease does not appear to occur at a greater frequency with HIV infection, when it does occur its natural history is more aggressive and an advanced presentation is common (198). In keeping with the oligoclonal gammopathies observed in HIV-infected patients, the B cell neoplasms appear to initiate in a multiclonal fashion, with eventual clonal selection due to the constitutive activation of c-*myc* (199–201). For both major types of lymphoma, the overall results of chemotherapy, including bone marrow transplantation (202), have been poor.

## REFERENCES


1. Spivak JL, Selonick SE, Quinn TC. Acquired immune deficiency syndrome and pancytopenia. JAMA 1983; 250:3084–7.
2. Durack DT. Opportunistic infections and Kaposi's sarcoma in homosexual men. N Engl J Med 1981; 308:125–9.
3. Centers for Disease Control. Possible transfusion-associated acquired immune deficiency syndrome (AIDS): California. MMWR 1982; 31:577–80.
4. Centers for Disease Control. Immunodeficiency among female sexual partners of males with acquired immune deficiency syndrome (AIDS): New York. MMWR 1982; 31:697–8.
5. Desforges JF. AIDS and preventive treatment in hemophilia. N Engl J Med 1983; 308:94–5.
6. Risdall RJ, McKenna RW, Nesbit ME, et al. Virus-associated hemophagocytic syndrome. Cancer 1979; 44:993–1002.
7. Spivak JL, Bender BS, Quinn TC. Hematologic abnormalities in the acquired immune deficiency syndrome. Am J Med 1984; 77:224–8.
8. Letvin NL, Eaton KA, Aldrich WR, et al. Acquired immunodeficiency syndrome in a colony of macaque monkeys. Proc Natl Acad U S A Sci 1983; 80:2718–22.
9. Anderson JH, Maul DH, Sever JL, Ellingsworth LR, Lowenstine LJ, Gardner MB. Epidemic of acquired immunodeficiency in rhesus monkeys. Lancet 1983; 1:388–90.
10. Letvin NL, Daniel MD, Sehgal PK, et al. Induction of AIDS-like disease in macaque monkeys with T-cell tropic retrovirus STLV-III. Science 1985; 230:71–3.
11. Teich N. Taxonomy of retroviruses. In: Weiss R, Teich N, Varmus H, Coffins J, eds. RNA tumor viruses. Cold Spring Harbor, NY: Cold Spring Harbor Laboratories, 1985; 25–207.
12. Teich N, Wyke J, Mak T. Pathogenesis of retrovirus-induced diseases. In: Weiss R, Teich N, Varmus H, Coffin J, eds. RNA tumor viruses. Cold Spring Harbor, NY: Cold Spring Harbor Laboratories, 1985; 785–998.
13. Desrosiers RC, Letvin NL. Animal models for acquired immunodeficiency syndrome. Rev Infect Dis 1987; 9:438–45.
14. Payne SL, Fang FD, Liu CP, et al. Antigenic variation and lentivirus persistence: variations in envelope gene sequences during EIAV infection resembles changes reported for sequential isolates of HIV. Virology 1987; 161:321–31.

15. Rice NR, Lequearre AS, Casey JW, Lahn S, Stephens RM, Edwards J. Viral DNA in horses infected with equine infectious anemia virus. J Virol 1989; 63: 5194–200.
16. Haase AT. Pathogenesis of lentivirus infections. Nature 1986; 322:130–6.
17. Chiu IM, Yaniv A, Dahlberg JE, et al. Nucleotide sequence evidence for relationship of AIDS retrovirus to lentiviruses. Nature 1985; 317:366–8.
18. Pedersen HC, Ho E, Brown MJ, Yamamoto K. Isolation of a T-lymphotropic virus from domestic cats with an immunodeficiency-like syndrome. Science 1987; 235:790–3.
19. Talbott RL, Sparger EE, Lovelace KM, et al. Nucleotide sequence and genomic organization of feline immunodeficiency virus. Biochemistry 1989; 86:5743–7.
20. Myers G, Rabson AB, Berzofsky JA, Smith TF, Wong-Staal F. Human retroviruses and AIDS: a compilation and analysis of nucleic acid and amino acid sequences. Los Alamos, NM: Theoretical Biology and Biophysics Group, Los Alamos National Laboratory, 1990.
21. Martin M, Weiss RA. Virology overview. AIDS 1989; 3:S3–4.
22. Cann AJ, Karn J. Molecular biology of HIV: new insights into the virus lifecycle. AIDS 1989; 3:S19–34.
23. Fenyo EM, Albert J, Asjo B. Replicative capacity, cytopathic effect and cell tropism of HIV. AIDS 1989; 3:S5–12.
24. York-Higgins D, Cheng-Mayer C, Bauer D, Levy JA, Dina D. Human immunodeficiency virus type 1 cellular host range, replication, and cytopathicity are linked to the envelope region of the viral genome. J Virol 1990; 64:4016–20.
25. Takeuchi Y, Akutsu M, Murayama K, Shimizu N, Hoshino H. Host range mutant of human immunodeficiency virus type 1: modification of cell tropism by a single point mutation at the neutralization epitope in the env gene. J Virol 1991; 65:1710–8.
26. Hwang SS, Boyle TJ, Lyerly HK, Cullen BR. Identification of the envelope V3 loop as the primary determinant of cell tropism in HIV-1. Science 1991; 253: 71–3.
27. Potts BJ, Hoggan MD, Lamperth L, Spivak J. Replication of HIV-1 and HIV-2 in human bone marrow cultures. Virology 1992; 188:840–49.
28. Potts BJ, Maury W, Martin MA. Replication of HIV-1 in primary monocyte cultures. Virology 1990; 175:465–76.
29. Daiv BR, Schwartz DH, Marx JC, et al. Absent or rare human immunodeficiency virus infection of bone marrow stem/progenitor cells in vivo. J Virol 1991; 65: 1985–90.
30. Wong-Staal F, Shaw GM, Hahn BH, Salahuddin SZ, Popovic M. Genomic diversity of human T-lymphotropic virus type III (HTLV-III). Science 1985; 229: 759–62.
31. Molina JM, Scadden DT, Sakaguchi M, Fuller B, Woon A, Grooperman JE. Lack of evidence for infection of or effect on growth of hematopoietic progenitor cells after in vivo or in vitro exposure to human immunodeficiency virus. Blood 1990; 76:2476–82.
32. Steinberg HN, Crumpacker CS, Chatis PA. In vitro suppression of normal human bone marrow progenitor cells by human immunodeficiency virus. J Virol 1991; 65:1765–9.
33. Watanabe M, Ringler DJ, Nakamura M, DeLong PA, Letvin NL. Simian im-

munodeficiency virus inhibits bone marrow hematopoietic progenitor cell growth. J Virol 1990; 64:656–63.

34. Gendelman HE, Narayan O, Molineaux S, Clements JE, Ghotbi Z. Slow persistent replication of lentiviruses: role of tissue macrophages and macrophage precursors in bone marrow. Proc Natl Acad Sci 1985; 82:7086–7090.
35. Sparger EE, Luciw PA, Elder JH, Yamamoto JK, Lowenstine LJ, Pedersen NC. Feline immunodeficiency virus is a lentivirus associated with an AIDS-like disease in cats. AIDS 1989; 3:S43–9.
36. Yamamoto JK, Sparger E, Ho EW, et al. Pathogenesis of experimentally induced feline immunodeficiency virus infection cats. Am J Vet Res 1988; 49:1246–62.
37. Murray HW, Rubin BY, Masur H, Roberts RB. Impaired production of lymphokines and immune (gamma) interferon in the acquired immunodeficiency syndrome. N Engl J Med 1984; 310:883–9.
38. Davis P. In: Adams DO, Edelson P, Koren H, eds. Methods for studying mononuclear phagocytes. New York: Academic Press, 1981; 549–59.
39. Leiderman IZ, Greenberg ML, Adelsberg BR, Siegel FP. Glycoprotein inhibitor of in vitro granulopoiesis associated with AIDS. Blood 1987; 70:1267–72.
40. Nathan CF, Murray HW, Cohn ZA. The macrophage as an effector cell. N Engl J Med 1980; 303:622–6.
41. Giulian D, Vaca K, Noonan CA. Secretion of neurotoxins by mononuclear phagocytes infected with HIV-1. Science 1990; 250:1593–6.
42. Navla BA, Cho E-S, Petito CK, Price RW. The AIDS dementia complex. II. Neuropathology 1986; 19:525–35.
43. Needlestick transmission of HTLV-III from a patient infected in Africa. *Lancet* 1984; 2:1376–7.
44. Cooper DA, Maclean P, Finlayson R, et al. Acute AIDS retrovirus infection. Lancet 1985; 1:537–40.
45. Buchanan JG, Goldwater PN, Somerfield SD, Tobias MI. Mononucleosis-like-syndrome associated with acute AIDS retrovirus infection. N Z Med J 1986; 99: 405–8.
46. Ho DD, Sarngadharan MG, Resnick L, Dimarzo-Veronese F, Rota TR, Hirsch MS. Primary human T-lymphotropic virus type III infection. Ann Intern Med 1985; 103:880–3.
47. Steeper TA, Horwitz CA, Hanson M, et al. Heterophil-negative mononucleosis-like illnesses with atypical lymphocytosis in patients undergoing seroconversions to the human immunodeficiency virus. Am J Clin Pathol 1988; 89:169–74.
48. Tucker J, Ludlam CA, Craig A, et al. HTLV-III infection associated with glandular-fever-like illness in a haemophiliac. Lancet 1985; 1:585.
49. Fox R, Eldred LJ, Fuchs EJ, et al. Clinical manifestations of acute infection with human immunodeficiency virus in a cohort of gay men. AIDS 1987; 1:35–8.
50. Evans AS. Infectious mononucleosis and related syndromes. Am J Med Sci 1978; 276:325.
51. Cohen JI, Corey GR. Cytomegalovirus infection in the normal host. Medicine (Baltimore) 1985; 64:100–4.
52. Horwitz CA, Henle W, Henle G, et al. Clinical and laboratory evaluation of cytomegalovirus-induced mononucleosis in previously healthy individuals. Report of 82 cases. Medicine (Baltimore) 1986; 65:124–34.

53. Hicks CB, Benson PM, Lupton GP, Tramont EC. Seronegative secondary syphilis in a patient infected with the human immunodeficiency virus (HIV) with Kaposi sarcoma. Ann Intern Med 1987; 107:492–5.
54. Metroka CE, Cunningham-Rundles S, Pollack MS, et al. Generalized lymphadenopathy in homosexual men. Ann Intern Med 1983; 99:585–91.
55. Morris L, Distenfeld A, Amorosi E, Karpatkin S. Autoimmune thrombocytopenic purpura in homosexual men. Ann Intern Med 1982; 96:714–7.
56. Ratnoff OD, Menitove JE, Aster RH, Lederman MM. Coincident classic hemophilia and "idiopathic" thrombocytopenic purpura in patients under treatment with concentrates of antihemophilic factor (factor VIII). N Engl J Med 1983; 308:439–442.
57. Savona S, Nardi MA, Lennette ET, Karpatkin S. Thrombocytopenic purpura in narcotics addicts. Ann Intern Med 1985; 102:737–41.
58. Karpatkin S, Nardi MA, Hymes KB. Immunologic thrombocytopenic purpura after heterosexual transmission of human immunodeficiency virus (HIV). Ann Intern Med 1988; 109:190–3.
59. Jost J, Tauber MG, Luthy R, Siegenthaler W. HIV-assoziierte thrombozytopenie. Schewiz Med Wocheschr 1988; 118:206–12.
60. Kaslow RA, Phair JP, Friedman HB, et al. Infection with the human immunodeficiency virus: clinical manifestations and their relationship to immune deficiency. Ann Intern Med 1987; 107:474–80.
61. Zon LI, Arkin C, Groopman JE. Haematologic manifestations of the human immune deficiency virus (HIV). Br J Haematol 1987; 66:251–6.
62. Ratner L. Human immunodeficiency virus-associated autoimmune thrombocytopenia purpura: a review. Am J Med 1989; 86:194–8.
63. Zucker-Franklin D, Cao Y. Megakaryocytes of human immunodeficiency virus-infected individuals express viral RNA. Proc Natl Acad Sci USA 1989; 86:5595–9.
64. Bello JL, Burgaleta C, Magallon M, Herruzo R, Villar JM. Hematological abnormalities in hemophilic patients with human immunodeficiency virus infection. Am J Hematol 1990; 33:230.
65. Schneider DR, Picker LJ. Myelodysplasia in the acquired immune deficiency syndrome. Am J Clin Pathol 1985; 84:144–52.
66. Zucker-Franklin D, Termin CS, Cooper MC. Structural changes in the megakaryocytes of patients infected with the human immune deficiency virus (HIV-1). Am J Pathol 1989; 134:1295–303.
67. Walsh CM, Nardi MA, Karpatkin S. On the mechanism of thrombocytopenic purpura in sexually active homosexual men. N Engl J Med 1984; 311:635–9.
68. Karpatkin S, Nardi MA. Immunologic thrombocytopenic purpura in human immunodeficiency virus-seropositive patients with hemophilia. J Lab Clin Med 1988; 111:441–8.
69. Murphy MF, Metcalfe P, Waters AH, et al. Incidence and mechanism of neutropenia and thrombocytopenia in patients with human immunodeficiency virus infection. Br J Haematol 1987; 66:337–40.
70. van der Lelie J, Lange JMA, Vos JJE, van Dalen CM, Canner SA, von dem borne AEGK. Autoimmunity against blood cells in human immunodeficiency-virus (HIV) infection. Br J Haematol 1987; 67:109–14.

71. Bender BS, Quinn TC, Spivak JL. Homosexual men with thrombocytopenia have impaired reticuloendothelial system Fc receptor-specific clearance. Blood 1987; 70:392–5.
72. Taaning E, Scheibel E, Laursen B, Ingerslev J. Pattern of immunoglobulin classes and IgG subclasses of platelet-associated immunoglobulin in HIV-seropositive haemophiliacs. Vox Sang 1988; 54:205–9.
73. Telen MJ, Roberts KB, Bartlett JA. HIV-associated autoimmune hemolytic anemia. J Acquired Immune Deficiency Syndromes 1990; 3:933–37.
74. Morrow WJW, Wharton M, Stricker RB, Levy JA. Circulating immune complexes in patients with acquired immune deficiency syndrome contain the AIDS-associated retrovirus. Clin Immunol Innumopathol 1986; 40:515–24.
75. Lange JMA, Paul DA, de Wolf F, Coutinho RA, Goudsmit J. Viral gene expression, antibody production and immune complex formation in human immunodeficiency virus infection. AIDS 1987; 1:15–20.
76. Karpatkin S, Nardi M, Lennette ET, Byrne B, Poiesz B. Anti-human immunodeficiency virus type 1 antibody complexes on platelets of seropositive thrombocytopenic homosexuals and narcotic addicts. Proc Natl Acad Sci U S A 1988; 85:9763–7.
77. Brand A, Witvliet M, Claas FHJ, Eernise JG. Beneficial effect of intravenous gammaglobulin in a patient with complement-mediated autoimmune thrombocytopenia due to IgM-anti-platelet antibodies. Br J Haematol 1988; 69:507–11.
78. Kelton JG, Carter CJ, Rodger C, et al. The relationship among platelet-associated IgG, platelet lifespan, and reticuloendothelial cell function. Blood 1984; 63:1434–8.
79. Heyns AP, Badenhorst PN, Lotter MG, Pieters H, Wessels P, Kotze HF. Platelet turnover and kinetics in immune thrombocytopenic purpura: results with autologous $^{111}$In-labeled platelets and homologous $^{51}$Cr-labeled platelets differ. Blood 1986; 67:86–92.
80. Bel-Ali Z, Dufour V, Najen Y. Platelet kinetics in human immunodeficiency induced thrombocytopenia. Am J Hematol 1987; 26:299.
81. Lane HC, Masur H, Edgar LC, Whalen G, Rook AH, Fauci AS. Abnormalities of B cell activation and immunoregulation in patients with the acquired immunodeficiency syndrome. N Engl J Med 1983; 309:453–8.
82. Bender BS, Frank MM, Lawley TJ, Smith WJ, Brickman CM, Quinn TC. Defective reticuloendothelial system Fc-receptor function in patients with acquired immunodeficiency syndrome. J Infect. Dis 1985; 152:409–12.
83. Walsh C, Krigel R, Lennette E, Karpatkin S. Thrombocytopenia in homosexual patients. Ann Intern Med 1985; 103:542–5.
84. Costello C, Treacy M, Lai L. Treatment of immune thrombocytopenic purpura in homosexual men. Scand J Haematol 1986; 36:507–10.
85. Goldsweig HG, Grossman R, William D. Thrombocytopenia in homosexual men. Am J Hematol 1986; 21:243–7.
86. Oksenhendler E, Bierling P, Farcet J-P, Rabian C, Seligmann M, Clauvel J-P. Response to therapy in 37 patients with HIV-related thrombocytopenic purpura. Br J Haematol 1987; 66:491–5.
87. Abrams DI, Kiprov DD, Goedert JJ, Sarngadharan MG, Gallo RC, Volberding PA. Antibodies to human T-lymphotropic virus type III and development of the

acquired immunodeficiency syndrome in homosexual men presenting with immune thrombocytopenia. Ann Intern Med 1986; 104:47–50.

88. Pollak AN, Janinis J, Green D. Successful intravenous immune globulin therapy for human immunodeficiency virus-associated thrombocytopenia. Arch Intern Med 1988; 148:695–7.
89. Bussel JF, Haimi JS. Isolated thrombocytopenia in patients infected with HIV: treatment. Am J Hematol 1988; 28:79–84.
90. Lynch EC, Huston DP. Immune thrombocytopenia in homosexual men. Ann Intern Med 1986; 104:583–4.
91. Oksenhendler E, Bierling P, Brossard Y, et al. Anti-RH immunoglobulin therapy for human immunodeficiency virus-related immune thrombocytopenic purpura. Blood 1988; 71:1499–502.
92. Ellis MD, Neal KR, Lean CLS, Newland AG. Alfa-2a recombinant interferon in HIV-associated thrombocytopenia. Br Med J 1987; 295:1519.
93. Lever AML, Brook MG, Yap I, Thomas HC. Treatment of thrombocytopenia with alfa interferon. Br Med J 1987; 295:1519–20.
94. Mintzer DM, Real FX, Jovin L, Krown SE. Treatment of Kaposi's sarcoma and thrombocytopenia with vincristine in patients with the acquired immunodeficiency syndrome. Ann Intern Med 1985; 102:200–2.
95. Hymes KB, Greene JB, Karpatkin S. The effect of azidothymidine on HIV-related thrombocytopenia. N Engl J Med 1988; 318:516–7.
96. Swiss Group for Clinical Studies on the Acquired Immunodeficiency Syndrome (AIDS). Zidovudine for the treatment of thrombocytopenia associated with human immunodeficiency virus (HIV). Ann Intern Med 1988; 109:718–21.
97. Pottage JC, Benson CA, Spear JB, Landay AL, Kressler HA. Treatment of human immunodeficiency virus-related thrombocytopenia with zidovudine. JAMA 1988; 260:3045–8.
98. Richman DD, Fischl MA, Grieco MH, et al. The toxicity of azidothymidine (AZT) in the treatment of patients with AIDS and AIDS-related complex. A double-blind, placebo-controlled trial. N Engl J Med 1987; 317:192–7.
99. Shafer RW, Offit K, Macris NT, Horbar GM, Ancona L, Hoffman IR. Possible risk of steroid administration in patients at risk for AIDS. Lancet 1985; 1:934–5.
100. Laurence J, Sellers MB, Sikder SK. Effect of glucocorticoids on chronic human immunodeficiency virus (HIV) infection and HIV promoter-mediated transcription. Blood 1989; 74:291–7.
101. Leaf AN, Laubenstein LJ, Raphael B, Hochster H, Baez L, Karpatkin S. Thrombotic thrombocytopenic purpura associated with human immunodeficiency virus type 1 (HIV-1) infection. Ann Intern Med 1988; 109:194–7.
102. Meisenberg BR, Robinson WL, Mosley CA, Duke MS, Rabetoy GM, Kosty MP. Thrombotic thrombocytopenic purpura in human immunodeficiency (HIV)-seropositive males. Am J Hematol 1988; 27:212–5.
103. Boccia RV, Gelman EP, Baker CC, Marti G, Longo DL. A hemolytic-uremic syndrome with the acquired immunodeficiency syndrome. Ann Intern Med 1984; 101:716–7.
104. Cohen AJ, Philips TM, Kessler CM. Circulating coagulation inhibitors in the acquired immunodeficiency syndrome. Ann Intern Med 1986; 104:175–80.

105. Bloom EJ, Abrams DI, Rodgers G. Lupus anticoagulant in the acquired immunodeficiency syndrome. JAMA 1986; 256:491–3.
106. Canoso RT, Zon LI, Groopman JE. Anticardiolipin antibodies associated with human T-lymphotrophic virus type III infection. Br J Haematol 1987; 65: 495.
107. Gupta S, Iman A, Locirish K. Serum ferritin in acquired immune deficiency syndrome. J Clin Lab Immunol 1986; 20:11–3.
108. Spivak JL. Serum immunoreactive erythropoietin in health and disease. Int J Cell Cloning 1990; 8:211–26.
109. Spivak JL, Barnes DC, Fuchs E, Quinn TC. Serum immunoreactive erythropoietin in HIV-infected patients. JAMA 1989; 261:3104–7.
110. McGinnis MH, Macher AM, Rook AH, Alter HJ. Red cell autoantibodies in patients with acquired immune deficiency syndrome. Transfusion 1986; 26: 405–9.
111. Toy PTCY, Reid ME, Burns M. Positive direct antiglobulin test associated with hyperglobulinemia in acquired immunodeficiency syndrome (AIDS). Am J Hematol 1985; 19:145–50.
112. Inada Y, Lange M, McKinley GF, et al. Hematologic correlates and the role of erythrocyte CR1 (C3b receptor) in the development of AIDS. AIDS Res Hum Retroviruses 1986; 2:235–47.
113. D'Onofrio G, Mancini S, Tamburrini E, Mango G, Ortona L. Giant neutrophils with increased peroxidase activity. Am J Clin Pathol 1987; 87:584–91.
114. Henochowicz S, Sahovic E, Pistole M, Rodrigues M, Macher A. Histoplasmosis diagnosed on peripheral blood smear from a patient with AIDS. JAMA 1985; 253:3148.
115. Tomita T, Chiga M. Disseminated histoplasmosis in acquired immunodeficiency syndrome: light and electron microscopic observations. Hum Pathol 1988; 19:438–41.
116. Lehmann LS, Spivak JL. Rapid and definitive diagnosis of infectious diseases using the peripheral blood smear: a report of three cases and a review of the literature. J Intensive Care Med 1992; 7:36–47.
117. Minchinton RM, Frazer I. Idiopathic neutropenia in homosexual men. Lancet 1985; 1:936–7.
118. Treacy M, Lai L, Costello C, Clark A. Peripheral blood and bone marrow abnormalities in patients with HIV related disease. Br J Haematol 1987; 65:289–94.
119. Abrams DI, Chin EK, Lewis BJ, Volberding PA, Conant MA, Townsend RM. Hematologic manifestations in homosexual men with Kaposi's sarcoma. Am J Clin Pathol 1984; 81:13–8.
120. Castella A, Croxson TS, Mildvan D, Witt DH, Zalusky R. The bone marrow in AIDS. Am J Clin Pathol. 1985; 84:425–32.
121. Geller SA, Muller R, Greenberg ML, Siegal FP. Acquired immunodeficiency syndrome. Arch Pathol Lab Med 1985; 109:138–41.
122. Osborne BM, Guarda LA, Butler JJ. Bone marrow biopsies in patients with the acquired immunodeficiency syndrome. Hum Pathol 1984; 15:1048–53.
123. Shenoy CM, Lin JH. Bone marrow findings in acquired immunodeficiency syndrome (AIDS). Am J Med Sci 1986; 292:372–5.

124. Sun NCJ, Shapshak P, Lachant NA, et al. Bone marrow examination in patients with AIDS and AIDS-related complex (ARC). Am J Clin Pathol 1989; 92:589–94.
125. Schneider DR, Picker LJ. Myelodysplasia in the acquired immune deficiency syndrome. Am J Clin Pathol 1985; 84:144–52.
126. Napoli VM, Stein SF, Spira TJ, Raskin D. Myelodysplasia progressing to acute myeloblastic leukemia in an HTLV-III virus-positive homosexual man with AIDS-related complex. Am J Clin Pathol 1986; 86:788–91.
127. Vogelsang GB, Spivak JL. Unusual case of acute leukemia. Am J Med 1984; 76:1144–50.
128. Kaelin WG Jr, Spivak JL. Systemic lupus erythematosus and myelofibrosis. Am J Med 1986; 81:935–8.
129. Reiner AP, Spivak JL. Hematophagic histiocytosis. Medicine (Baltimore) 1988; 67:369–88.
130. Little BJ, Spivak JL, Quinn TC, Mann RB. Case report. Kaposi's sarcoma with bone marrow involvement: occurrence in a patient with the acquired immunodeficiency syndrome. Am J Med Sci 1986; 29:44–6.
131. Farhi DC, Mason UG, Horsburgh CR Jr. The bone marrow in disseminated mycobacterium avium-intracellulare infection. Am J Clin Pathol 1985; 83: 463–8.
132. Bonner JR, Alexander WJ, Dismukes WE, et al. Disseminated histoplasmosis in patients with the acquired immune deficiency syndrome. Arch Intern Med 1984; 144:2178–81.
133. Kurtin PJ, McKinsey DS, Gupta MR, Driks M. Histoplasmosis in patients with acquired immunodeficiency syndrome. Am J Clin Pathol 1990; 93:367–72.
134. Berengner J, Morena S, Cercenado E, Bernaldo de Quiros JCL, Garcia de la Fuente A, Bouza E. Visceral leishmaniasis in patients infected with human immunodeficiency virus (HIV). Ann Intern Med 1989; 111:129–32.
135. Heyman MR, Rasmussen P. *Pneumocystis carinii* involvement of the bone marrow in acquired immunodeficiency syndrome. Am J Clin Pathol 1987; 87: 780–3.
136. Frickhofen N, Abkowitz JL, Safford M, et al. Persistent B19 parvovirus infection in patients infected with human immunodeficiency virus type 1 (HIV-1): a treatable cause of anemia in AIDS. Ann Intern Med 1990; 113:926–33.
137. Gordin FM, Simon GL, Wofsy CB, Mills J. Adverse reactions to trimethoprim-sulfamethoxazole in patients with the acquired immunodeficiency syndrome. Ann Intern Med 1984; 100:495–9.
138. Wormser GP, Krupp LB, Hanrahan JP, Gavis G, Spira TJ, Cunningham-Rundles S. Acquired immunodeficiency syndrome in male prisoners. Ann Intern Med 1983; 98:297–303.
139. Walker RE, Parker RI, Kovacs JA, et al. Anemia and erythropoiesis in patients with the acquired immunodeficiency syndrome (AIDS) and Kaposi sarcoma treated with zidovudine. Ann Intern Med 1988; 108:372–6.

140. Pedersen C, Ingeberg S, Teglbjaerg LS. Serum thymidine kinase—a marker of bone marrow toxicity during treatment with zidovudine. AIDS 1989; 3:743–6.
141. Burkes RL, Cohen H, Krailo M, Sinow RM, Carmel R. Low serum cobalamin levels occur frequently in the acquired immune deficiency syndrome and related disorders. Eur J Haematol 1987; 38:141–7.
142. Gill PS, Rarick M, Brynes RK, Causey D, Loureiro C, Levine AM. Azidothymidine associated with bone marrow failure in the acquired immunodeficiency syndrome (AIDS). Ann Intern Med 1987; 107:502–5.
143. Chow F-PR, Sutton PA, Hamburger AW. Sensitivity of erythroid progenitor colonies to erythropoietin in azidothymidine treated immunodeficient mice. Br J Haematol 1991; 77:139–44.
144. Fischl M, Galpin JE, Levine JD, et al. Recombinant human erythropoietin for patients with AIDS treated with zidovudine. N Engl J Med 1990; 322:1488–93.
145. DaCosta NA, Hultin MB. Effective therapy of human immunodeficiency virus-associated anemia with recombinant human erythropoietin despite high endogenous erythropoietin. Am J Hematol 1991; 36:71–2.
146. Dainiak N, Worthington M, Riordan MA, Kreczko S, Goldman L. 3′-Azido-3′-deoxythymidine (AZT) inhibits proliferation in vitro of human haematopoietic progenitor cells. Br J Haematol 1988; 69:299–304.
147. Ganser A, Greher J, Volkers B, Staszewski S, Hoelzer D. Inhibitory effect of azidothymidine, 2′3′-dideoxyadenosine, and 2-′3′-dideoxycytidine on in vitro growth of hematopoietic progenitor cells from normal persons and from patients with AIDS. Exp Hematol 1989; 17:321–5.
148. Sommadossi J-P, Carlisle R. Toxicity of 3′-azido-3′-deoxythymidine and 9-(1,3-dihydroxy-2-propoxymethyl)guanine for normal human hematopoietic progenitor cells in vitro. Antimicrob Agents Chemother 1987; 31:452–4.
149. Johnson M, Caiazzo T, Molina J-M, Donahue R, Groopman J. Inhibition of bone marrow myelopoiesis and erythropoiesis in vitro by anti-retroviral nucleoside derivatives. Br J Haematol 1988; 70:137–41.
150. Bhalla K, Birkhofer M, Grant S, Graham G. The effect of recombinant human granulocyte-macrophage colony-stimulating factor (rGM-CSF) on 3′-azido-3′-deoxythymidine (AZT)-mediated biochemical and cytotoxic effects on normal human myeloid progenitor cells. Exp Hematol 1989; 17:17–20.
151. Hochster H, Dieterich D, Bozzette S, et al. Toxicity of combined gancyclovir and zidovudine for cytomegalovirus disease associated with AIDS. Ann Intern Med 1990; 113:111–7.
152. Abraham NG, Bucher D, Niranjan U, et al. Microenvironmental toxicity of azidothymidine: partial sparing with hemin. Blood 1989; 74:139–44.
153. Bogliolo G, Lerza R, Mencoboni M, Saviane A, Pannacciulli I. Azidothymidine-induced depression of murine hemopoietic progenitor cells. Exp Hematol 1988; 16:938–40.
154. Stella CC, Ganser A, Hoelzer D. Defective in vitro growth of the hemopoietic progenitor cells in the acquired immunodeficiency syndrome. J Clin Invest 1987; 80:286–93.

155. Bagnara GP, Zauli G, Giovannini M, Re MC, Furlini G, La Placa M. Early loss of circulating hemopoietic progenitors in HIV-1-infected subjects. Exp Hematol 1990; 18:426–30.
156. Donahue RE, Johnson MM, Zon LI, Clark SC, Groopman JE. Suppression of in vitro haematopoiesis following human immunodeficiency virus infection. Nature 1987; 326:200–3.
157. Burgaleta C, Bello JL, Magallon M. Granulopoietic precursors in hemophiliac patients infected by HTLV-III/LAV. Am J Clin Pathol 1987; 88:121.
158. Watanabe M, Reimann KA, DeLong, PA, Liu T, Fisher RA, Letvin NL. Effect of recombinant soluble CD4 in rhesus monkeys infected with simian immunodeficiency virus of macaques. Nature 1989; 337:267–70.
159. Dalgleish AG, Beverley PCL, Clapham PR, Crawford DH, Greaves MF, Weiss RA. The CD4 (T4) antigen is an essential component of the receptor for the AIDS retrovirus. Nature 1984; 312:763–7.
160. Klatzmann D, Champagne E, Chamaret S, et al. T-lymphocyte T4 molecule behaves as the receptor for human retrovirus LAV. Nature 1984; 312:767–8.
161. Gartner S, Markovitz P, Markovitz DM, Kaplan MH, Gallo RC, Popovic M. The role of mononuclear phagocytes in HTLV-III/LAV infection. Science 1986; 233:215–8.
162. Ho DD, Sarngadharan MG, Resnick L, Dimarzo-Veronese F, Rota TR, Hirsch MS. Primary human T-lymphotropic virus type III infection. Ann Intern Med 1985; 103:880–3.
163. Nicholson JKA, Cross GD, Callaway CS, McDougal JS. In vitro infection of human monocytes with human T lymphotropic virus type III/lymphadenopathy-associated virus (HTLV-III/LAV). J Immunol 1986; 137:323–9.
164. Zucker-Franklin D, Seremetis S, Zheng ZY. Internalization of human immunodeficiency virus type I and other retroviruses by megakaryocytes and platelets. Blood 1990; 75:1920–3.
165. Sakaguchi M, Sato T, Groopman JE. Human immunodeficiency virus infection of megakaryocytic cells. Blood 1991; 77:481–5.
166. Folks TM, Kessler SW, Orenstein JM, Justement JS, Jaffe ES, Fauci AS. Infection and replication of HIV-1 in purified progenitor cells of normal human bone marrow. Science 1988; 242:919–22.
167. Kitano K, Abboud CN, Ryan DH, Quan SG, Baldwin GC, Golde DW. Macrophage-active colony-stimulating factors enhance human immunodeficiency virus type 1 infection in bone marrow stem cells. Blood 1991; 77:1699–705.
168. McCune JM. HIV-1: The infective process in vivo. Cell 1991; 64:351–63.
169. von Laer D, Hufert FT, Fenner TE, et al. $CD34^+$ hematopoietic progenitor cells are not a major reservoir of the human immunodeficiency virus. Blood 1990; 76:1281–6.
170. Scadden DT, Zeira M, Woon A, et al. Human immunodeficiency virus infection of human bone marrow stromal fibroblasts. Blood 1990; 76:317–22.
171. Miles SA, Mitsuyasu RT, Lee K, et al. Recombinant human granulocyte colony-stimulating factor increases circulating burst forming unit-erythron and red

blood cell production in patients with severe human immunodeficiency virus infection. Blood 1990; 75:2137–42.

172. Roberts DE, Berman SM, Nakasato S, Wyle FA, Wishnow RM, Segal GP. Effect of lithium carbonate on zidovudine-associated neutropenia in the acquired immunodeficiency syndrome. Am J Med 1988; 85:428–31.
173. Hufert FT, Laer DV, Schramm C, Tarnok A, Schmitz H. Detection of HIV-1 DNA in different subsets of human peripheral blood mononuclear cells using the polymerase chain reaction. Arch Virol 1989; 106:341–5.
174. McElrath MJ, Pruett JE, Cohn ZA. Mononuclear phagocytes of blood and bone marrow: comparative roles as viral reservoirs in human immunodeficiency virus type 1 infections. Proc Natl Acad Sci USA 1989; 86:675–9.
175. Lucey DR, Dorsky DI, Nicholson-Weller A, Weller PF. Human eosinophils express CD4 protein and bind human immunodeficiency virus 1 gp120. J Exp Med 1989; 169:327–32.
176. Baldwin GC, Fleischmann J, Chung Y, Koyanagi Y, Chen ISY, Golde DW. Human immunodeficiency virus causes mononuclear phagocyte dysfunction. Proc Natl Acad Sci U S A 1990; 87:3933–7.
177. Smith PD, Ohura K, Masur H, Lane HC, Fauci AS, Wahl SM. Monocyte function in the acquired immune deficiency syndrome. J Clin Invest 1984; 74:2121–8.
178. Poli G, Bottazzi B, Acero R, et al. Monocyte function in intravenous drug abusers with lymphadenopathy syndrome: selective impairment of chemotaxis. Clin Exp Immunol 1985; 62:136–47.
179. Baldwin GC, Gasson JC, Quan SG, et al. Granulocyte-macrophage colony-stimulating factor enhances neutrophil function in acquired immunodeficiency syndrome patients. Proc Natl Acad Sci U S A 1988; 85:2763–6.
180. Kitano K, Baldwin GC, Raines MA, Golde DW. Differentiating agents facilitate infection of myeloid leukemia cell lines by monocytotropic HIV-1 strains. Blood 1990; 76:1980–8.
181. Folks TM, Justement J, Kinter A, Dinarello CA, Fauci AS. Cytokine-induced expression of HIV-1 in a chronically infected promonocyte cell line. Science 1987; 238:800.
182. Perno C-F, Yarchoan R, Cooney DA, et al. Replication of human immunodeficiency virus in monocytes. J Exp Med 1989; 169:933–51.
183. Koyanagi Y, O'Brien WA, Zhao JQ, Golde DW, Gasson JD, Chen ISY. Cytokines alter production of HIV-1 from primary mononuclear phagocytes. Science 1988; 241:1673–5.
184. Hammer SM, Gillis JM, Groopman JE, Rose RM. In vitro modification of human immunodeficiency virus infection in granulocyte-macrophage colony-stimulating factor and g interferon. Proc Natl Acad Sci U S A 1986; 83:8734–8.
185. Hammer SM, Gillis JM, Pinkson P, Rose RM. Effect of zidovudine and granulocyte-macrophage colony-stimulating factor on human immunodeficiency virus replication in alveolar macrophages. Blood 1990; 75:1215–9.

186. Schuitemaker H, Kootstra NA, van Oers, MHJ, van Lambalgen R, Tersmette M, Miedema F. Induction of monocyte proliferation and HIV expression by IL-3 does not interfere with antiviral activity of zidovudine. Blood 1990; 76: 1490–3.
187. Crapper RM, Deam DR, Mackay IR. Paraproteinemias in homosexual men with HIV infection. Am J Clin Pathol 1987; 88:348–51.
188. Blumenfeld W, Beckstead JH. Angioimmunoblastic lymphadenopathy with dysproteinemia in homosexual men with acquired immune deficiency syndrome. Arch Pathol Lab Med 1983; 107:567–9.
189. Steinberg AD, Seldin MF, Jaffe ES, et al. Angioimmunoblastic lymphadenopathy with dysproteinemia. Ann Intern Med 1988; 108:575–84.
190. Gold JWM, Weikel CL, Godbold J, et al. Unexplained persistent lymphadenopathy in homosexual men and the acquired immune deficiency syndrome. Medicine (Baltimore) 1985; 64:203–13.
191. Murray HW, Godbold JH, Jurica KB, Roberts RB. Progression to AIDS in patients with lymphadenopathy or AIDS-related complex: reappraisal of risk and predictive factors. Am J Med 1989; 86:533–8.
192. Biggar RJ, Horm J, Goedert JJ, Melbye M. Cancer in the group at risk of acquired immunodeficiency syndrome (AIDS) through 1984. Am J Epidemiol 1987, 126:578–86.
193. Moore RD, Kessler H, Richman DD, Flexner C, Chaisson RE. Non-Hodgkin's lymphoma in patients with advanced HIV infection treated with zidovudine. JAMA 1991; 265:2208–11.
194. Kaplan LD, Abrams DI, Feigal E, et al. AIDS-associated non-Hodgkin's lymphoma in San Francisco. JAMA 1989; 261:719–24.
195. Knowles DM, Chamulak GA, Subar M, et al. Lymphoid neoplasia associated with the acquired immunodeficiency. Ann Intern Med 1988; 108:744–53.
196. Ciobanu N, Andreeff M, Safai B, Koziner B, Mertelsmann R. Lymphoblastic neoplasia in a homosexual patient with Kaposi's sarcoma. Ann Intern Med 1983; 98:151–5.
197. Presant CA, Gala K, Wiseman C, et al. Human immunodeficiency virus-associated T-cell lymphoblastic lymphoma in AIDS. Cancer 1987; 60:1459–61.
198. Serrano M, Bellas C, Campo E, et al. Hodgkin's disease in patients with antibodies to human immunodeficiency virus. Cancer 1990; 65:2248–54.
199. Knowles DM. Malignant lymphomas occurring in association with acquired immunodeficiency syndrome. Lab Med 1986; 17:674–8.
200. Lippman SM, Volk JR, Spier CM, Grogan TM. Clonal ambiguity of human immunodeficiency virus-associated lymphomas. Arch Pathol Lab Med 1988; 112:128–32.
201. Subar M, Neri A, Inghirami G, Knowles DM, Dalla-Favera R. Frequent c-*myc* oncogene activation and infrequent presence of Epstein-Barr virus genome in AIDS-associated lymphoma. Blood 1968; 72:667–71.

202. Holland HK, Saral R, Rossi JJ, et al. Allogeneic bone marrow transplantation, zidovudine, and human immunodeficiency virus type 1 (HIV-1) infection. Ann Intern Med 1989; 111:973–81.

# 10

# Friend Spleen Focus-Forming Virus

**Sandra K. Ruscetti**

*National Cancer Institute*
*Frederick, Maryland*

## INTRODUCTION

The Friend virus complex induces an acute erythroleukemia in susceptible strains of both adult and newborn mice. It consists of two components: the defective spleen focus-forming virus (SFFV), which is responsible for the acute pathogenicity of the complex, and the Friend murine leukemia virus (MuLV), which acts as a helper virus for the defective SFFV. Since it was first described by Friend in 1957 (1), Friend virus has been the subject of numerous studies by both hematologists and virologists (for earlier reviews, see Refs. 2–4). It is interesting from a hematologic standpoint because SFFV exclusively affects the erythroid pathway and alters the requirements of erythroid precursor cells for the erythroid hormone erythropoietin (Epo). Virologically, the SFFV component of the viral complex is an intriguing virus because it causes an acute leukemia in the absence of a classic oncogene. Instead, the virus possesses a unique envelope gene that is responsible for the early effects of the virus on erythroid cell growth. Finally, SFFV-induced disease is a good model for studying tumor progression because the disease consists of well-defined stages, from the hyperplasia of erythroid cells to the outgrowth of autonomously proliferating cells. Recent technological advances have provided us with the tools not only for dissecting the virus complex to understand the pathogenic elements for the various stages but also for characterizing the components of the erythroid pathway with which the viral gene products may interact to alter cell growth. This review covers studies carried out by a number of laboratories to determine the effects of the Friend virus complex on erythroid cells and the role of specific viral genes in this process.

## EFFECTS OF THE SPLEEN FOCUS-FORMING VIRUS ON HEMATOPOIETIC CELLS

### Erythroid Hyperplasia

The Friend spleen-focus-forming virus induces an acute erythroleukemia in adult mice that is manifested by foci on the surface of the spleen at 9–10 days and a greatly enlarged spleen and liver at 2–3 weeks after injection (see Table 1) (1,5,6). The animals generally die within 6 weeks, often as a result of splenic rupture. This represents the hyperplastic phase of the disease and is the direct result of virus infection. Two variants of SFFV have been described that have somewhat different effects in the animal: $SFFV_P$ and $SFFV_A$ (see Fig. 1). Mice infected with $SFFV_P$ develop erythroleukemia associated with polycythemia (7–10). Although Epo levels in these mice are undetectable, erythropoiesis does not cease. Within 2 days of virus infection, spleen cells from these mice show a large increase in late erythroid colonies (colony-forming units-erythroid, CFU-E) that are Epo independent (11–13) and proliferate to high levels in a [$^3$H]thymidine assay in the absence of Epo (14). In contrast, mice infected with $SFFV_A$ develop erythroleukemia without polycythemia, and erythropoiesis in these mice is sensitive to normal physiologic controls (15,16). Although $SFFV_A$-infected mice show an overall increase in erythrocyte production, the hematocrit is slightly decreased as a result of an increased plasma volume (16). Spleen cells from these mice, like those from mice infected with $SFFV_P$, also show a large increase in CFU-E, but development of these colonies depends upon the presence of Epo (15, 17). Spleen cells from $SFFV_A$-infected mice can proliferate in a [$^3$H]thymidine

**Table 1** SFFV-Induced Leukemia

| |
|---|
| Exclusively erythroid: predominant cell is a progenitor erythroblast |
| Induced in newborn or adult mice |
| Early onset (9 days, splenic foci) |
| Rapid acute phase (beginning at 2 weeks) |
| Grossly enlarged spleen and liver |
| High hematocrit ($SFFV_P$) or mild anemia ($SFFV_A$) |
| Death (2½–5 weeks) |

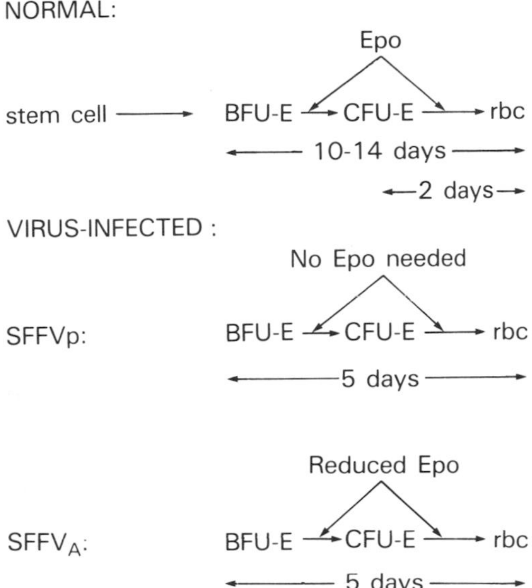


**Figure 1** Early effects of SFFV on erythroid cell growth. Normal cells require Epo, but cells infected with SFFV can proliferate and differentiate in the presence of low amounts of Epo or in its absence. BFU-E, burst-forming units, erythroid; CFU-E, colony-forming units, erythroid; rbc, red blood cells.

assay in the absence of Epo, but in contrast to cells from $SFFV_P$-infected animals, the level of proliferation is greatly enhanced by addition of the hormone (14).

The target for SFFV appears to be a late erythroid precursor cell that is Epo responsive (10,18). Studies using cell separation techniques have suggested that the target cell for SFFV is located in a compartment between the day 8 BFU-E and the day 2 CFU-E. These cells are in a state of active cellular DNA synthesis, which may be required for the proper integration of the SFFV genome into the host cellular DNA (19,20).

In addition to studying the effects of SFFV in mice, the results of in vitro infection of erythroid cells with SFFV can also be measured. When erythroid precursor cells are inoculated with $SFFV_P$ and plated in methylcellulose, large clusters of erythroid bursts (vBFU-E) form after 5–6 days in the absence of Epo (21). Uninfected cells or cells infected with helper virus alone do not form erythroid bursts in the absence of Epo. vBFU-E can also be detected 5–6 days after infection with $SFFV_A$ (22), but the cells in these colonies do not differentiate into mature red blood cells unless a small amount of Epo is added to the culture, an amount too low to induce differentiation of uninfected erythroid precursor cells.

SFFV can also induce changes in long-term bone marrow suspension cultures if the cultures are grown under conditions that favor erythropoiesis (23). Like mice infected with $SFFV_P$, these cultures show an accumulation of Epo-independent CFU-E and eventually develop into autonomous erythroid cell lines.

The ability of $SFFV_P$ to abrogate factor dependence has been dramatically shown after infection of an Epo-dependent erythroleukemia cell line from a mouse infected with Friend MuLV (24). The SFFV-infected, factor-independent cell lines offer an advantage over spleen cells from virus-infected mice in that they are a homogeneous population of cells that have an uninfected counterpart for comparison. Expression of an SFFV gene product is the only event necessary for transformation of the Epo-dependent cells: the lines can be generated at high frequency (approximately 10% of the cells become factor independent), and the factor-independent cells express high levels of the SFFV envelope glycoprotein. $SFFV_P$ appears to be unique in its ability to abrogate the factor dependence of these cells, since infection with other retroviruses carrying a variety of different oncogenes does not have this effect. Factor-independent cell lines can also be generated after infection with $SFFV_A$, but consistent with previous data on the biologic effects of the virus, they are generated at a much lower efficiency (approximately 0.04% of the cells become Epo independent) than after infection with $SFFV_P$. The ability of $SFFV_P$ to induce factor independence is unique to the erythroid pathway, since infection of interleukin-3 (IL-3)-dependent cells with the virus has no effect (24,25). However, $SFFV_P$ has induced factor independence in an IL-3-dependent lymphoid cell line when it was coexpressed with the Epo receptor gene (25).

## Malignant Transformation of Erythroid Cells

Erythroid cells proliferating in the early stages of SFFV-induced disease have a limited self-renewal capacity and fail to grow when transplanted to syngeneic mice or as established cell lines in vitro. However, around 3 weeks after infection with $SFFV_P$ and 7–8 weeks after infection with $SFFV_A$, spleens of SFFV-infected mice contain more autonomous cells, which represents a second stage in the transformation process (see Fig. 2) (16,26). These cells, unlike those in the first stage, are monoclonal and probably represent the progeny of a single cell that has undergone a secondary genetic event. Cells in this stage can be detected by their ability to grow in the omentum of sublethally irradiated mice (27) or in the spleens of $Sl/Sl^d$ mice, which have a defect in their hematopoietic microenvironment (28), as well as by their ability

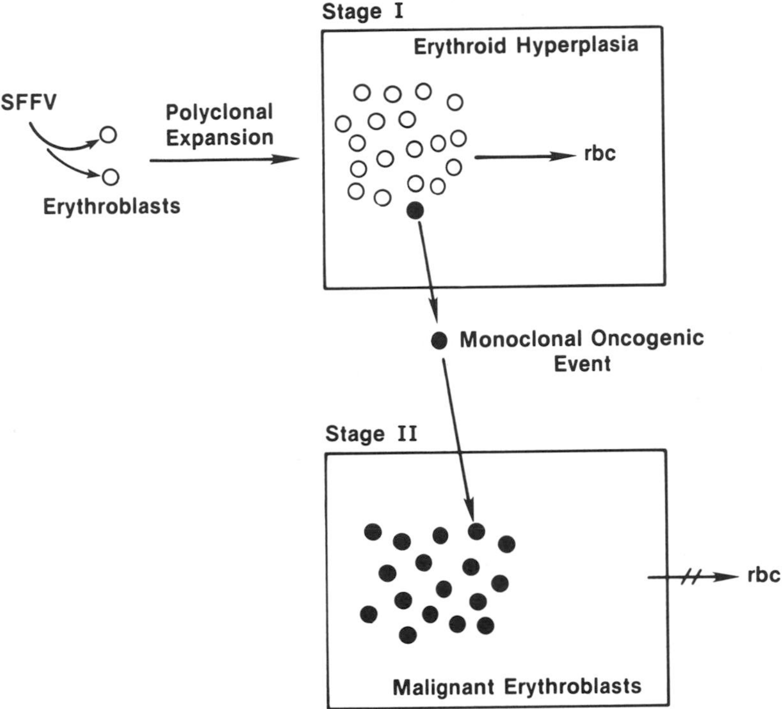


**Figure 2** Progressive stages of transformation of erythroid cells by SFFV. Infection of erythroblasts with SFFV leads to erythroid hyperplasia without blocking differentiation (stage I). These cells have a limited self-renewal capacity and fail to grow when transplanted to syngeneic mice or in vitro. A rare cell in this proliferating population becomes transformed as a result of a secondary genetic event (stage II). These cells, which are blocked in differentiation, can be transplanted to syngeneic mice and grow in vitro.

to form macroscopic colonies in methylcellulose (29). These cells have an unlimited self-renewal capacity and can grow as subcutaneous tumors in syngeneic mice and as continuous erythroleukemia cell lines (the classic MEL lines) (30–32). Unlike cells in the first stage of SFFV-induced disease, these cells are blocked in their ability to differentiate but can be induced to do so with certain chemicals, such as dimethylsulfoxide (33).

## Indirect Effects of SFFV

Mice infected with SFFV can also exhibit changes in hematopoietic cells that are not due to a direct effect of the virus. Whether these changes play a role in the pathogenic process or whether they occur in response to the erythroid hyperplasia induced by the virus is not known. For example, SFFV infection leads to both an increase in the production of and hypersensitivity of cells to burst-promoting activity, later shown to be IL-3, a factor involved in the proliferation of early erythroid as well as myeloid precursor cells (34). Also, macrophage-like cells from SFFV-infected mice produce high levels of a factor that inhibits normal erythroid differentiation but stimulates the differentiation of erythroid precursor cells from SFFV-infected mice (35). Both these effects may lead to an increase in the number of target cells for the virus. In other studies, infection of long-term bone marrow cultures with $SFFV_P$ pseudotyped with Friend MuLV led to the frequent isolation of IL-3-dependent myeloid cell lines (36). It was later shown that IL-3-dependent myeloid cell lines can be obtained from the spleens of mice infected with helper-free $SFFV_P$ (37). These in vivo derived cell lines do not contain virus and are thought to be a host response to leukemogenesis. Finally, infection of Fv-2-resistant mice with SFFV, which does not result in the development of erythroleukemia, leads to extended self-renewal of pluripotent hematopoietic stem cells (38), whereas injection of SFFV into $W/W^v$ mice, which are deficient in hematopoietic stem cells and resistant to SFFV-induced erythroleukemia, restored the spleen colony-forming capacity of the $W/W^v$ stem cells but left their self-renewal defective (39).

## GENETIC STRUCTURE OF SFFV

Once SFFV was cloned free of its helper virus it was possible to study its structure and compare it with other MuLV. SFFV appears to have arisen by recombination of Friend MuLV, which induces no acute disease in adult mice, with envelope (*env*) gene sequences present in mouse DNA, sequences related to those found in mink cell focus-inducing (MCF) viruses (40,41). As shown in Figure 3, this results in a virus that differs from Friend MuLV in that it contains deletions in all its structural genes and a unique envelope gene. A typical mouse retrovirus, such as Friend MuLV, consists of three structural genes: the *gag* gene, which encodes proteins that make up the core of the virus particle; the *pol* gene, which encodes the RNA-dependent DNA polymerase used to convert the viral RNA into a DNA copy to be integrated into the host DNA; and the *env* gene, which encodes the proteins that make up the outside envelope of the virus. These genes are flanked by regulatory sequences called long terminal repeat (LTR) sequences. Unlike the typical retroviral genome, the SFFV genome encodes two products: a 45 kD protein encoded by the deleted *gag* sequences, which is not produced by all isolates of SFFV (42), and a gp52/55 that is encoded by the deleted *env* gene (43–45). SFFV is unique compared to other acutely transforming retroviruses

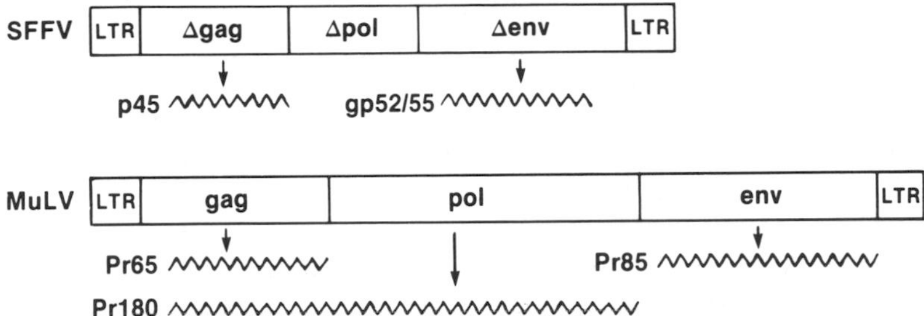


**Figure 3** Comparison of the genomes of SFFV and a typical murine leukemia virus (MuLV). SFFV contains deletions Δ in all its structural genes and a unique envelope gene. It codes for a 45 kD gag-related protein and a 52/55 kD envelope glycoprotein.

in that it consists entirely of retroviral sequences and does not carry a classic oncogene to which one could attribute its biologic activity. Since SFFV lacks functional *gag, pol,* and *env* proteins, it is defective for replication and requires helper virus-encoded proteins that act in trans to allow the SFFV genome to enter and integrate into the DNA of the host cell. Thus, studies with SFFV have traditionally been carried out in the presence of a helper virus.

## LOCALIZATION OF SEQUENCES IN SFFV RESPONSIBLE FOR PATHOGENICITY AND TARGET CELL SPECIFICITY

In an effort to understand the molecular basis for the transforming nature of SFFV, studies have been carried out by a number of laboratories to dissect the viral genome to determine the location of the pathogenic elements. Early studies using subgenomic fragments of the SFFV genome, as well as deletion mutants, showed that the pathogenic region of SFFV could be entirely localized to a 1.5 kb region encompassing both the *env* gene and a portion of the LTR sequences and that *gag* and *pol* sequences are not required to produce disease (46,47). In subsequent studies, it was shown that substitution of the LTR sequences with analogous sequences from other retroviruses, including those from lymphoma-inducing viruses, had no effect on the nature of the disease (48). This lent support to the idea that the *env* gene, which encodes gp52/55, may be the gene responsible for the initiation of erythroid hyperplasia by the virus. That the *env* gene is sufficient and essential for pathogenicity was most conclusively demonstrated in studies utilizing a Moloney MuLV-based retroviral vector that expressed only the *env* gene product from SFFV (49). When the vector containing the SFFV *env* gene in the correct orientation was introduced along with helper virus into fibroblasts, the resulting virus complex induced a rapid erythroid disease in mice that was indistinguishable from that induced by the entire SFFV genome. Spleen cells from the diseased mice expressed the SFFV *env* gene product but not the *gag* gene product. Mice that were given virus that contained the SFFV *env* gene in the reverse orientation did not express the SFFV envelope protein or develop erythroleukemia. Consistent with these results, transgenic mice expressing the SFFV *env* gene under control of either the SFFV LTR or the cytoplasmic $\beta$-actin transcriptional regulatory unit were shown to develop erythroleukemia (50). Thus, the envelope gene product of SFFV is responsible for the acute effects of this virus on erythroid cell growth.

Because SFFV is defective for replication, most studies of the virus are carried out with a complex consisting of SFFV and certain replication-competent helper viruses. Erythroleukemia can be induced by helper-free SFFV (51–53), however, and the disease is progressive in animals that are pretreated with the chemical phenylhydrazine to increase the number of erythroid target cells for the virus (51). This suggests that helper virus does not contribute directly to the erythroid hyperplasia induced by the SFFV complex but allows the spread of virus to a critical number of erythroid target cells. Not all replication-competent MuLV, however, can act as helper viruses for SFFV. Akv, the endogenous ecotropic virus of AKR mice, is one such virus (54). The failure of Akv to act as a helper for SFFV is not due to the inability of Akv to package SFFV RNA (54) but may be due to the failure of the Akv envelope protein to recognize specific receptors on erythroid cells.

## CHARACTERIZATION OF THE SFFV ENVELOPE GENE AND ITS PRODUCT

### Comparison with the Envelope Genes of Other Murine Leukemia Viruses

The SFFV *env* gene product, although related to those of other retroviruses, has certain unique features that are conserved in every strain and may be important for pathogenicity (see Fig. 4). A typical retroviral envelope gene encodes an 85 kD precursor protein that is cleaved into gp70, p15E, and an R peptide (55). The SFFV envelope gene contains three major changes compared to the envelope gene of a typical retrovirus, such as Friend MuLV (56–58). First, the SFFV *env* gene contains 5′ sequences that are related to the *env* gene sequences of MCF viruses, which like SFFV carry envelope genes derived from mouse DNA. Second, the *env* gene of SFFV contains a centrally located, 585 base pair deletion in the open reading frame of the

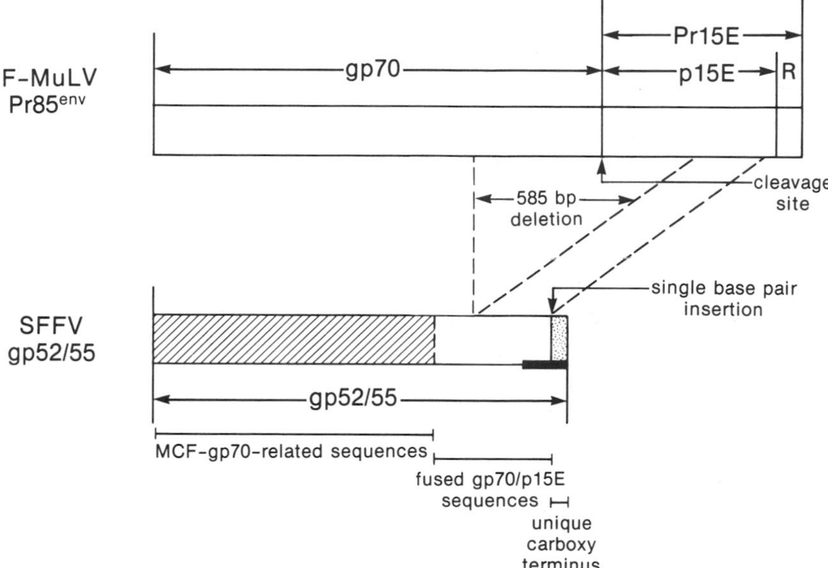


**Figure 4** Comparison of the envelope proteins of Friend MuLV and SFFV. SFFV contains three basic changes in its envelope protein compared to Friend MuLV. In the SFFV envelope protein, the hatched area represents the region related to the gp70 of mink cell focus-inducing (MCF) viruses and the open area is that derived from F-MuLV. The dotted area is the unique sequence caused by the single base pair insertion and the resulting shift in reading frame, and the heavy bar represents the p15E-related transmembrane domain of the SFFV envelope protein.

gene, resulting in a gene product, gp52/55, which is considerably smaller than the standard retroviral envelope precursor and has covalently linked terminal portions of gp70 and p15E. Finally, the gene has a single base pair insertion in the p15E-coding region, which results in a changed reading frame, translation of a short unique sequence, and premature termination 34 base pairs before the termination codon in MuLV p15E. Thus, compared with the envelope protein of Friend MuLV, the envelope protein encoded by SFFV lacks a cytoplasmic tail.

## Importance of Conserved Changes for Pathogenicity

To determine which changes in the envelope gene are essential for rendering SFFV an acutely pathogenic virus, several laboratories prepared recombinants between SFFV and F-MuLV to restore the large deletion or remove the base pair insertion that resulted in a truncated protein. A requirement for the single base pair insertion occurring at the 3′ end of the SFFV *env* gene was shown by construction of a chimeric envelope gene that codes for a molecule with the amino-terminal two-thirds derived from the SFFV envelope gene and the carboxy-terminal domain derived from F-MuLV p15E (59,60). The protein encoded by this chimeric envelope gene still contains the large deletion present in the wild-type SFFV envelope protein but now has a cytoplasmic tail. Unlike the wild-type SFFV, a complex of this chimeric virus with helper virus failed to induce erythroleukemia in mice. However, passage of the chimeric virus through newborn mice gave rise to weakly pathogenic variants of the injected SFFV (60). When the variant SFFV were cloned and sequenced, it was found that they had regained the single base pair insertion, indicating that the 3′ insertion was essential for the biologic activity of SFFV. In further studies (61), chimeric *env* genes were also made to determine the biologic significance of the 585 bp deletion in the SFFV *env* gene. When the *env* deletion in SFFV was filled with the corresponding *env* sequences of Friend MCF virus, leaving the single base pair insertion in the 3′ end of the SFFV *env* gene intact, the resulting virus was nonpathogenic in adult mice. The failure of this virus to cause disease does not appear to be due to the cleavage of the protein at the gp70/p15E cleavage site (which is missing in SFFV), since modification of this site to prevent cleavage failed to restore the pathogenicity of the virus. Pathogenic variants of the injected virus could be recovered after passage in newborn mice, however, and each had a distinct deletion within the *env* gene that was similar but not identical to that in the wild-type SFFV *env* gene. These combined results indicate that both the large deletion in the *env* gene of SFFV as well as a single base pair insertion in the p15E-coding region are required for the pathogenic activity of the envelope protein. This is consistent with earlier studies in which spontaneous mutants of SFFV were used to show that different nonoverlapping mutations throughout the *env* gene can eliminate pathogenicity (62). Thus, proper folding or tertiary structure of the protein may be crucial for allowing a biologically significant interaction of the envelope glycoprotein with its target.

In addition to studying the importance of certain SFFV *env* gene sequences for pathogenicity, studies have also been carried out to identify those changes that are necessary for distinct biologic effects of the virus on erythroid cells. As mentioned earlier, variants of SFFV exist that cause erythroleukemia but have different effects on erythroid cell growth. $SFFV_P$ renders erythroid cells Epo independent, but cells infected with $SFFV_A$ still require some Epo for proliferation and differentiation. These different biologic phenotypes conferred by each virus are due to the slightly different envelope genes that they carry (63). To localize the sequences in $SFFV_P$ responsible for its ability to confer Epo independence, recombinants between the envelope genes of the two viruses were prepared (64,65). The results indicated that a 113 bp region from $SFFV_P$, which encodes the p15E-related transmembrane region, was necessary and sufficient to confer the Epo-independent phenotype. Recombinants that lacked this transmembrane region from $SFFV_P$, even if they were expressed well on the cell surface, failed to confer Epo independence. Thus, the membrane-anchoring region of the envelope protein of $SFFV_P$ is important not only for pathogenicity but because particular sequences within this region determine the consequences of virus infection for erythroid cell growth.

## Biochemical Features of the SFFV Envelope Glycoprotein

The changes that have occurred in the envelope gene of SFFV result in a unique envelope glycoprotein (see Table 2). Unlike other retroviral envelope proteins, the SFFV envelope protein does not function as a structural protein in the virion (43,45). Most of the SFFV envelope protein is associated with the endoplasmic reticulum within the cell. A small percentage (3–5%) of envelope protein is further modified in the Golgi apparatus by the addition of complex carbohydrates and is transported as a 65 kD protein to the cell surface (43,66–69). The large deletion in the envelope gene of SFFV appears to be responsible for this inefficient transport to the cell surface (59,60,70), perhaps because of the poor formation of homodimers, which are needed for export from the endoplasmic reticulum to the Golgi apparatus (71–73). The envelope glycoprotein encoded by $SFFV_A$ is even more deficient in transport to the cell surface than the envelope protein of $SFFV_P$ (74), a quality apparently unrelated to the failure of $SFFV_A$ to induce Epo independence (65).

**Table 2** Properties of the SFFV-Encoded Transforming Protein

| |
|---|
| Contains exclusively MuLV envelope sequences |
| Highly homologous to MCF envelope protein at its amino terminus |
| Never becomes part of viral envelope |
| Poorly processed |
| Major species, gp52/55 |
| Associated with internal cellular membranes |
| Contains exclusively high-mannose oligosaccharides |
| Minor species, gp65 |
| Associated with cell surface membrane |
| Contains complex carbohydrate |
| Secreted from cell |

The cell surface form of the envelope proteins of $SFFV_P$ and $SFFV_A$ is efficiently released into the culture medium (75,76), the extracellular form being approximately 3 kD smaller than the cell-associated form (72,76). This would be consistent with cleavage of the protein at a site at the plasma membrane surface immediately preceding the transmembrane region, resulting in the transmembrane region of the envelope protein remaining embedded in the membrane. It is not known whether cleavage of the extracellular domain is important for pathogenicity.

## POSSIBLE MECHANISMS OF SFFV-INDUCED PATHOGENESIS

The primary effect of SFFV is to cause Epo-independent erythroid hyperplasia, apparently as a direct result of the expression of the envelope protein of the virus. The majority of the cells within this proliferating, virus-infected population are not transformed, but propagation of the rare, malignant cell is favored. Although these latter cells are infected with SFFV, their malignant nature is not due to expression of the SFFV envelope glycoprotein. Studies have therefore been carried out to try to determine the mechanisms by which SFFV can cause both hyperplasia and malignant transformation of erythroid cells.

### Erythroid Hyperplasia

Erythroid cells from mice infected with $SFFV_P$ differ from normal cells in that they can proliferate and differentiate in the absence of Epo. The mechanism by which the $SFFV_P$ envelope protein alters the growth and differentiation of erythroid cells is of obvious interest. Unlike the products of other acute leukemia-inducing retroviruses, the SFFV envelope protein has not been shown to be a protein kinase or a DNA binding protein. Several years ago it was proposed that the SFFV envelope protein contains an active site in its MCF-specific domain that binds to MCF-MuLV receptors on erythroid cells and that this interaction triggers their proliferation (77). This idea was based on the observation that pathogenic, but not nonpathogenic, SFFV cause a weak interference to superinfection by MCF MuLV. This model, however, does not explain why SFFV affects only erythroid cell growth, since MCF-MuLV receptors are present on many cell types, including lymphoid cells and fibroblasts. Since the SFFV envelope protein can be expressed in a variety of cell types but exerts its effect only on Epo-dependent erythroid cells, it is more likely that the SFFV envelope protein is mimicking, inducing, or interacting with a component of the Epo signal transduction pathway.

In recent years, much new information has emerged on erythropoietin and its receptor (for review, see Ref. 78). Erythropoietin is a 35–40 kD glycoprotein that is produced by the kidney in response to hypoxia. It interacts with its receptor on the surface of erythroid cells and transmits a signal through an unknown second messenger system. Once the gene was molecularly cloned (79–82), it was possible to study its interaction with receptors on the cell surface. Using iodinated Epo, it was shown that two classes of binding sites exist on erythroid cells: high-affinity receptors that bind Epo with a $K_d$ of 40–80 pM and lower affinity receptors that bind Epo with a $K_d$ of around 500 pM (83–87). Chemical cross-linking studies have indicated that the Epo receptor exists as 105 and 90 kD proteins on the cell surface (88–95), the 90 kD protein being a proteolytic cleavage product of the larger protein (96). Once Epo binds to its receptor on the cell surface, the complex is taken into the cell by endocytosis (83,84,97). Epo, and probably its receptor, are eventually degraded. In 1989, a cDNA clone of the Epo receptor was prepared (98). The sequence of the gene predicted that the receptor would be a 55 kD protein with a single membrane-spanning region. Unlike many growth factor receptors, the Epo receptor does not contain a tyrosine kinase domain. When expressed in COS cells, the Epo receptor cDNA generates both high and lower affinity binding sites and chemical cross-linking reveals binding to 105 and 65 kD proteins on the cell surface. Antisera to the Epo receptor can detect a 66 kD protein in erythroid cells but fails to detect a 105 kD protein (25,78). The 105 kD protein does not appear to be a homodimer of the smaller protein or a heavily glycosylated 66 kD protein (89,99). It is possible that the 105 kD protein represents a second component of the Epo receptor that is unrelated to the receptor that has been cloned. The cloned Epo receptor gene belongs to a family of growth factor receptors that include the receptors for IL-2$\beta$, IL-3, IL-4, IL-6, IL-7, and granulocyte-macrophage colony-stimulating factor (GM-CSF), as well as the receptors for prolactin and growth hormone (100–104).

There are a number of ways that expression of the SFFV envelope glycoprotein in erythroid cells could affect the Epo signal transduction pathway. The viral envelope protein could be a constitutively produced analog of Epo or its receptor, analogous to the products of a number of other acute leukemia-inducing retroviruses (55). However, the envelope protein of SFFV shares no homology to either Epo or the Epo receptor (81,82,98). Although the SFFV envelope protein is not related to Epo, it could be stimulating the production of Epo in erythroid cells, leading to autocrine growth in the absence of added Epo. Against this hypothesis is the lack of evidence that the SFFV-infected cells secrete or express Epo or depend upon it for their growth (24, 105). Finally, the SFFV envelope protein could be interacting with the Epo receptor or with a component involved in a postreceptor step in the Epo signal transduction pathway.

That the SFFV envelope protein is interacting with and triggering the Epo receptor is supported by several recent studies. Comparison of Epo-dependent erythroleukemia cells with those that were rendered factor independent by infection with $SFFV_P$ showed that the SFFV-infected cells had considerably fewer (four to sixfold) Epo receptors available for binding Epo (24). This suggested that the viral protein may be inhibiting Epo from binding to the receptor at the cell surface or may be preventing its transport to the cell surface. Once the Epo receptor gene was cloned and antiserum was prepared against its gene product, it was possible to carry out more direct studies to determine if the SFFV envelope protein is interacting with the Epo receptor. When both the SFFV *env* gene and the Epo receptor gene were coexpressed in fibroblasts, it was shown that the two proteins could be coprecipitated using double immune precipitation with anti-MuLV gp70 and anti-Epo sera (25). These data strongly suggested that the two proteins were tightly associated. The same association was seen when both the Epo receptor and the SFFV envelope protein were coexpressed in an IL-3-dependent lymphoid cell line (106). It will be important to determine if the same association can be detected in *erythroid* cells expressing the $SFFV_P$ envelope glycoprotein as well as in cells expressing the envelope protein of $SFFV_A$, which does not render erythroid cells Epo independent.

Most of the SFFV envelope glycoprotein expressed in erythroid cells exists as a gp52/55 protein that is associated with the endoplasmic reticulum, but a small percentage is further processed in the Golgi apparatus and transported to the cell surface, where it can be proteolytically cleaved proximal to the transmembrane domain and secreted from the cell. It is not known which form of the protein is important for determining the biologic activity of the virus, and the laboratory data are conflicting. On the one hand, studies using a series of *env* gene mutants suggested that the cell surface component of the SFFV glycoprotein was required for pathogenesis (77). In other studies, the SFFV envelope protein was found to be physically associated with the Epo receptor within the endoplasmic reticulum, at least in nonerythroid cells (106). It has also been suggested that the extracellular form of the SFFV envelope protein may be directly responsible for stimulating proliferation not only of virus-infected erythroid cells but also of adjacent cells (75,76). However, recent data (72,76) have shown that the extracellular form of the SFFV envelope protein lacks the transmembrane domain, which has been shown to be crucial for determining Epo independence (65). Thus, it is more likely that the transmembrane portion that remains embedded in the membrane, rather than the extracellular form of the protein, is responsible for the biologic activity of the virus.

## Malignant Transformation of Erythroid Cells

The progression from the early polyclonal proliferation of SFFV-infected erythroid cells to the appearance of monoclonal malignant erythroleukemic cells is thought to require additional molecular events. That these events are mediated by SFFV is supported by the findings that helper-free SFFV can lead to the generation of the malignant cells (107) and that similar cell lines have never been generated by any other MuLV, even Friend MuLV. It should also be noted that transformed cells derived from SFFV-infected mice are always erythroid in nature. Thus, the mechanism by which SFFV transforms cells is unique to erythroid cells.

Insertional mutagenesis has been proposed as a common mechanism for transformation of hematopoietic cells by retroviruses. Examination of erythroleukemia cells transformed by SFFV for common sites of SFFV integration showed that the virus integrated into a specific region of mouse DNA in 95% of the erythroid tumors studied (108). This integration led to rearrangement and enhanced transcription of the *spi*-1 gene (109), which is expressed at low levels in normal mouse spleen. No *spi*-1 gene rearrangement was detected in other virally induced myeloid, lymphoid, or erythroid tumors tested. The *spi*-1 gene is identical to the PU.1 gene (110,111), a mouse gene that encodes a sequence-specific DNA binding protein that binds to the PU box, a purine-rich sequence that can act as a lymphoid-specific enhancer. The PU.1 protein is normally expressed in macrophages and B cells, where it has no malignant potential. This suggests that inappropriate expression of the spi-1/PU.1 protein may activate cell division in erythroid cells by stimulating expression of other gene products involved in cell proliferation. Erythroleukemia cell lines from SFFV-infected mice, but not those from F-MuLV-infected mice, have been shown to synthesize a growth factor, similar to IL-3, which may allow the cells to grow in an autocrine fashion (112). Perhaps the gene encoding the growth factor can be activated by the *spi*-1 gene product. Independent studies utilizing a derivative of SFFV tagged with simian virus 40 DNA sequences (113) also identified a common site of SFFV integration, designated *imi*-1, which is probably identical to the *spi*-1 gene.

SFFV was also found to commonly integrate into the p53 gene (114–117), resulting either in overexpression of the p53 protein or in its inactivation. The p53 gene was inactivated in 20–40% of the SFFV-transformed erythroleukemia cell lines, lending support to the idea that the p53 gene is a tumor suppressor gene (116,117). Although p53 is overexpressed in the majority of SFFV-transformed cell lines, it is thought that the p53 protein in these cells is functionally inactive and inhibits the normal activity of p53 in the cells. Inactivation of the p53 gene does not appear, however, to be sufficient to induce the late stage of SFFV-induced disease but probably acts in conjunction with the *spi*-1 gene product.

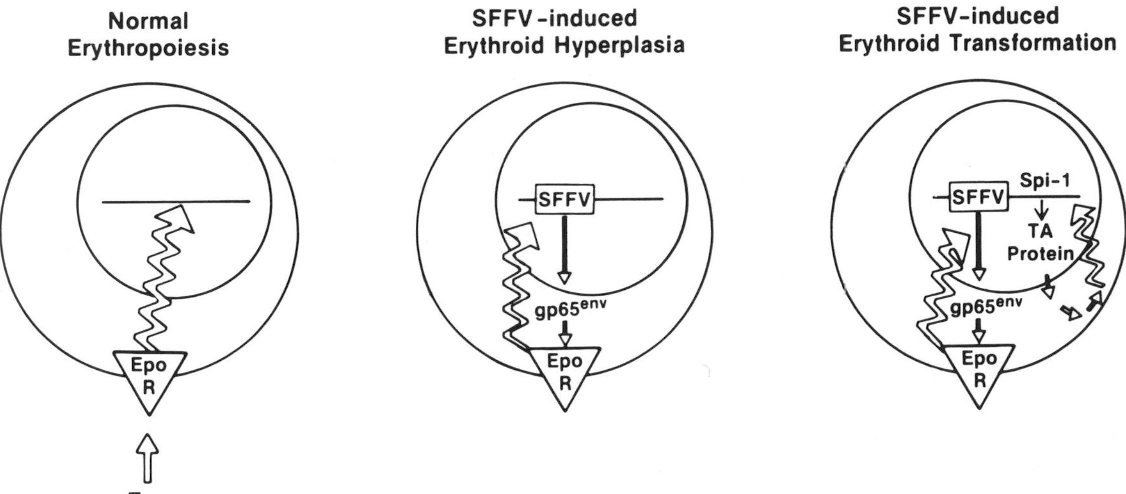


**Figure 5** Putative mechanisms for the biologic effects of SFFV on erythroid cells. Proliferation of normal erythroid cells requires Epo to bind to the Epo receptor (Epo R). Cells expressing the $SFFV_P$ envelope protein ($gp65^{env}$) can proliferate (jagged arrows) in the absence of Epo, perhaps by binding to and triggering the Epo receptor. SFFV integrates into host DNA near the Spi-1 gene and activates the expression of its trans-activating (TA) protein. This protein either directly or indirectly activates genes involved in transforming the cell.

## SUMMARY

Friend spleen focus-forming virus-induced erythroleukemia provides an excellent model system for studying various stages of retrovirus-induced diseases. Infection of a single erythroid cell with SFFV can lead to both hyperplasia and malignant transformation (see Fig. 5). The hyperplasia is due to expression of the unique envelope glycoprotein encoded by SFFV, which appears to bind to and trigger the Epo receptor. Malignant transformation is due to specific integration of SFFV into the host DNA and activation of the spi-1/Pu.1 gene, which encodes a transactivating protein that either directly or indirectly leads to immortalization of the cell. It is not known whether expression of the SFFV envelope protein is still needed in conjunction with the spi-1/Pu.1 gene product to induce transformation. SFFV-transformed erythroleukemia cell lines always continue to express the SFFV envelope glycoprotein, even though they often fail to express the envelope protein of the helper virus they contain (118).

SFFV is unique among acute leukemia-inducing mouse viruses in that it lacks a classic oncogene. Rather, its acute pathogenicity is associated with a modified viral structural protein. There are other examples of pathogenic retroviruses whose pathogenicity is associated with modified viral structural proteins. These include the Laterjet-Duplan strain of the radiation leukemia virus (the murine acquired immunodeficiency MAIDS, virus), which causes a severe immunodeficiency disease in mice as a result of expression of an altered *gag* gene (119,120); Cas-Br-E, an ecotropic virus from wild mice that causes hindlimb paralysis due to a unique envelope gene (121,122); FeLV-FAIDS, an isolate of the feline leukemia virus that causes a severe immunodeficiency syndrome in cats due to alterations in its envelope gene (123, 124); and mink cell focus-inducing viruses, which have altered envelope genes, related to those of SFFV, which are thought to be responsible for their ability to induce or accelerate leukemia in mice (for review, see Ref. 125). The human retroviruses, human T cell leukemia virus type I and human immunodeficiency virus, which cause T cell leukemia and an immunodeficiency syndrome, respectively, may also exert their effects through altered viral structural genes.

Because mouse DNA contains many copies of MCF viral envelope gene sequences, which are highly related to the SFFV *env* gene, it has not been possible to detect a normal cellular counterpart of the pathogenic gene. Thus, it is still conceivable that the SFFV envelope glycoprotein is an analog of a normal cellular protein. If a normal counterpart of the SFFV *env* gene exists, the role of its product may be to interact with the Epo receptor. However, it may not interact with the receptor in its native state, but only after Epo binding has induced a conformational change in the receptor. The $SFFV_P$ envelope protein may be able to interact with the Epo receptor in its native state and induce proliferation in the absence of Epo. The $SFFV_A$ envelope protein, because of changes in its transmembrane domain, may not be able to stimulate proliferation in the absence of Epo because it interacts less efficiently. As we learn more about the events that occur after Epo binds to its receptor, we will be able to design experiments to determine if the SFFV envelope protein has a normal counterpart in the Epo signal transduction pathway.

## ACKNOWLEDGMENTS

I thank Karen Cannon for her assistance in the preparation of this manuscript and Rose Aurigemma, Michiaki Masuda, and Frank Ruscetti for helpful comments and suggestions.

## REFERENCES

1. Friend C. Cell-free transmission in adult Swiss mice of a disease having the character of a leukemia. J Exp Med 1957; 105:307–18.
2. Ruscetti S, Wolff L. Spleen focus-forming virus: relationship of an altered envelope gene to the development of a rapid erythroleukemia. Curr Top Microbiol Immunol 1984; 112:21–44.
3. Ostertag W, Stocking C, Johnson GR, et al. Transforming genes and target cells of murine spleen focus-forming viruses. Adv Cancer Res 1987; 48:193–355.
4. Kabat D. Molecular biology of Friend viral erythroleukemia. Curr Top Microbiol Immunol 1989; 148:1–42.
5. Axelrad AA, Steeves RA. Assay for Friend leukemia virus: rapid quantitative method based on enumeration of macroscopic spleen foci in mice. Virology 1964; 24:513–8.
6. Mirand EA, Steeves RA, Ayila L, Grace JT. Spleen focus formation by polycythemic strains of Friend leukemia virus. Proc Soc Exp Biol Med 1968; 127:900–4.
7. Mirand EA. Virus-induced erythropoiesis in hypertransfused polycythemic mice. Science 1967; 156:832–3.
8. Mirand EA, Steeves RA, Lang RD, Grace JT. Virus-induced polycythemia in mice: erythropoiesis without erythropoietin. Proc Soc Exp Biol Med 1968; 128:844–9.
9. Sassa S, Takaku F, Nakao K. Regulation of erythropoiesis in the Friend leukemia mouse. Blood 1968; 31:758–65.
10. Tambourin P, Wendling F. Malignant transformation and erythroid differentiation by polycythaemia-inducing Friend virus. Nature 1971; 234:230–3.
11. Horoszewicz JS, Leong SS, Carter WA. Friend leukemia: rapid development of erythropoietin-independent hematopoietic precursors. J Natl Cancer Inst 1975; 54:265–7.

12. Liao S, Axelrad AA. Erythropoietin-independent erythroid colony formation in vitro by hematopoietic cells of mice infected with Friend virus. Int J Cancer 1975; 15:467–82.
13. Hankins WD, Krantz SB. In vitro expression of erythroid differentiation induced by Friend polycythemia virus. Nature 1975; 253:731–2.
14. Ruscetti SK. Employment of a ($^3$H) thymidine-incorporation assay to distinguish the effects of different Friend erythroleukemia-inducing retroviruses on erythroid cell proliferation. J Natl Cancer Inst 1986; 77:241–5.
15. Steinheider G, Seidel HJ, Kreja L. Comparison of the biological effects of anemia inducing and polycythemia inducing Friend virus complex. Experientia 1979; 35:1173–5.
16. Tambourin PE, Wendling F, Jasmin C, Smadja-Joffe F. The physiopathology of Friend leukemia. Leuk Res 1979; 3:117–29.
17. MacDonald ME, Reynolds FH, Van de Ven WJM, Stephenson JR, Mak TW, and Bernstein A. Anemia- and polycythemia-inducing isolates of Friend spleen focus-forming virus. Biological and molecular evidence for two distinct viral genomes. J Exp Med 1980; 151:1447–92.
18. Tambourin P, Wendling F. Target cell for oncogenic action of polycythaemia-inducing Friend virus. Nature 1975; 256:320–2.
19. Kost TA, Koury MJ, Hankins WD, Krantz SB. Target cells for Friend virus-induced erythroid bursts in vitro. Cell 1979; 18:145–52.
20. Kost TA, Koury MJ, Krantz SB. Mature erythroid burst forming units are target cells for Friend virus-induced erythroid bursts. Virology 1981; 108:309–17.
21. Hankins WD, Kost TA, Koury MJ, Krantz SB. Erythroid bursts produced by Friend leukemia virus in vitro. Nature 1978; 276:506–8.
22. Hankins WD, Troxler D. Polycythemia- and anemia-inducing erythroleukemia viruses exhibit differential erythroid transforming effects in vitro. Cell 1980; 22:693–9.
23. Dexter TM, Allen TD, Testa NG, Scolnick E. Friend disease in vitro. J Exp Med 1981; 154:594–608.
24. Ruscetti SK, Janesch NJ, Chakraborti A, Sawyer ST, Hankins WD. Friend spleen focus-forming virus induces factor independence in an erythropoietin-dependent erythroleukemia cell line. J Virol 1990; 63:1057–62.
25. Li J, D'Andrea AD, Lodish HF, Baltimore D. Activation of cell growth by binding of Friend spleen focus-forming virus gp55 glycoprotein to the erythropoietin receptor. Nature 1990; 343:762–4.
26. Tambourin P, Wendling F, Moreau-Gachelin F, Charon M, Bucau-Varlet P. Friend leukemia: a multi-step malignant disease. In: Rossi GB, ed. In vivo and in vitro erythropoiesis: the Friend system. Amsterdam, Elsevier, 1980, 127–38.
27. Wendling F, Moreau-Gachelin F, Tambourin P. Emergence of tumorigenic cells during the course of Friend virus leukemias. Proc Natl Acad Sci U S A 1981; 78: 3614–8.
28. Mager D, Mak TW, Bernstein A. Friend leukemia virus-transformed cells, unlike normal stem cells, form spleen colonies in $S1/S1^d$ mice. Nature 1980; 288: 592–4.

29. Mager DL, Mak TW, Bernstein A. Quantitative colony method for tumorigenic cells transformed by two distinct strains of Friend leukemia virus. Proc Natl Acad Sci U S A 1981; 78:1703–7.
30. Friend C, Haddad JR. Tumor formation with transplants of spleen or liver from mice with virus-induced leukemia. J Natl Cancer Inst. 1960; 25:1279–89.
31. Friend C, Patuleia MC, deHarven E. Erythrocytic maturation in vitro of murine (Friend) virus-induced leukemia cells. Natl Cancer Inst Monogr 1966; 288:505–20.
32. Marks PA, Rifkind RA. Erythroleukemic differentiation. Annu Rev Biochem 1978; 47:419–48.
33. Friend C, Sher W, Holland JG, Sato T. Hemoglobin synthesis in murine virus-induced leukemia cells in vitro: stimulation of erythroid differentiation by dimethylsulfoxide. Proc Natl Acad Sci U S A 1971; 68:378–82.
34. Peschle C, Colletta G, Covelli A, Ciccariello R, Migliaccio G, Rossi GB. The erythropoietic component of Friend virus erythroleukemias: role of erythropoietic hormones and SFFV genome. In: Revoltella R, Pontieri G, Rovera G, Basilico C, Gallo RC, Subak-Sharpe J, eds. Expression of differentiated functions in cancer cells. New York: Raven Press, 1981; 311–21.
35. Johnson CS, Marcelletti J, Longley C, Furmanski P. Inhibition of normal erythropoiesis in mice with Friend virus induced erythroleukemia. Exp Hematol 1982; 10:743–53.
36. Greenberger JS, Eckner RJ, Ostertag W, et al. Release of spleen focus-forming virus (SFFV) from differentiation inducible promyelocytic leukemia cell lines transformed in vitro by Friend leukemia virus. Virology 1980; 105:425–35.
37. Spiro C, Gliniak BC, Kabat D. Splenic accumulation of interleukin-3-dependent hematopoietic cells in Friend erythroleukemia. J Virol 1989; 63:4434–7.
38. Eckner RJ, Hettrick KL, Greenberger JS, Bennett M. Extended self-renewal capacity of pluripotent hematopoietic stem cells: association with persistent Friend spleen focus-forming virus. Cell 1982; 31:732–8.
39. Merchav S, Wagemaker G, van Bekkum DW. Reconstitution of the W/W$^v$ stem cell differentiation defect by infection with Rauscher leukemia virus. J Natl Cancer Inst 1985; 75:361–8.
40. Troxler DH, Boyars JK, Parks WP, Scolnick EM. Friend strain of spleen focus-forming virus: a recombinant between mouse type C ecotropic viral sequences and sequences related to xenotropic virus. J Virol 1977; 22:361–72.
41. Troxler DH, Lowy D, Howk R, Young H, Scolnick EM. Friend strain of spleen focus-forming virus is a recombinant between ecotropic murine type C virus and the *env* gene region of xenotropic type C virus. Proc Natl Acad Sci U S A 1977; 74:4671–5.
42. Ruscetti S, Troxler D, Linemeyer D, Scolnick E. Three laboratory strains of spleen focus-forming virus: comparison of their genomes and translational products. J Virol 1980; 33:140–51.
43. Ruscetti S, Linemeyer D, Feild J, Troxler D, Scolnick EM. Characterization of a protein found in cells infected with the spleen focus-forming virus that shares immunological cross-reactivity with the gp70 found in mink cell focus-inducing virus particles. J Virol 1979; 30:787–98.

44. Ikawa Y, Yoshida M, Yoshikura H. Identification of proteins specific to Friend strain of spleen focus forming virus (SFFV). Proc Jpn Acad 1978; 54:651-6.
45. Dresler S, Ruta M, Murray MJ, Kabat D. Glycoprotein encoded by the Friend spleen focus-forming virus. J Virol 1979; 30:564–75.
46. Linemeyer DL, Ruscetti SK, Scolnick EM, Evans LH, Duesberg PH. Biological activity of the spleen focus-forming virus is encoded by a molecularly cloned subgenomic fragment of spleen focus-forming virus DNA. Proc Natl Acad Sci U S A 1981; 78:1401-5.
47. Linemeyer DL, Menke JG, Ruscetti SK, Evans LH, Scolnick EM. Envelope gene sequences which encode the gp52 protein of spleen focus-forming virus are required for the induction of erythroid cell proliferation. J Virol 1982; 43:223–33.
48. Wolff L, Ruscetti S. Tissue tropism of a leukemogenic murine retrovirus is determined by sequences outside of the long terminal repeats. Proc Natl Acad Sci U S A 1986; 83:3376–80.
49. Wolff L, Ruscetti S. The spleen focus-forming virus (SFFV) envelope gene, when introduced into mice in the absence of other SFFV genes, induces acute erythroleukemia. J Virol 1988; 62:2158–63.
50. Aizawa S, Suda Y, Furuta Y, et al. *Env*-derived gp55 gene of Friend spleen focus-forming virus specifically induces neoplastic proliferation of erythroid progenitor cells. EMBO J 1990; 9:2107–16.
51. Wolff L, Ruscetti S. Malignant transformation of erythroid cells in vivo by introduction of a nonreplicating retrovirus vector. Science 1985; 228:1549–52.
52. Berger SA, Sanderson N, Bernstein A, Hankins WD. Induction of the early stages of Friend erythroleukemia with helper-free Friend spleen focus-forming virus. Proc Natl Acad Sci U S A 1985; 82:6913–7.
53. Bestwick RK, Hankins WD, Kabat D. Roles of helper and defective retroviral genomes in murine erythroleukemia: studies of spleen focus-forming virus in the absence of helper. J Virol 1985; 56:660–4.
54. Jones KS, Ruscetti S, Lilly F. Loss of pathogenicity of spleen focus-forming virus after pseudotyping with Akv. J Virol 1988; 62:511–8.
55. Weiss R, Teich N, Varmus H, Coffin J, eds. RNA tumor viruses. Cold Spring Harbor, NY: Cold Spring Harbor Laboratory, 1982.
56. Wolff L, Scolnick E, Ruscetti S. Envelope gene of the Friend spleen focus-forming virus: deletion and insertions in 3′ gp70/p15E-encoding region have resulted in unique features in the primary structure of its protein product. Proc Natl Acad Sci U S A 1983; 80:4718-22.
57. Amanuma H, Akiko K, Obata M, Sagata N, Ikawa Y. Complete nucleotide sequence of the gene for the specific glycoprotein (gp55) of Friend spleen focus-forming virus. Proc Natl Acad Sci U S A 1983; 80:3913–7.
58. Clark SP, Mak TW. Complete nucleotide sequences of an infectious clone of Friend spleen focus-forming provirus: gp55 is an envelope fusion glycoprotein. Proc Natl Acad Sci U S A 1983; 80:5037–41.
59. Srinivas RV, Kilpatrick DR, Compans RW. Intracellular transport and leukemogenicity of spleen focus-forming virus envelope glycoprotein with altered transmembrane domains. J Virol 1987; 61:4007–11.

60. Amanuma H, Watanabe N, Nishi M, Ikawa Y. Requirement of the single base insertion at the 3′ end of the *env*-related gene of Friend spleen focus-forming virus for pathogenic activity and its effect on localization of the glycoprotein product (gp55). J Virol 1989; 63:4824–33.
61. Watanabe N, Nishi M, Ikawa Y, Amanuma H. A deletion in the Friend spleen focus-forming virus *env* gene is necessary for its product (gp55) to be leukemogenic. J Virol 1990; 64:2678–86.
62. Ruta M, Bestwick R, Machida C, Kabat D. Loss of leukemogenicity caused by mutations in the membrane glycoprotein structural gene of Friend spleen focus-forming virus. Proc Natl Acad Sci U S A 1983; 80:4704–8.
63. Kaminchik J, Hankins WD, Ruscetti SK, Linemeyer DL, Scolnick EM. Molecular cloning of biologically active proviral DNA of the anemia-inducing strain of spleen focus-forming virus. J Virol 1982; 44:922–31.
64. Chung S-W, Wolff L, Ruscetti S. Sequences responsible for the altered Epo responsiveness in $SFFV_P$-infected cells are localized to a 678-bp region at the 3′ end of the envelope gene. J Virol 1987; 61:1661–4.
65. Chung S, Wolff L, Ruscetti SK. Transmembrane domain of the envelope gene of a polycythemia-inducing retrovirus determine erythropoietin-independent growth. Proc Natl Acad Sci U S A 1989; 86:7957–60.
66. Ruta M, Kabat D. Plasma membrane glycoproteins encoded by cloned Rauscher and Friend spleen focus-forming viruses. J Virol 1980; 35:844–53.
67. Ruta M, Clarke S, Boswell B, Kabat D. Heterogeneous metabolism and subcellular localization of a potentially leukemogenic membrane glycoprotein encoded by Friend erythroleukemia virus. J Biol Chem 1982; 257:126–34.
68. Srinivas RV, Compans RW. Glycosylation and intracellular transport of spleen focus-forming virus glycoproteins. Virology 1983; 125:274–86.
69. Srinivas RV, Compans RW. Membrane association and defective transport of spleen focus-forming virus glycoproteins. J Biol Chem 1983; 258:14718–24.
70. Kilpatrick DR, Srinivas RV, Stephens EB, Compans RW. Effects of deletion of the cytoplasmic domain upon surface expression and membrane stability of a viral envelope glycoprotein. J Biol Chem 1987; 262:16116–21.
71. Kilpatrick DR, Srinivas RV, Compans RW. The spleen focus-forming virus envelope glycoprotein is defective in oligomerization. J Biol Chem 1989; 264: 10732–7.
72. Gliniak BC, Kabat D. Leukemogenic membrane glycoprotein encoded by Friend focus-forming virus: transport to cell surfaces and shedding are controlled by disulfide-bonded dimerization and by cleavage of a hydrophobic membrane anchor. J Virol 1989; 63:3561–8.
73. Yang Y, Tojo A, Watanabe N, Amanuma H. Oligomerization of Friend spleen focus-forming virus (SFFV) *env* glycoproteins. Virology 1990; 177:312–6.
74. Ruscetti SK, Feild JA, Scolnick EM. Polycythemia- and anaemia-inducing strains of spleen focus-forming virus differ in post-translational processing of envelope-related glycoprotein. Nature 294:663–5.
75. Pinter A, Honnen WJ. The mature form of the Friend spleen focus-forming virus envelope protein, gp65, is efficiently secreted from cells. Virology 1985; 143:646–50.

76. Pinter A, Honnen WJ. Biochemical characterization of cell-associated and extracellular products of the Friend spleen focus-forming virus *env* gene. Virology 1989; 173:136–43.
77. Li J, Bestwick RK, Spiro C, Kabat D. The membrane glycoprotein of Friend spleen focus-forming virus: evidence that the cell surface component is required for pathogenesis and that it binds to a receptor. J Virol 1987; 61:2782–92.
78. Sawyer ST. Erythropoietin: synthesis of the hormone and its interaction with receptors on erythroid progenitors. Clin Biotech 1990; 2:77–85.
79. Jacobs K, Shoemaker C, Rudersdorf R, et al. Isolation and characterization of genomic and cDNA clones of human erythropoietin. Nature 1985; 313:806–10.
80. Lin F-K, Suggs S, Lin C-H, et al. Cloning and expression of the human erythropoietin gene. Proc Natl Acad Sci U S A 1985; 82:7580–4.
81. McDonald JD, Lin F, Goldwasser E. Cloning, sequencing and evolutionary analysis of the mouse erythropoietin gene. Mol Cell Biol 1986; 6:842–8.
82. Shoemaker CB, Mistock LD. Murine erythropoietin gene: cloning, expression and human gene homology. Mol Cell Biol 1986; 6:849–58.
83. Sawyer ST, Krantz SB, Goldwasser E. Binding and receptor-mediated endocytosis of erythropoietin in Friend virus infected erythroid cells. J Biol Chem 1987; 262:5554–62.
84. Sawada K, Krantz SB, Sawyer ST, Civin CI. Quantitation of specific binding of erythropoietin to human erythroid colony-forming cells. J Cell Physiol 1988; 137:337–45.
85. Landschulz KT, Noyes AV, Rodgers D, Boyer S. Erythropoietin receptors on murine colony-forming units; natural history. Blood 1989; 73:1476–86.
86. Fukamachi H, Saito T, Tojo A, Kitamura T, Urabe A, Takaku F. Binding of erythropoietin to CFU-E derived from fetal mouse liver cells. Exp Hematol 1987; 15:833–7.
87. Tojo A, Fukamachi H, Kasuga M, Urabe A, Takaku F. Identification of erythropoietin receptors on fetal liver erythroid cells. Biochem Biophys Res Commun 1987; 148:443–8.
88. Sawyer ST, Krantz SB, Luna J. Identification of the receptor for erythropoietin by cross-linking to Friend-virus-infected erythroid cells. Proc Natl Acad Sci U S A 1987; 84:3690–4.
89. Hosoi T, Sawyer ST, Krantz SB. Identification of erythropoietin receptor in a ligand-free form with $^{125}$I-labeled, photoreactive, cleavable cross-linker (Denny-Jaffe reagent). Exp Hematol 1989; 17:224a.
90. Sasaki R, Yanagawa S, Hitomi K, Chiba H. Characterization of erythropoietin receptor of murine erythroid cells. Eur J Biochem 1987; 168:43–8.
91. Takanashi T, Imura H. Erythropoietin receptor of a human leukemic cell line with erythroid characteristics. Biochem Biophys Res Commun 1988; 154:902–9.
92. Hitomi K, Masuda S, Ito K, Ueda M, Sasaki R. Solubilization and characterization of erythropoietin receptor from transplantable mouse erythroblastic leukemic cells. Biochem Biophys Res Commun 1989; 160:1140–8.
93. Broudy VC, Lin N, Egrie J, et al. Identification of the receptor for erythropoietin on human and murine erythroleukemia cells and modulation by phorbol ester and dimethyl sulfoxide. Proc Natl Acad Sci U S A 1988; 85:6513–7.

94. Mayeux P, Billat C, Jacquot R. The erythropoietin receptor of rat erythroid progenitor cells. J Biol Chem 1987; 262:13985–90.
95. Todokoro K, Kanazawa S, Amanuma H, Ikawa Y. Specific binding of erythropoietin to its receptor on responsive mouse erythroleukemia cells. Proc Natl Acad Sci U S A 1987; 84:4126–30.
96. Sawyer ST. The two proteins of the erythropoietin receptor are structurally similar. J Biol Chem 1989; 264:13343–7.
97. Sawyer ST, Hankins WD. Metabolism of erythropoietin in erythropoietin-dependent cell lines. Blood 1988; 72:440.
98. D'Andrea AD, Lodish HF, Wong GG. Expression cloning of the murine erythropoietin receptor. Cell 1989; 57:277–85.
99. Hosoi T, Sawyer ST, Krantz SB. The receptor for erythropoietin lacks detectable glycosylation. Exp Hematol 1988; 16:118.
100. D'Andrea AD, Fasman GD, Lodish HF. Erythropoietin receptor and interleukin-2 receptor $\beta$ chain: a new receptor family. Cell 1989; 58:1023–4.
101. Bazan JF. A novel family of growth factor receptors: a common binding domain in the growth hormone, prolactin, erythropoietin, and IL-6 receptors, and the p75 IL-2 receptor beta chain. Biochem Biophys Res Commun 1989; 164:788–95.
102. Gearing DP, King JA, Gough NM, Nicole NA. Expression cloning of a receptor for human granulocyte-macrophage colony-stimulating factor. EMBO J 1989; 8:3667–76.
103. Itoh N, Yonehara S, Schureurs J, et al. Cloning of an interleukin 3 receptor gene, a member of a distinct receptor gene family. Science 1990; 247:324–7.
104. Goodwin RG, Friend D, Ziegler SF, et al. Cloning of the human and murine interleukin-7 receptors: demonstration of a soluble form and homology to a new receptor superfamily. Cell 1990; 60:941–51.
105. Ruscetti SK, Ruscetti FW. Apparent Epo-independence of erythroid cells infected with the polycythemia-inducing strain of Friend spleen focus-forming virus is not due to Epo production or change in number or affinity of Epo receptors. Leukemia 1989; 3:703–7.
106. Yoshimura A, D'Andrea AD, Lodish HF. Friend spleen focus-forming virus glycoprotein gp55 interacts with the erythropoietin receptor in the endoplasmic reticulum and affects receptor metabolism. Proc Natl Acad Sci U S A 1990; 87:4139–43.
107. Wolff L, Tambourin P, Ruscetti S. Induction of the autonomous stage of transformation in erythroid cells infected with SFFV: helper virus is not required. Virology 1986; 152:272–6.
108. Moreau-Gachelin F, Tavitian A, Tambourin P. Spi-1 is a putative oncogene in virally induced murine erythroleukemias. Nature 1988; 331:277–80.
109. Moreau-Gachelin F, Ray D, Mattei M, Tambourin P, Tavitian A. The putative oncogene Spi-1: murine chromosomal localization and transcriptional activation in murine acute erythroleukemias. Oncogene 1989; 4:1449–56.
110. Goebl MG, Moreau-Gachelin F, Ray D, et al. The PU.1 transcription factor is the product of the putative oncogene Spi-1 (letter to the editor). Cell 1990; 61:1165–6.

111. Klemsz MJ, McKercher SR, Celada A, Van Beveren C, Maki RA. The macrophage and B-cell-specific transcription factor PU.1 is related to the *ets* oncogene. Cell 1990; 61:113–24.
112. Migliaccio G, Migliaccio AR, Ruscetti S, Adamson JW. The growth of Rauscher erythroleukemia cells is mediated by autocrine production of a factor with biological activity similar to interleukin-3. Blood 1989; 73:1770–7.
113. Paul R, Schuetze S, Kozak SL, Kabat D. A common site for immortlizing proviral integrations in Friend erythroleukemia: molecular cloning and characterization. J Virol 1989; 63:4958–61.
114. Ruscetti SK, Scolnick EM. Expression of a transformation-related protein (p53) in the malignant stage of Friend virus-induced diseases. J Virol 1983; 46:1022–6.
115. Mowat M, Cheng A, Kimura N, Bernstein A, Benchimol S. Rearrangements of cellular p53 gene in erythroleukemic cells transformed by Friend virus. Nature 1985; 314:633–6.
116. Ben David Y, Prideaux VR, Chow V, Benchimol S, Bernstein A. Inactivation of the p53 oncogene by internal deletion or retroviral integration in erythroleukemic cell lines induced by Friend leukemia virus. Oncogene 1988; 3:179–85.
117. Munroe DG, Peacock JW, Benchimol S. Inactivation of the cellular p53 gene is a common feature of Friend virus-induced erythroleukemia: relationship of inactivation to dominant transforming alleles. Mol Cell Biol 1990; 10:3307–13.
118. Anand R, Ruscetti SK, Lilly F. Viral protein expression in producer and nonproducer clones of Friend erythroleukemia cell lines. J Virol 1981; 37:654–60.
119. Chattopadhyay SK, Morse HC III, Makino M, Ruscetti SK, Hartley JW. Defective virus is associated with induction of murine retrovirus-induced immunodeficiency syndrome. Proc Natl Acad Sci U S A 1989; 86:3862–6.
120. Huang M, Jolicoeur P. Characterization of the gag/fusion protein encoded by the defective Duplan retrovirus inducing murine acquired immunodeficiency syndrome. J Virol 1990; 64:5764–72.
121. DesGroseillers L, Barrette N, Jolicoeur P. Physical mapping of the paralysis-inducing determinant of a wild mouse ecotropic neurotropic virus. J Virol 1984; 52:356–63.
122. Rassart E, Nelbach L, Jolicoeur P. Cas BrE murine leukemia virus: sequencing of the paralytogenic region of its genome and derivation of specific probes to study its origin and the structure of its recombinant genomes in leukemic tissues. J Virol 1986; 60:910–9.
123. Overbaugh J, Donahue PR, Quackenbush SL, Hoover EA, Mullins JI. Molecular cloning of a feline leukemia virus that induces fatal immunodeficiency disease in cats. Science 1988; 239:906–10.
124. Poss ML, Quackenbush SL, Mullins JI, Hoover EA. Characterization and significance of delayed processing of the feline leukemia virus FeLV-FAIDS envelope glycoprotein. J Virol 1990; 64:4338–45.
125. Famulari NG. Murine leukemia viruses with recombinant env genes: a discussion of their role in leukemogenesis. Curr Top Microbiol Immunol 1983; 103: 78–108.

# 11

# Hematologic Consequences of Feline Leukemia Virus Infection

**Michael L. Linenberger and Janis L. Abkowitz**

*University of Washington*
*Seattle, Washington*

## INTRODUCTION

Feline leukemia virus (FeLV) is an important pathogen in the outbred domestic cat population. Among cats, the majority of lethal infections and a high percentage of malignancies are associated with FeLV (1,2). Of equal importance, FeLV provides an animal model to study the mechanisms of retrovirally induced neoplastic and nonneoplastic disorders (3–5). Because the marrow in chronically viremic cats is infected, both hematopoietic cells and cells of the hematopoietic microenvironment may be involved in the pathogenesis of the hematologic abnormalities associated with FeLV.

## HISTORICAL PERSPECTIVES

In 1964, Jarrett and colleagues reported that inoculation of homogenized, freeze-thawed tumor cells obtained from a cat with a multicentric lymphosarcoma induced similar lymphosarcomas in four kittens (6). A viral etiology was suggested by the demonstration of C-type particles on electron microscopy of the secondary tumors and of primary tumor cells cultured in vitro (7). Similar C-type particles were subsequently identified in the tissue and plasma of cats with spontaneous (8–10) and experimentally induced (8,11–14) lymphoid and myeloid neoplasms. Epidemiologic data revealed a high incidence of lymphosarcoma in cats (15) and clusters of this disease in households with many pet cats (16), suggesting that the etiologic agent was infectious and horizontally transmitted. The presumptive virus was designated feline leukemia virus. By 1971, three groups had reported the experimental transmission of fibrosarcoma by cell-free tumor extracts from cats bearing spontaneous, multiple subcutaneous fibrosarcomas (17–19). Although there was no evidence of horizontal transmission in this disease, these tumors also contained intracellular C-type particles, designated feline sarcoma virus (FeSV).

By the mid-1970s, immunologic reagents were developed to identify FeLV group-specific antigens (viral *gag* gene products), which are produced in great excess in infected cells (20–22). As a result, indirect immunofluorescence assay provided a simple, rapid, and sensitive test to identify infected tissues and cells (22). Subsequent studies showed excellent correlation between the presence of *gag* proteins in peripheral blood cells and infectious virus in serum (23). This assay not only provided an important veterinary test to identify FeLV-infected pet cats but also facilitated studies of the epidemiology, immunology, and pathology of FeLV-induced diseases (24–28). These studies demonstrated that cats infected with FeLV have short life expectancies and develop neoplastic or, more frequently, nonneoplastic abnormalities of the lymphohematopoietic system (1,24).

Over the past two decades the pathophysiologic mechanisms of several disorders have been characterized in cats experimentally infected with biologic clones of natural FeLV isolates; these clones were derived through in vitro passage in tissue culture at limiting dilutions. Within the last 10 years, full-length proviral genomes have been molecularly cloned and sequenced. Regions from different cloned proviruses have been combined to form full-length chimeric viruses. Proviral sequence data have revealed the genetic origin of some FeLV strains, and in vitro and in vivo studies using infectious proviral clones and chimeric viruses have identified the FeLV genes and sequences involved in disease pathogenesis.

## VIROLOGY

### Taxonomy and Classification of Feline Retroviruses

Feline leukemia virus is a member of the virus family Retroviridae because of its single-stranded RNA genome and RNA-dependent DNA polymerase (reverse transcriptase). Based on its oncogenic potential and characteristic morphologic, biochemical, and physical properties, it is further classified in the subfamily Oncornavirinae (29). Infectious viruses representing the two other subfamilies of retroviruses have been identified in domestic cats (Table 1) and include the nonpathogenic feline syncytia-forming virus (FeSFV; subfamily Spumavirinae) (30) and feline immunodeficiency virus (FIV; sub-

**Table 1** Classification of Feline Retroviruses

| Virus | Subfamily |
|---|---|
| Feline leukemia virus (FeLV) | Oncornavirinae |
| Exogenous replication-competent FeLV | |
| Exogenous replication-defective FeLV | |
| Endogenous FeLV (enFeLV) | |
| RD-114 endogenous xenotropic retroviruses | Oncornavirinae |
| Feline syncytia-forming virus (FeSFV) | Spumavirinae |
| Feline immunodeficiency virus (FIV) | Lentivirinae |

family Lentivirinae) (31). FIV is biologically similar to human immunodeficiency virus (HIV) (31). Infection with FIV is associated with an immunodeficiency syndrome in domestic cats (31–33), an increased risk of lymphomas (34), and hematologic abnormalities (35).

## Endogenous Feline Retroviruses

Like many animal species, the germ line cat genome contains multiple copies of endogenous retroviral sequences. One class of endogenous feline retroviruses, the RD-114 group, is genomically unrelated to FeLV (36–38). The RD-114 proviruses encode full-length retroviral genomes that can replicate complete infectious virus, but these viruses are xenotropic (i.e., cannot infect feline cells), and thus they do not play a role in disease pathogenesis (36). A second class of endogenous retrovirus, designated enFeLV, is homologous to exogenous FeLV (39). The enFeLV proviral sequences are diverse in length and copy number and variable in their distribution from cat to cat. No complete infectious virus has been induced or detected from enFeLV proviruses, but enFeLV genes are transcriptionally active during stages of development in certain tissues (40,41) and in tumors (42). Additionally, enFeLV genes participate in recombination events with exogenous FeLV (43) to generate potentially pathogenic recombination viruses.

## Exogenous Replication-Competent FeLV

Infectious FeLV virions are 110–120 nm diameter particles. Each is composed of a core of structural proteins, reverse transcriptase, and dimeric, single-stranded genomic RNA as a ribonucleoprotein complex packaged within a host cell membrane-derived coat that is studded with FeLV envelope proteins. Within an infected cell, FeLV gene products and genomic RNA assemble at the cell membrane, where progeny virions arise by budding from the membrane (Fig. 1).

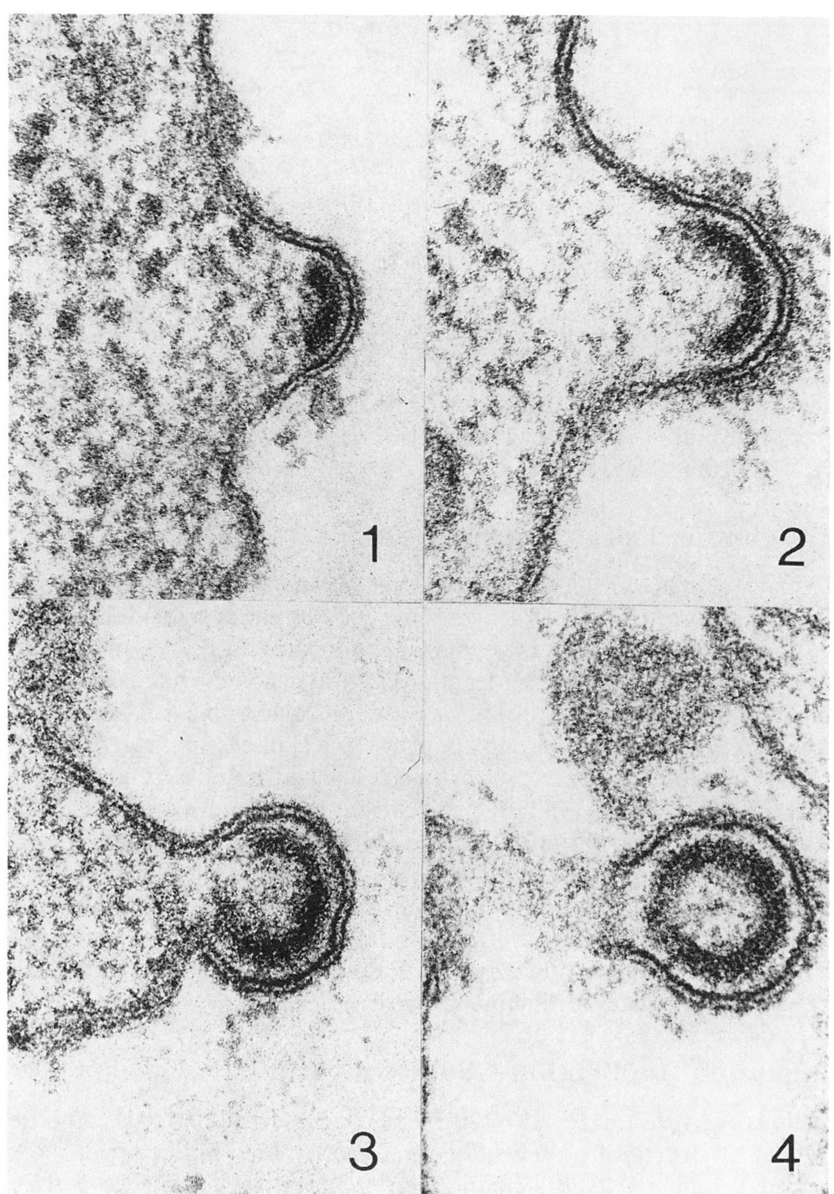


**Figure 1** Electron photomicrographs depicting sequential stages of virion budding from the membrane of an FeLV-infected cell, producing a typical, extracellular C-type particle. (Published with permission of Appleton-Lange, Norwalk, CT.)

The RNA genome of replication-competent FeLV strains is plus stranded and is approximately 8.5 kb in length. Similar to retroviruses from other species, FeLV contains three major genes, *gag-pol-env*, flanked by unique (U) and redundant (R) sequences at the 5′ and 3′ ends (Fig. 2) (3). During viral DNA synthesis, the U3 and U5 sequences are duplicated, resulting in identical U3-R-U5 long terminal repeat (LTR) regions on both ends of the proviral DNA (Fig. 2). The LTR contains sequences that act as promoters and enhancers of transcription. They also direct initiation and termination of transcription and polyadenylation of RNA transcripts. The leader region next to the 5′ LTR contains sequences that are probably important for the packaging of genomic RNA into maturing virions and for the splicing of precursor RNA into subgenomic mRNA. The *gag, pol,* and env genes encode information for the core proteins, reverse transcriptase, and envelope proteins, respectively. Sequences at the 5′ end of the *pol* gene encode for an enzyme with protease activity (44). By analogy with other retroviruses, additional gene product(s) of the 3′ end of the *pol* gene provide integrase and endonuclease functions. There is no identifiable regulatory gene in FeLV, such as the *tax* gene found in human T cell leukemia (lymphotropic) virus type I (HTLV-I).

FeLV proviral DNA may be integrated into the host cell genome in several copies. The site of integration can involve host regions of importance in tumorigenesis, as found in certain lymphosarcomas (45–48). Expression of proviral genes and production of infectious viral particles rely on the structural integrity of the integrated genome and regulatory influences from the

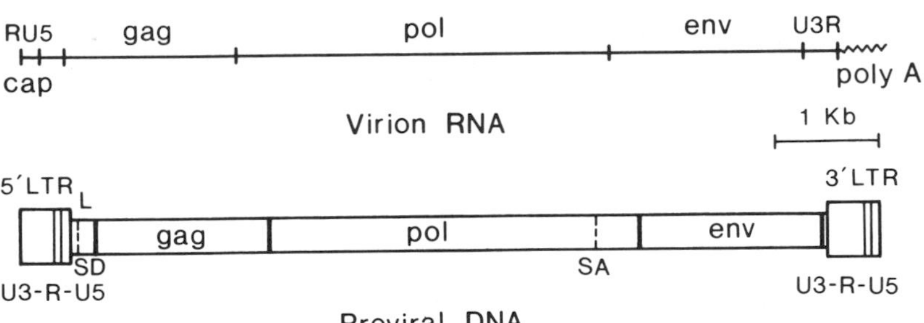


**Figure 2** A typical FeLV genome and proviral DNA. The RNA viral genome is flanked by redundant (R) regions that contain the cap site at the 5′ end and the signal for polyadenylation at the 3′ end. The proviral DNA is approximately 8.4 kb in length. The locations of the splice donor (SD) and splice acceptor (SA) sites and the relative sizes of the unique (U3 and U5) long terminal repeat (LTR), leader (L), redundant, and *gag*, *pol*, and *env* regions were derived from sequence data published in Reference 59.

viral LTR and host cell signals. The transcription enhancer region within the LTR contains sequences that can be recognized by both general and tissue-specific host cell-derived nuclear binding factors (49). The LTR-mediated activation of transcription not only regulates proviral gene expression but may activate or alter the transcription of host cell genes (47,50). In some cases, intact FeLV provirus is transcriptionally silent. Such nonreplicating proviral DNAs may be inherently defective or their expression may be regulated by host cell factors (51), but reactivation of viral replication may occur under certain conditions (52–55).

The FeLV provirus is transcribed into genomic-length RNA, which is polyadenylated and utilized as either infectious virion RNA or as a template for expression of the *gag* and *gag-pol* precursor proteins (Fig. 3). Alter-

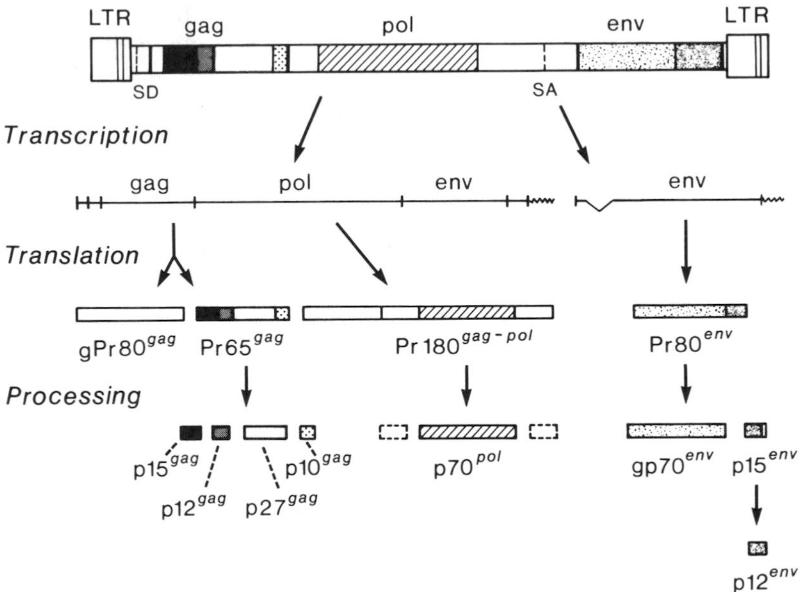


**Figure 3** Synthetic pathway of FeLV gene products. Shaded regions of proviral DNA denote sequences encoding the major precursor proteins and respective final gene products. The two major transcription products include a genomic-length RNA and a spliced *env* messenger RNA. The hatched boxes represent the putative protease and endonuclease-integrase proteins, encoded at the 5′ and 3′ ends, respectively, of the *pol* gene. Further details of the gene products are given in the text. Abbreviations are the same as those used in Figure 2. Proviral gene regions were derived from sequence data published in Reference 59. (This scheme was adapted from a figure in Ref. 3, with permission of the author.)

natively, primary transcripts are processed and spliced to subgenomic *env* mRNA for translation into the *env* precursor protein (3). The major products of the *gag* gene are a glycosylated protein (gPr80*gag*) and a nonglycosylated precursor protein (Pr65*gag*). Pr65*gag* is modified to generate core proteins (p15*gag*, p12*gag*, p27*gag*, and p10*gag*), which are important in the assembly and budding of the immature virion. The *pol* gene products arise from a *gag-pol* precursor protein (Pr180*gag-pol*), which is ultimately processed into the reverse transcriptase (p70*pol*) and the putative protease and endonuclease-integrase proteins (Fig. 3). The *env* gene product is a precursor protein (Pr80*env*) that is cleaved into the major envelope glycoprotein (gp70*env*) and a transmembrane anchoring protein (p15*env*), which in turn generates a smaller protein (p12*env*; Fig. 3).

Many of the *gag* proteins and p15*env* (p15E) are antigenically similar to equivalently sized core and transmembrane envelope proteins of other animal retroviruses. The gp70 molecule, however, is specific to FeLV. Furthermore, the 5′ portion of the *env* gene encodes the distinct antigenic epitopes of gp70 that identify three subgroups (A, B, and C) of FeLV (56–59). There is 98% homology among the *env* gene sequences of different FeLV subgroup A strains (59), but the 5′ region of the FeLV subgroup B *env* gene is quite divergent from subgroup A (56) and subgroup C *env* genes (57,58). The *env* gene of the Gardner-Arnstein strain of FeLV subgroup B is homologous to enFeLV *env* gene sequences and suggests that subgroup B viruses arise by recombination of exogenous FeLV subgroup A with enFeLV *env* gene sequences (57).

The gp70 molecule serves as the ligand for attachment to the virus receptor and penetration of FeLV into susceptible cells. It therefore dictates the range of host cell susceptibility. For example, FeLV subgroup A infects only feline and canine cells, but subgroup B and C viruses infect feline, human, bovine, and canine cells or cell lines in vitro (60,61). Only FeLV subgroup C can infect guinea pig cells in vitro (60,61). After infection of a cell, gp70 molecules interact with the subgroup-specific viral receptors to prevent superinfection of that cell by FeLV of the same subgroup. This interference does not prevent coinfection with FeLV from other subgroups, and there is in vivo evidence suggesting that primary infection by FeLV subgroup A may enhance coinfection by subgroup B or C viruses (62,63).

## Exogenous Replication-Defective FeLV

Replication of infectious viral progeny requires an intact complement of proviral structural genes and the functional integrity of the proviral LTR. Proviruses that contain mutations, deletions, or a transduced cellular gene may still actively express native or altered viral genes, but such viruses often lack the combined machinery necessary to fully construct, assemble, and bud mature virions. Replication-defective viruses are therefore only packaged and transmitted to other cells when coinfecting, replication-competent "helper" virus provides the missing machinery and/or vehicle (the virion). To coinfect the cell, either the helper virus must express a gp70 molecule different from the defective FeLV gp70 (to bypass the subgroup-specific interference), or the defective FeLV must not express intact gp70. This process ultimately results in the production of infectious pseudotype virions that contain the genome of the defective virus packaged in a coat expressing the helper virus gp70 (and possibly the defective virus gp70, if it is expressed in the cell). Pseudotype virion production also probably takes place in feline cells coinfected with two replication-competent FeLV strains of different subgroups, as commonly found in nature.

Many replication-defective viruses have been identified in isolates of pathogenic FeLV strains. The majority of these viruses are defective because cellular genes have been transduced into the viral genome and replaced viral structural genes. For example, replication-defective viruses have been isolated from T cell lymphosarcomas that contain a transduced c-*myc* (45,64, 65) or a T cell antigen receptor β-chain gene (66). A second, larger group of replication-defective isolates, the feline sarcoma viruses, have been obtained from spontaneous multicentric fibrosarcomas in young cats (reviewed in Refs. 3 and 67–69). These FeSV strains contain transduced cellular protooncogenes (e.g., *abl, fes, fgr, fms,* K-*ras, kit,* and *sis*) that in turn are expressed as *gag-onc* fusion protein gene products (67). As a result, FeSV inoculation induces tumors after a short time period.

Some FeLV strains are replication defective as a result of deletions or other mutations but do not contain transduced oncogenes. Defective FeLV variants have been molecularly cloned from proviral sequences in tissues or cells infected with FeLV strains associated with feline acquired immunodeficiency syndrome (FAIDS) (70), myeloid leukemia (71), and large granular lymphoma (72). These variant proviruses are important in the pathogenesis of disease, as demonstrated by in vivo studies using molecular clones of defective variants (70,71).

## EPIDEMIOLOGY

### Transmission

Cats chronically infected with FeLV maintain a high titer of infectious virus in the plasma and saliva (73) due to persistent, productive infection of marrow, mucosal, and glandular epithelial cells (24,25,28). Virus is horizontally transmitted from animal to animal, from saliva and respiratory secretions of the infected host to the oronasal passage of the recipient, by mutual grooming, shared feeding, and sneezing (24,25). Transmission of virus in blood, urine, and feces probably accounts for very few cases of natural infection. Queen cats can transmit FeLV to the fetus and kitten transplacentally and in milk (74).

Studies of FeLV transmission among cats within colonies (75) and studies of experimental infection by artificial exposure and inoculation (76) have revealed that many factors affect host susceptibility to infection by FeLV. The strain of virus used, its in vitro or in vivo passage history, and the route of exposure (intraperitoneal, intranasal, and intramedullary) are important variables (75–78). Neonatal kittens (77) and immunocompromised cats are most easily infected (76,79,80).

## Prevalence of Natural Infection

Adult community cats from urban areas are exposed to FeLV frequently, as indicated by the 50% prevalence of serum antibodies against FeLV cell membrane antigens (27). However, significant exposure resulting in protective immunity with viral neutralizing antibody is much less frequent (74). Chronic infection with FeLV is found in less than 1% of stray cats in large cities (81). In contrast, persistent viremia occurs in 28% of healthy pet cats exposed to an FeLV-infected cat in a multiple-cat household (74), suggesting that chronic exposures are required for efficient transmission.

In clinical studies, in vitro interference and viral neutralization patterns have been used to identify the three FeLV subgroups (82). Among naturally infected cats, FeLV subgroup A is found in 100% of all isolates. Subgroup A virus is found alone in 65–70% of isolates from healthy, viremic cats, the remainder being mixtures of FeLV subgroups A and B (74,83). In comparison, mixtures of FeLV subgroup B and subgroup A are found in 60% of cats with clinical disease. FeLV subgroup C is also always found in a mixture with FeLV subgroup A and occasionally with both A and B (83). Viruses containing FeLV subgroup C account for only 1% of isolates from infected cats and are found in cats with pure red cell aplasia (61,74,83). The combination of subgroup A with the other two subgroups may reflect the enhanced in vivo infectivity of subgroup B or subgroup C after subgroup A infection (62,63). Alternatively, subgroup A alone may account for most primary, natural infections, and recombination events with enFeLV *env* gene sequences may yield replication-competent strains of subgroup B and C that then propagate as phenotypic mixture viruses with the original FeLV subgroup A (43,57).

# IMMUNOBIOLOGY

## Immune Response to FeLV Infection

After exposure, FeLV initially replicates in a local lymph node and then spreads sequentially to other lymphoid tissue, the marrow, intestinal crypt epithelial cells, and finally to mucosal and glandular epithelial cells (28). By 2–3 weeks, when marrow cells become infected, antibodies appear against multiple FeLV antigens and against putative tumor-associated antigen(s), designated feline oncornavirus-associated cell membrane antigen (FOCMA) (84). It is unclear whether FOCMA determinant(s) are derived from oxogenous FeLV or, in some cases, are products of enFeLV genes (42,85). By 6 weeks after exposure, most cats mount an immune response that is sufficient to limit further spread of FeLV, and the virus is subsequently cleared from the plasma and all tissues (28). These "regressor" cats have protective immunity, high titers of antibody against FOCMA, and neutralizing antibodies against gp70.

Some regressor cats reactivate FeLV after administration of corticosteroids (52). Also, infectious virus may be demonstrated in vitro when marrow from recently exposed, regressor cats is cultured in the presence of corticosteroids (53–55). The percentage of cats that demonstrate this in vitro reactivation declines to less than 10% by 6–7 months after exposure (55). Spontaneous reactivation of latent FeLV infection rarely occurs in naturally exposed, regressor cats (3). However, the transmission of virus from a latently infected queen to a kitten has been described (53).

Approximately 28% of cats exposed to FeLV do not develop an adequate immune response, and they become persistently viremic (81). Among these cats, 25% develop FOCMA antibody titers >1:32, which are believed to be "protective" against the development of lymphosarcoma (81). This immunologic response is often unstable and may either evolve to full protective immunity with additional production of viral neutralizing antibody (with subsequent clearance of virus) or revert to a state of low anti-FOCMA antibody titers (84,86). Persistently viremic cats with little or no virus-neutralizing or anti-FOCMA antibodies frequently develop FeLV-associated neoplastic and/or nonneoplastic diseases and have an 83% mortality over the next 3–4 years (87).

## FeLV-Related Immunosuppression

Most cats viremic with FeLV have abnormal immune function. Chronically viremic cats that are otherwise healthy have a delayed and decreased antibody response after challenge with synthetic antigen (88). FeLV-infected cats frequently develop thymic atrophy, lymphoid depletion, lymphopenia, and chronic, recurrent infections (4,89). Thus, a feline acquired immunodeficiency syndrome may result from infection with FeLV (4,89), and this is similar to the clinical syndrome associated with FIV infection (31).

Lymphocytes and neutrophils from FeLV-infected cats function abnormally in assays in vitro. Mitogen-induced lymphocyte blastogenesis (89,

90), mitogen-induced T cell interleukin-2 production (91), and neutrophil chemotaxis (92) are impaired. Because normal, uninfected cat lymphocytes and neutrophils exhibit similar abnormal in vitro responses after exposure to ultraviolet (UV)-inactivated FeLV or the FeLV transmembrane protein p15E (93–96), the in vivo abnormalities may be mediated by p15E. Of note, neutrophil function is also impaired in FeLV-exposed, regressor cats (97,98), and regressor cats have a higher incidence of infectious disease than cats never exposed to FeLV (99).

## MARROW DISORDERS ASSOCIATED WITH FeLV INFECTION

### General Considerations

All subgroups of FeLV infect rapidly dividing cells of hematopoietic lineages. Kittens are particularly susceptible to progressive FeLV infection because they have an immature immune system and an abundance of target cells in the thymus, marrow, and foci of extramedullary hematopoiesis in liver and spleen (100). The early viremic phase of naturally transmitted FeLV infection is often associated with marrow hypoplasia and variable degrees of anemia, leukopenia, and thrombocytopenia (75). As the infection becomes chronic these cytopenias may persist, worsen in severity, or resolve, depending on the strain of FeLV, the cellular immune response, and the development of subsequent neoplastic or nonneoplastic diseases.

When FeLV infection persists for months to years, specific hematologic syndromes develop (1,101). These disorders have been classified in the veterinary literature according to hematopathologic criteria previously used for human diseases (1,101–103). Table 2 lists this veterinary terminology and a classification scheme for FeLV-associated hematologic disorders based on current human nomenclature (104–106). In individual cats, overlapping and/or transitions between syndromes may be observed.

### Anemia

Anemia alone is the cause of death in 8% of FeLV-infected cats (24), but over 50% of cats dying of nonneoplastic FeLV-related diseases are anemic (2). Among all cats presenting with chronic anemia, 75% are associated with FeLV infection (107).

A hypoproliferative anemia is found in 80–85% of FeLV-infected cats with isolated, chronic anemia (107–109). It is characterized by normocytic red blood cells (RBC), a low reticulocyte index, and usually a normal white blood cell (WBC) count and platelet count. There is marrow erythroid hypoplasia with an increased myeloid-erythroid (M/E) ratio (108). Iron studies

**Table 2** Hematologic Disorders Associated with FeLV

| Human terminology | Veterinary terminology | Clonal, neoplastic | Comment | References |
|---|---|---|---|---|
| Anemia | | | | |
| Hypoproliferative anemia | Nonregenerative anemia | — | May reflect an inflammatory block of iron utilization | 1, 107, 108, 110, 117 |
| Pure red cell aplasia | Erythroblastopenia, aplastic anemia | No | Associated with FeLV subgroup C | 110, 114, 138, 139 |
| Hemolytic anemia | Regenerative anemia | — | May result from *Hemobartonella felis* infection; rarely, associated with antierythrocyte antibodies | 1, 107, 108, 110, 117 |
| Leukopenia | | | | |
| Leukopenia with enteropathy | Panleukopenialike syndrome | — | Clinically resembles panleukopenia (parvovirus) infection | 1, 24, 101, 118 |
| Cyclic neutropenia | Cyclic neutropenia | — | Responds to corticosteroids | 119–121 |
| Aplastic anemia | Pancytopenia | — | | 1 |

| | | | | |
|---|---|---|---|---|
| Myelodysplastic syndromes | Myeloproliferative disorders, reticuloendotheliosis, erythremic myelosis (erythroleukemia) | Yes | Associated with megaloblastic erythropoiesis; nonerythroid blasts comprise $<30\%$ of nucleated marrow cells (106) | 1, 71, 100, 111–113 |
| Acute non-lymphocytic leukemia | Myeloproliferative disorders, erythroleukemia, myeloid leukemias | Yes | Nonerythroid blasts comprise $\geqslant 30\%$ of nucleated marrow cells; erythroleukemia diagnosed with erythroblasts $\geqslant 50\%$ of nucleated marrow cells *and* blasts comprise $\geqslant 30\%$ of nonerythroid cells (106) | 1, 14, 71, 100, 113, 124, 125, 128–131, 134 |
| Acute lymphocytic leukemia | Lymphosarcoma | Yes | Lymphoblasts comprise $\geqslant 30\%$ of all nucleated marrow cells; includes secondary marrow involvement with extramedullary lymphosarcoma | 1, 132, 133, 167 |
| Myelofibrosis | Myelofibrosis | — | Associated with aplastic anemia, pure red cell aplasia, myelodysplasia, and myeloid leukemias | 1, 123, 125, 135, 136 |
| Medullary osteosclerosis | Medullary osteosclerosis | — | Associated with FeLV subgroup C; osteocytes are infected with FeLV | 109, 115 |

are normal, and the anemia does not respond to vitamin $B_{12}$ or folate administration (108). Because of the frequent occurrence of opportunistic and secondary infections in FeLV-infected, immunosuppressed cats, it is likely that hypoproliferative anemias result from an inflammatory block of iron utilization. Hypoproliferative anemia also occurs in up to 68% of FeLV-infected cats with lymphosarcoma (in the absence of marrow involvement) (1,110). Occasionally, megaloblastic erythropoiesis with circulating nucleated RBC (NRBC) (108), and splenomegaly with extramedullary hematopoiesis (EMH) (110) have been reported with FeLV-associated hyporoliferative anemia. It is possible that, in these animals, the anemia is a clinical manifestation of a myelodysplastic syndrome (111–113) and the progeny of the neoplastic stem cell are unable to complete erythroid differentiation.

Pure red cell aplasia (PRCA) is a progressively severe and fatal anemia that occurs in less than 1% of FeLV-infected cats (109). Reticulocytes are absent and the marrow reveals no hemoglobinized cells, but the myeloid and megakaryocyte precursors are normal in morphology and number (114). Medullary osteosclerosis and, less frequently, myelofibrosis have been associated with this anemia (see later) (115). Splenic EMH is characteristically not found. Pure red cell aplasia in community cats is associated with FeLV isolates containing subgroup C virus (116), and PRCA is inducible by inoculation of kittens or immunosuppressed adults with biologic or molecular clones of FeLV subgroup C/Sarma (58,78,110,114).

Up to 20% of anemic, FeLV-infected cats have a hyperproliferative anemia characterized by macrocytosis, reticulocytosis, circulating peripheral NRBC, and normal WBC and platelet counts (107–109). Other findings include splenomegaly with EMH, marrow erythroid hyperplasia, and a decreased M/E ratio. This anemic syndrome is presumably due to hemolysis (in the absence of blood loss) and has rarely been associated with an antierythrocyte antibody (117). In other cases, hemolysis may be secondary to *Hemobartonella felis* infection, since 40% of cats infected with this red cell parasite are viremic with FeLV (107). Because hyperproliferative anemia has been reported to progress to a hypoproliferative process or to leukemia over time (1,107), this clinical syndrome may include cats with myelodysplasia.

## Leukopenia

A panleukopenialike syndrome, clinically similar to feline distemper caused by the parvovirus feline panleukopenia virus (see Chap. 6), may occur in FeLV-infected cats (1). This syndrome causes 9% of deaths in FeLV-infected cats, including cats that have been immunized against panleukopenia virus (1,24). It may be precipitated by physiologic stress, such as cat fights and hospitalization. Although WBC counts are 300–3000, platelet counts and hematocrits are generally normal. The cats die with hemorrhagic necrosis of the small intestine, and the marrow reveals myeloid hypoplasia (101,109, 118).

Cyclic hematopoiesis affecting neutrophils and other cell lines has been reported in three FeLV-infected cats and in one latently infected cat that reactivated FeLV after corticosteroid administration (119–121). The neutrophil counts varied from as low as zero (120) to normal over an 8–14 day cycle. Clinical improvement was noted with corticosteroid administration in three of these cats (119,120). Corticosteroids have been reported to reverse neutropenia in other FeLV-infected cats (122).

## Myelodysplastic Syndromes

A number of FeLV-infected cats have peripheral blood cytopenias and ineffective hematopoiesis. Marrow morphologic features include megaloblastic erythroid maturation and a shift toward immature or "undifferentiated" marrow cells. EMH in the spleen and liver commonly accompanies these blood and marrow abnormalities, and there is a tendency to progress to frank leukemia (1,71,100,107,111–114,123–125). These disorders have been referred to as myeloproliferative diseases (107,123–125), reticuloendotheliosis, erythremic myelosis, and erythroleukemia (1,101–103,125), but in fact they fulfill the French-American British (FAB) diagnostic criteria for myelodysplastic syndromes (105). A recent 5 year retrospective study of peripheral blood and marrow smears from cats presenting with peripheral blood cytopenias, macrocytosis, or blast cells identified 21 cases of myelodysplasia and 39 cases of myeloid leukemia (113). Of the cats with myelodysplasia and those with leukemia, 71 and 90%, respectively, were FeLV infected (113), and all exhibited morphologic features that permitted their classification according to FAB criteria (105,106). Clinically, approximately one-half to two-thirds of cats with FeLV-associated myelodysplastic syndromes have significant pancytopenia (111–113). These cats die from anemia, infection, or hemorrhage with or without progression to either acute lymphocytic or nonlymphocytic leukemia (111,112).

## Acute Nonlymphocytic Leukemia

Cytochemical characterization of normal and leukemic feline blood and marrow cells has facilitated the classification of feline leukemias into acute lymphocytic (ALL) and acute nonlymphocytic (ANLL) (126,127). Acute nonlymphocytic leukemia comprised only 10% of all hematopoietic neoplasms in FeLV-infected cats in one earlier survey (1); however, the work of other investigators suggests that the true prevalence may be higher (113,128).

Histologically, the majority of naturally occurring and experimentally induced ANLL have been myeloblastic (1,107,113,128,129), with fewer cases of erythroleukemia (M6 leukemia by FAB criteria) (113) and rare reports of myelomonocytic (100,130), basophilic (1), and megakaryocytic leukemias (1,107). All cats with ANLL have severe hypoproliferative anemia, and many are thrombocytopenic. Presentation with a high WBC count is unusual (113), and therefore the diagnosis may be missed on screening the complete blood count. The marrow, by definition, contains over 30% blasts (14,100,113, 129–131). The liver and spleen are frequently infiltrated with leukemic cells and/or EMH.

### Acute Lymphocytic Leukemia

Primary involvement of the marrow by neoplastic lymphoid cells, without nodal or tumor involvement elsewhere, occurs in a minority of cats with FeLV-associated lymphoproliferative diseases (1,132). One survey reported primary ALL in 40% of all such cases (132); another found that 8% of FeLV-associated lymphoid malignancies present as primary ALL (1). Roughly 70% of all ALL cases occur in FeLV-infected cats (133).

Peripheral blood leukocytosis is seen in only 10% of primary ALL cases, although 40% have lymphocytosis (132). Neutropenia is present in one-third and severe hypoproliferative anemia in over two-thirds of cats presenting with ALL (132). All affected cats have 30% or more lymphoblasts in the marrow (132). Circulation of high numbers of peripheral blood neoplastic lymphocytes occurs in 15% of cats with FeLV-associated lymphosarcoma outside the marrow (134). Secondary marrow involvement with lymphosarcoma (with or without peripheral blood lymphocytosis) occurs in 33% of FeLV-positive cases (1).

### Effects of FeLV Infection on Nonhematopoietic Marrow Elements

Myelofibrosis, or an abnormal proliferation of marrow fibroblasts with reticulin and collagen deposition, has been reported with FeLV infection associated with nonneoplastic anemias (1,135), pancytopenias (1), myelodysplasias (123,125,136), and myeloid leukemias (137). Careful histologic staining for reticulin reveals increased amounts in marrow sections from over one-half of cats with myelodysplasia and ANLL (136), and smaller series have reported myelofibrosis in 30–40% of cats with various myelodysplastic syndromes (123,125). One case of myelofibrosis was examined by electron microscopy for the presence of C-type viral particles, and no virus was seen in the fibroblasts (125). Virus is found, however, in hematopoietic marrow cells in such cases of myelofibrosis (123,125).

Some naturally infected cats with severe anemia and cats experimentally infected with strains of FeLV that induce pure red cell aplasia develop medullary osteosclerosis (1,115). This disorder is characterized by a proliferation of bony trabeculae into the marrow cavity and is particularly noted in long bones. In the most advanced stage the entire medullary cavity is obliterated. Intracellular C-type viral particles have been identified in the proliferative osteocytes by electron microscopy (115). It is not known if this is a primary or reactive process of infected osteocytes, but the development or severity of osteosclerosis is not directly related to the development or severity of anemia in these cats (115).

## CELLULAR AND MOLECULAR MECHANISMS OF FeLV-ASSOCIATED DISEASES

### Pathogenesis of Pure Red Cell Aplasia Induced by FeLV Subgroup C

The syndrome of feline PRCA requires FeLV subgroup C infection. Isolates from cats with community-acquired disease contain subgroup C virus (116), and PRCA results from experimental infection with all strains containing FeLV subgroup C (63,114,135,137,138). The Sarma strain of FeLV subgroup C (FeLV-C/Sarma) has been molecularly cloned (58), and the cloned virus induces fatal PRCA in newborn specific pathogen-free (SPF) cats (58). Chimeric viruses have been constructed with genomic sequences from molecular clones of FeLV-C/Sarma and a nonpathogenic strain of FeLV subgroup A (FeLV-61E) (139). With this approach, Riedel et al. determined that an 886 base pair sequence, encompassing the 3′ end of the *pol* gene through the 5′ end of the *env* gene (including the region that encodes 241 amino acids of the N terminus of gp70), was both necessary and sufficient to induce PRCA (139). This region was also required for infection of guinea pig cells, a property unique to FeLV-C/Sarma (139). Part of this sequence is predicted to encode for hydrophilic amino acids in the gp70 molecule, which may function as a viral receptor recognition site (139).

The mechanism by which the gp70 of FeLV-C/Sarma induces PRCA is not known. Several studies have demonstrated that the pathogenesis of this disease is not similar to mechanisms for human PRCA. First, virus has been demonstrated in spleen tissue (58), granulocytes, platelets (114), and erythroid and myeloid progenitor cells (140,141) of cats with PRCA. Because both burst-forming erythroid progenitors (BFU-E) and granulocyte-macrophage progenitors (colony-forming units, CFU-GM) are infected, the selective infection and lysis of erythroid cells (the mechanism of human PRCA associated with parvovirus B19 infection) is not relevant. Also, erythroid progenitors may be infected 8–20 weeks before the onset of anemia (140) and remain infected after suramin therapy, even when erythropoiesis improves (142). Second, when cats heterozygous for the X-linked enzyme glucose-6-phosphate dehydrogenase (G-6-PD) develop PRCA, there is no change from the baseline ratios of G-6-PD isoenzyme types among myeloid or erythroid progenitor cells (138) or peripheral blood lymphocytes (143). These results suggest that PRCA does not arise from a clonal hematopoietic stem cell defect or as a consequence of a clonal lymphoproliferative process. Therefore, in contrast to some cases of human PRCA, this disease is not a manifestation of a myelodysplastic syndrome or lymphoid malignancy. Finally, there is no suppression of in vitro erythropoiesis by antibody or T cells from cats that develop PRCA (143), suggesting that feline PRCA is not immunologically mediated.

All anemic cats infected with FeLV subgroup C have a marked depletion of erythroid progenitors (58,78,135,137,139,144,145). Marrow cultures done under optimal growth conditions (with added cat serum) reveal that BFU-E are preserved but the more mature colony-forming erythroid progenitors (CFU-E) are lost (138,144). In prospective studies, the decrease in CFU-E occurs 2–3 weeks before severe anemia (Fig. 4) (138,144), and therefore it is likely that PRCA reflects in vivo inhibition of differentiation from BFU-E to CFU-E. Since BFU-E mature in methylcellulose cultures to form hemoglobinized bursts, these data further imply that the abnormality in differentiation is at least partially overcome by conditions of culture (e.g., less cell motility or cell-cell interactions from semisolid medium, altered growth factors and nutrients, or different extracellular concentrations of viral proteins). Studies by some investigators suggest that biologically cloned (146), UV-inactivated (147), and molecularly cloned (148) strains of FeLV that contain subgroup C impair in vitro erythroid differentiation when added to cultures of BFU-E from normal, uninfected cats. In contrast, exposure of normal cat marrow cells to heat-inactivated FeLV subgroup C does not suppress erythropoiesis in vitro (146,149).

Infected BFU-E from cats with PRCA have several abnormal characteristics. Thymidine suicide studies reveal that twice the normal percentage of BFU-E are in active cell cycle (144). Also, infected BFU-E are susceptible to lysis by exposure to heterologous complement in vitro (140). This complement sensitivity was found to be mediated by activation of the classic pathway and therefore is different from the hemolysis in paroxysmal nocturnal hemoglobinuria, which is mediated by activation of the alternate complement pathway. BFU-E from cats with PRCA require cat serum for optimal growth in culture (144), and they fail to respond to the hematopoietic growth factors present in the conditioned medium from feline embryonic fibroblast cells infected with FeLV-A/Glasgow-1 (FEF-A CM) (144), but their response to erythropoietin remains normal (142). In contrast, infected granulocyte-macrophage progenitors (CFU-GM) from anemic cats do not exhibit complement sensitivity (140), a change in cell cycle kinetics, or a change in the response to cat serum or hematopoietic growth factors in vitro (138,144).

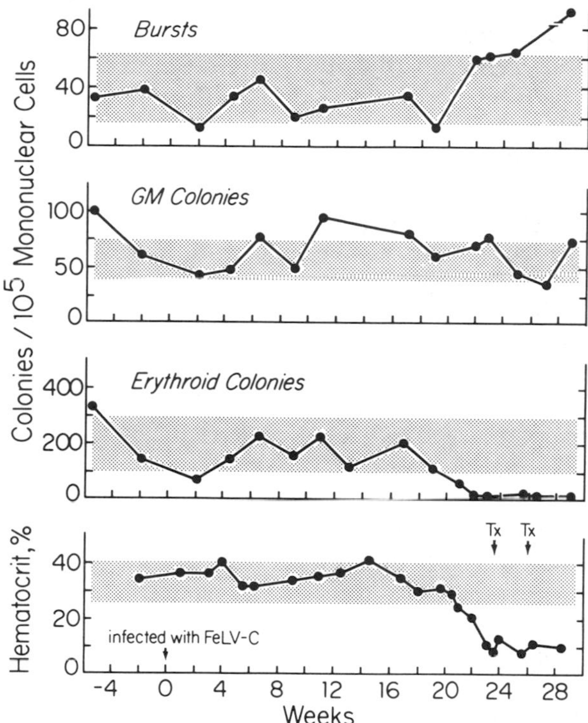


**Figure 4** Studies of pure red cell aplasia induced by FeLV-C/Sarma. This cat received FeLV-C/Sarma at week 0. Severe anemia requiring transfusions (Tx) developed by week 24. At week 22, erythroid colonies (from CFU-E) became undetectable in marrow culture, but the frequencies of erythroid bursts (from BFU-E) and GM (granulocyte-macrophage) colonies (from CFU-GM) did not change. Shaded areas represent the ranges of each value in control cats (Reproduced from the *Journal of Clinical Investigation*, 1985; 75:133–40; by copyright permission of the American Society of Clinical Investigation.)

In prospective, sequential studies of marrow from cats inoculated with FeLV-C/Sarma, infected BFU-E lost their responsiveness to FEF-A CM in vitro at the same time that the frequency of CFU-E markedly decreased (2–3 weeks before severe anemia) (142). These observations, along with the information that PRCA is mediated by gp70, have led to the hypothesis that the cell surface receptor for FeLV-C/Sarma is also a receptor that is necessary for the differentiation of BFU-E to CFU-E. One candidate receptor is the transferrin receptor, which is present on many different cells but is of critical importance in erythroid progenitors for the increased iron transport required for hemoglobin formation. Impairment of transferrin receptor function or intracellular cycling by gp70 may explain the specific erythroid effects of FeLV subgroup C. Alternatively, the gp70 of FeLV-C/Sarma could interfere with the receptor for hematopoietic growth factor(s) present in FEF-A CM or with signal transduction pathways unique to erythroid cells. It seems likely that further studies of this disorder will provide insights to mechanisms controlling normal early erythropoiesis as well as the pathogenesis of PRCA.

## Pathogenesis of Myeloid Leukemia Induced by FeLV-AB/GM1

One strain of FeLV (FeLV-AB/GM1) induces myelodysplasia and myeloid leukemia in neonatal kittens (100). Serial studies of viremic kittens reveal anemia with trilineage morphologic abnormalities of marrow cells within 2 weeks of infection. By 3–5 weeks, the cats develop pancytopenia, marrow erythroid and myeloid hyperplasia, and an increased percentage (20–24%) of blasts. Myeloid or myelomonocytic leukemia (≥ 30% marrow blasts) develops within 7 weeks of infection (100). In vitro marrow culture studies on cats experimentally infected with FeLV-AB/GM1 reveal an increase in the frequency of CFU-GM detected as early as 2 weeks after infection (5). Serum-containing cultures seeded at low cell density ($10^4$ marrow mononuclear cells per ml) and in the absence of colony-stimulating factors (CSF) reveal up to a 100-fold increase in the number of CFU-GM-derived colonies compared to similar cultures of marrow from uninfected cats (5). These results suggest an increased sensitivity of the infected CFU-GM to the low levels of CSF present in the serum. By 3 months after infection, the frequency of CFU-GM decreases and marrow cultures from cats with increased numbers of marrow blasts grow large numbers of small cell clusters (5). Long-term marrow cultures established from cats with myelodysplasia induced by FeLV-AB/GM1 demonstrate subnormal production of CFU-GM and granulocytes (5).

Proviruses in feline embryonic fibroblasts infected with FeLV-AB/GM1 have been recently cloned and characterized (71). These include a replication-competent FeLV subgroup A as well as replication-defective strains of FeLV subgroup B type (71). Two of the replication-defective proviruses have deletions in the *gag* and/or *pol* regions and contain sequences in the *gag* and *env* genes that are highly homologous with enFeLV sequences. Mixtures of the molecularly cloned viruses cause persistent viremia in newborn cats and an early (3 weeks after infection) polyclonal expansion in the number of CFU-GM per $10^5$ marrow cells cultured in vitro (71). Similar to the effects of the biologically cloned virus (5), the frequency of CFU-GM declined at 47 weeks after infection, and small cell clusters grew in marrow cultures of most cats. Only one cat inoculated with the molecularly cloned FeLV-AB/GM1 complex developed myeloid leukemia, and the leukemic clone was infected with FeLV subgroup A only (71). Despite the in vitro culture abnormalities, the five long-term survivors maintained normal peripheral blood counts and marrow morphologies. In an additional experiment, only two of six newborn kittens inoculated with the replication-competent clone FeLV-A/GM1 alone became persistently viremic, but one of the two developed myelodysplasia (71).

Taken together, these data suggest that a multistep progression of disease occurs after infection with FeLV-AB/GM1. The early, polyclonal expansion of CFU-GM occurs in all viremic cats, but leukemia develops infrequently and most likely as a result of a second event in a single infected cell. The replication-defective subgroup B viruses probably arise from a recombination event with enFeLV sequences, and their role in pathogenesis appears to be indirect. The pathophysiology of the myeloid neoplasia resulting from FeLV-AB/GM1 has conceptual similarities to that described for a nononcogene-containing murine retrovirus (150).

## Nonneoplastic Effects of FeLV and FeLV p15E

Productive infection with replication-competent FeLV generally does not result in obvious morphologic or phenotypic changes in the host feline cells. Effects on proliferation or cell function may occur, however. T lymphocytes (89–91) and neutrophils (92,151) taken from cats viremic with FeLV demonstrate a variety of functional defects (see section on immunobiology). Similar functional abnormalities are induced in normal feline lymphocytes and neutrophils (93–96) and in human lymphocytes (reviewed in Ref. 152) exposed in vitro to UV-inactivated FeLV or purified p15E protein (purified by liquid column chromatography). Growth of erythroid progenitors (147) and fibroblast colony-forming cells (153) is decreased in vitro by exposure to purified FeLV p15E. Furthermore, inoculation of cats with p15E results in suppression of both cytotoxic antibody production and resistance to challenge with FeSV (93). It has been hypothesized that FeLV p15E may affect cellular function by interference with the protein kinase C-mediated signal transduction pathway (154) and/or the accompanying intracellular free calcium level (155).

In addition to the effects of FeLV on cell growth or response, direct cytopathic effects have been implicated in the pathogenesis of disease caused by the FeLV-FAIDS strain. This strain, isolated from a spontaneous thymic lymphoma, causes severe lymphopenia and fatal immunodeficiency in experimentally infected cats (89). A prospective study of circulating T lymphocyte progenitors (T-CFU-lc) in cats viremic with FeLV-FAIDS revealed a decrease in the frequency of these progenitors before the onset of acute immunodeficiency syndrome (wasting, diarrhea, and opportunistic infections) at 6–22 weeks after infection (156). This decrease preceded the lymphopenia and functional lymphocyte defects associated with later disease but was temporally associated with the appearance of unintegrated, variant FeLV DNA in marrow cells (156,157). Because high levels of unintegrated viral DNA have been associated with the cytopathogenicity of other retroviruses (158, 159), it was hypothesized that a similar mechanism may occur with FeLV-FAIDS (156).

Recently, proviral DNAs have been cloned from tissues of cats infected with FeLV-FAIDS, and a number of replication-defective FeLV variants were identified (70). Viral chimeras, consisting of sequences from a defective variant clone combined with sequences from a nonpathogenic FeLV subgroup A clone, were able to induce disease in vivo and demonstrated that the *env* gene region of the replication-defective variant virus was responsible for the pathogenicity of FeLV-FAIDS (70). Additional studies utilizing a T lymphocyte cell line infected with the FeLV-FAIDS chimeric virus demonstrated that the posttranslational processing of the variant *env* gene precursor product (gp80) is defective and that this is associated with in vitro cell killing (160,161). Although abnormal gp80 processing and unintegrated viral DNA accumulation have been demonstrated in different infected cell types under different conditions, they may be linked pathophysiologically. One theory is that defective envelope protein expression may permit cell superinfection and result in cytotoxicity due to high levels of unintegrated viral DNA. Alternatively, it is possible that accumulation of unprocessed gp80 alone is directly cytotoxic.

## Indirect Effects of FeLV on Hematopoietic Cells

Normal hematopoiesis requires a supportive microenvironment. The hematopoietic microenvironment within the marrow includes accessory cells of hematopoietic (T lymphocytes and macrophages) and nonhematopoietic (endothelial cells and fibroblasts) origin, humoral signals that regulate proliferation and differentiation (hematopoietic growth factors and inhibitors), and a structural framework that organizes these cells and humoral factors (the extracellular matrix). The extracellular matrix products and regulatory growth signals are supplied by the microenvironmental cells (162,163). Alterations in the number or function of these accessory cells may contribute to deficient hematopoiesis or, alternatively, be the source of growth stimulatory signals promoting preferential growth of an abnormal hematopoietic clone.

Medullary osteosclerosis occurs in cats with FeLV-associated pure red cell aplasia and can result in complete obliteration of the marrow cavity. Although C-type particles are visualized in the osteocytes in these marrows, it is unclear if their proliferation is a direct result of infection or a reactive process (115). Myelofibrosis is associated with FeLV-induced myelodysplasia and myeloid leukemia (123,125,136) but is also seen in cases of myelodysplasia and myeloid leukemia not associated with FeLV infection (136). Therefore, it is likely that the fibroblast proliferation associated with these disorders is not a direct result of FeLV infection but, as in human clonal stem cell diseases (164,165), is a reactive process.

Our in vitro culture studies of marrow from viremic and regressor cats suggest that feline marrow fibroblasts are infected with FeLV in vivo and may be a reservoir of latent virus in regressor cats (166). Furthermore, infection of feline fibroblasts (Ref. 149 and Abkowitz, unpublished data) by nonpathogenic strains of FeLV results in a significant increase in the constitutive production of hematopoietic colony-stimulating factor(s). Infected fibroblasts in the hematopoietic microenvironment may therefore be similarly altered to release factors that modulate hematopoiesis.

FeLV infection may affect the number of marrow cells that give rise to fibroblast colonies in vitro. For example, decreased numbers of fibroblast colony-forming cells per $10^6$ marrow mononuclear cells have been reported in cats viremic with a strain of FeLV associated with pure red cell aplasia (FeLV-KT) (153), but marrow from regressor cats (153) or cats viremic with FeLV-AB/GM1 (5) have normal or increased numbers. Despite increased frequencies of fibroblast colony-forming cells, long-term marrow culture adherent layers are difficult to establish from cats viremic with FeLV-AB/GM1 and they support hematopoiesis poorly (5). This suggests that there is also a functional defect in the hematopoietic microenvironment of cats infected with FeLV-AB/GM1.

## Molecular Mechanisms of FeLV-Induced Neoplasia

Lymphoid neoplasms arising outside the marrow account for most of the FeLV-associated malignancies (167). Much of our current knowledge of the molecular mechanisms of FeLV-induced neoplasia has come from the study of proviruses found in lymphoid tumors. FeLV-associated multicentric fibrosarcomas occur much less frequently, but the strains of replication-defective FeSV that cause these tumors have also been studied extensively (reviewed in Ref. 67). Although these viruses are not germane to a discussion of the hematologic consequences of FeLV, their mechanism of disease is relevant to that of lymphoid neoplasia. All FeSV genomes contain an oncogene, and two of the seven oncogenes identified to date have been found in multiple, unrelated FeSV isolates (reviewed in Refs. 67–69). The viral oncogene product (often a *gag-onc* fusion protein) promotes direct transformation of infected cells and rapid disease progression.

Transduction of the *myc* cellular protooncogene into the FeLV genome has been implicated as part of the pathogenesis of up to 15% of naturally occurring T cell lymphosarcomas (69). The recombinant proviruses, designated FeLV *myc*, are replication-defective, but when mixed with replication-competent helper FeLV, they induce clonal or oligoclonal T cell lymphosarcomas in cats (168,169). Like FeSV, FeLV *myc* is not horizontally transmitted, although the requisite helper virus is passed by contact among animals (169). These defective viruses may arise de novo in FeLV-infected cats and then lead to lymphosarcomas.

That isolates from T cell lymphosarcomas from different cats involve the same oncogene (*myc*) suggests a lineage-specific role for *myc* in tumorigenesis. Three FeLV *myc* isolates have been cloned and partially sequenced (170–172). These viruses contain complete coding sequences of c-*myc* exons 2 and 3 (171,172), with a single point mutation detected in one (170). Two of the proviruses contain the integrated *myc* gene near the splice acceptor site of the *env* gene (170,172) and should express a v-*myc* gene product very similar to the c-*myc* protein. In the third cloned provirus, v-*myc* is integrated adjacent to the *gag* gene, replacing the *pol* gene, and the predicted gene product is a *gag-myc* fusion protein (171).

FeLV *myc* isolates, unlike FeSV, do not cause the rapid onset of multiclonal tumors in inoculated animals, nor do they transform infected cells in vitro (168–170,173). In vivo tumorigenesis therefore likely requires additional events. For example, two recombinant proviruses were detected in a naturally occurring T cell lymphosarcoma (66). One provirus contained a transduced *myc* gene, and the other contained the gene encoding the T cell antigen receptor $\beta$-chain (designated *tcr*) (66). It is hypothesized that the v-*tcr* gene product contributes to neoplastic transformation if it functions as a component of the T cell-receptor complex and leads to constitutive activity (i.e., in the absence of antigen) or continuous stimulation by ubiquitous antigens (perhaps FeLV antigens). In this setting, the v-*tcr* gene product would provide a proliferative signal that, in concert with v-*myc*-mediated inhibition of differentiation, generates the full neoplastic phenotype (174).

In other lymphoid tumors, analysis of FeLV proviral integration sites has suggested that insertional mutagenesis of specific host genes (proto-oncogenes) may be related to neoplastic growth. In many FeLV-associated lymphosarcomas, an FeLV provirus is integrated near c-*myc* (46,47). The insertion site is usually upstream of exon 1, the proviral genome is in the opposite orientation, and there is overexpression of the adjacent c-*myc* gene (47,50). The overexpression is likely due to activation of the c-*myc* promoter by an enhancer in the proviral LTR (46,47,50,69). Only 7% of naturally occurring T cell lymphosarcomas involve insertional mutagenesis of the *myc* gene, whereas 75% of experimentally induced tumors involve *myc* (46,47, 69). This difference may reflect laboratory selection of FeLV strains that induce tumors because of high LTR enhancer activity (69). Increased enhancer activity has been further implicated in tumorigenesis by the observations that frequent duplications are found in the LTR enhancer regions of proviruses cloned from naturally occurring lymphosarcomas compared to proviruses cloned from other sources (49,50). The FeLV LTR enhancer sequences contain nuclear protein binding sites (49); therefore, host cell gene regulatory proteins may also modulate their function.

Insertional mutagenesis may also play a role in the physiology of splenic non-T cell lymphosarcomas associated with FeLV (48). A common proviral integration site, designated *flvi*-1, has been identified in the genome of tumor cells from four unrelated animals with splenic lymphosarcomas (48). The function of this gene and/or the presence of adjacent protooncogenes have not yet been defined. Other potential, but as yet rarely identified, mechanisms of FeLV insertional mutagenesis involve the integration of the proviral LTR promoter within a cellular oncogene or proviral insertion within a repressor region of a gene. Either event could result in gene overexpression.

## CONCLUSIONS

Much remains unknown about the pathophysiologic mechanisms underlying the hematologic disorders associated with FeLV. Infection of hematopoietic progenitors and/or high concentrations of FeLV envelope proteins may suppress hematopoiesis, as exemplified by the pathogenesis of pure red cell aplasia associated with FeLV subgroup C. Because FeLV also infects lymphocytes, macrophages, and marrow fibroblasts, both neoplastic and nonneoplastic disorders may be influenced by alterations in the structural integrity of the hematopoietic microenvironment or in the production of growth factors by microenvironmental cells. Finally, it is not known if myelodysplasia or ANLL results from insertional mutagenesis or recombination events involving genes important in the proliferation and differentiation of myeloid cells, analogous to events described in FeLV-induced lymphoid neoplasms. Certainly, further studies of these FeLV-induced marrow disorders will provide insights to the molecular and cellular events important in hematopoiesis and in leukemogenesis.

## ACKNOWLEDGMENTS

The authors thank Julie Overbaugh for her thoughtful review of the virology data, William Hardy, Jr. for assistance in obtaining a copy of Figure 1, James Neil for his suggestions for Figure 3, and Zeny Sisk for her help in the preparation of this manuscript. This work was supported by Grants HL02396 and HL31823 from the National Institutes of Health.

## REFERENCES


1. Hardy WD Jr. Feline leukemia virus diseases. In: Hardy WD Jr, Essex M, McClelland AJ, eds. Feline leukemia virus. New York: Elsevier-North Holland, 1980; 3–31.
2. Reinacher M. Diseases associated with spontaneous feline leukemia virus (FeLV) infection in cats. Vet Immunol Immunopathol 1989; 21:85–95.
3. Neil JC, Onions DE. Feline leukaemia viruses: molecular biology and pathogenesis. Anticancer Res 1985; 5:49–64.
4. Hardy WD Jr. Feline acquired immune deficiency syndrome: a feline retrovirus-induced syndrome of pet cats. In: Salzman LA, ed. Animal models of retrovirus infection and their relationship to AIDS. New York: Academic Press, 1986; 75–93.
5. Testa NG, Onions DE, Lord BI. A feline model for the myelodysplastic syndrome: pre-leukaemic abnormalities caused in cats by infection with a new isolate of feline leukaemia virus (FeLV), AB/GM1. Haematologica 1988; 73:317–20.
6. Jarrett WFH, Martin WB, Crighton GW, Dalton RG, Stewart MF. Leukaemia in the cat. Nature 1964; 202:566–7.
7. Jarrett WFH, Crawford EM, Martin WB, Davie F. A virus-like particle associated with leukaemia (lymphosarcoma). Nature 1964; 202:567–8.
8. Kawakami TG, Theilen GH, Dungworth DL, Munn RJ, Beall SG. "C"-Type viral particles in plasma of cats with feline leukemia. Science 1967; 158:1049–50.
9. Rickard CG, Barr LM, Noronha F, Dougherty E III, Post JE. C-type virus particles in spontaneous lymphocytic leukemia in a cat. Cornell Vet 1967; 57:302–7.
10. Laird HM, Jarrett WFH, Jarrett JO, Crighton GW. Virus-like particles in three field cases of feline lymphosarcoma. Vet Rec 1967; 80:606.
11. Laird HM, Jarrett O, Crighton GW, Jarrett WFH, Hay D. Replication of leukemogenic-type virus in cats inoculated with feline lymphosarcoma extracts. J Natl Cancer Inst 1968; 41:879–93.
12. Theilen GH, Kawakami TG, Dungworth DL, Switzer JW, Munn RJ, Harrold JB. Current status of transmissible agents in feline leukemia. J Am Vet Med Assoc 1968; 153:1864–72.
13. Rickard CG, Post JE, Noronha F, Barr LM. A transmissible virus-induced lymphocytic leukemia of the cat. J Natl Cancer Inst 1969; 42:987–1014.
14. Mackey LJ, Jarrett WFH, Jarrett O, Laird HM. An experimental study of virus leukemia in cats. J Natl Cancer Inst 1972; 48:1663–70.
15. Dorn CR, Taylor DON, Schneider R, Hibbard HH, Klauber MR. Survey of animal neoplasms in Alameda and Contra Costa counties, California. II. Cancer morbidity in dogs and cats from Alameda County. J Natl Cancer Inst 1968; 40:307–18.
16. Schneider R, Frye FL, Taylor DON, Dorn CR. A household cluster of feline malignant lymphoma. Cancer Res 1967; 27:1316–22.
17. Snyder SP, Theilen GH. Transmissible feline fibrosarcoma. Nature 1969; 221: 1074–5.

18. Gardner MB, Rongey RW, Arnstein P, et al. Experimental transmission of feline fibrosarcoma to cats and dogs. Nature 1970; 226:807–9.
19. McDonough SK, Larsen S, Brodey RS, Stock ND, Hardy WD Jr. A transmissible feline fibrosarcoma of viral origin. Cancer Res 1971; 31:953–6.
20. Hardy WD Jr, Geering G, Old LJ, De Harven E, Brodey RS, McDonough S. Feline leukemia virus: occurrence of viral antigen in the tissues of cats with lymphosarcoma and other diseases. Science 1969; 166:1019–21.
21. Hardy WD Jr. Immunodiffusion studies of feline leukemia and sarcoma. J Am Vet Med Assoc 1971; 158:1060–9.
22. Hardy WD Jr, Hirshaut Y, Hess P. Detection of the feline leukemia virus and other mammalian oncornaviruses by immunofluorescence. In: Unifying concepts of leukemia, Bibl. haemat., No. 39. Edited by Dutcher RM, Chieco-Bianchi L, eds. Basel: Karger, 1973; 778–99.
23. Jarrett O, Golder MC, Weijer K. A comparison of three methods of feline leukaemia virus diagnosis. Vet Rec 1982; 110:325–8.
24. Hardy WD Jr, Old LJ, Hess PW, Essex M, Cotter S. Horizontal transmission of feline leukaemia virus. Nature 1973; 244:266–9.
25. Jarrett W, Jarret O, Mackey L, Laird H, Hardy WD Jr, Essex M. Horizontal transmission of leukemia virus and leukemia in the cat. J Natl Cancer Inst 1973; 51:833–41.
26. Essex M, Sliski A, Cotter SM, Jakowski RM, Hardy WD Jr. Immunosurveillance of naturally occurring feline leukemia. Science 1975; 190:790–2.
27. Rogerson P, Jarrett W, Mackey L. Epidemiological studies on feline leukaemia virus infection. I. A serological survey in urban cats. Int J Cancer 1975; 15:781–5.
28. Rojko JL, Hoover EA, Mathes LE, Olsen RG, Schaller JP. Pathogenesis of experimental feline leukemia virus infection. J Natl Cancer Inst 1979; 63:759–68.
29. Teich N. Taxonomy of retroviruses. In: Weiss R, Teich N, Varmus H, Coffin J, eds. RNA tumor viruses: molecular biology of tumor viruses, 2nd ed. Cold Spring Harbor, NY: Cold Spring Harbor Laboratory, 1984; 25–209.
30. Shroyer EL, Shalaby MR. Isolation of feline syncytia-forming virus from oropharyngeal swab samples and buffy coat cells. Am J Vet Res 1978; 39:555–60.
31. Pedersen NC, Ho EW, Brown ML, Yamamoto JK. Isolation of a T-lymphotropic virus from domestic cats with an immunodeficiency-like syndrome. Science 1987; 235:790–3.
32. Ishida T, Washizu T, Toriyabe K, Motoyoshi S, Tomoda I, Pedersen NC. Feline immunodeficiency virus infection in cats of Japan. J Am Vet Med Assoc 1989; 194:221–5.
33. Pedersen NC, Yamamoto JK, Ishida T, Hansen H. Feline immunodeficiency virus infection. Vet Immunol Immunopathol 1989; 21:111–29.
34. Shelton GH, Grant CK, Cotter SM, Gardner MB, Hardy WD Jr, DiGiacomo RF. Feline immunodeficiency virus and feline leukemia virus infections and their relationships to lymphoid malignancies in cats: a retrospective study (1968–1988). AIDS 1990; 3:623–30.
35. Shelton GH, Linenberger ML, Grant CK, Abkowitz JL. Hematologic manifestations of feline immunodeficiency virus infection. Blood 1990; 76:1104–9.

36. Livingston DM, Todaro GJ. Endogenous type C virus from a cat cell clone with properties distinct from previously described feline type C virus. Virology 1973; 53:142–51.
37. Fischinger PJ, Peebles PT, Nomura S, Haapala DK. Isolation of an RD-114-like oncornavirus from a cat cell line. J Virol 1973; 11:978–85.
38. Neiman PE. Measurement of RD114 virus nucleotide sequences in feline cellular DNA. Nature (New Biol) 1973; 244:62–4.
39. Okabe H, Twiddy E, Gilden RV, Hatanaka M, Hoover EA, Olsen RG. FeLV-related sequences in DNA from a FeLV-free cat colony. Virology 1976; 69:788–801.
40. Niman HL, Akhavi M, Gardner MB, Stephenson JR, Roy-Burman P. Differential expression of two distinct endogenous retrovirus genomes in developing tissues of the domestic cat. J Natl Cancer Inst 1980; 64:587–94.
41. Busch MP, Devi BG, Soe LH, Perbal B, Baluda MA, Roy-Burman P. Characterization of the expression of cellular retrovirus genes and oncogenes in feline cells. Hematol Oncol 1983; 1:61–75.
42. Neil JC, McDougall A, Rojko J, Terry A, Stewart M, Jarrett O. High expression of endogenous FeLV-related proviral sequences in feline leukemia cell lines and virus-infected lymphoid tissues (abstract). In: Cold Spring Harbor Conference on RNA tumor viruses. Cold Spring Harbor, NY: Cold Spring Harbor Laboratory, 1990; 109.
43. Overbaugh J, Riedel N, Hoover EA, Mullins JI. Transduction of endogenous envelope genes by feline leukaemia virus in vitro. Nature 1988; 332:731–4.
44. Yoshinaka Y, Katoh I. Copeland TD, Oroszlan S. Translational readthrough of an amber termination codon during synthesis of feline leukemia virus protease. J Virol 1985; 55:870–3.
45. Neil JC, Hughes D, McFarlane R, et al. Transduction and rearrangement of the *myc* gene by feline leukaemia virus in naturally occurring T-cell leukaemias. Nature 1984; 308:814–20.
46. Miura T, Tsujimoto H, Fukasawa M, et al. Structural abnormality and over-expression of the *myc* gene in feline leukemias. Int J Cancer 1987; 40:564–9.
47. Forrest D, Onions D, Lees G, Neil JC. Altered structure and expression of c-*myc* in feline T-cell tumours. Virology 1987; 158:194–205.
48. Levesque KS, Bonham L, Levy LS. flvi-1, a common integration domain of feline leukemia virus in naturally occurring lymphomas of a particular type. J Virol 1990; 64:3455–62.
49. Fulton R, Plumb M, Shield L, Neil JC. Structural diversity and nuclear protein binding sites in the long terminal repeats of feline leukemia virus. J Virol 1990; 64:1675–82.
50. Miura T, Shibuya M, Tsujimoto H, Fukasawa M, Hayami M. Molecular cloning of a feline leukemia provirus integrated adjacent to the c-*myc* gene in a feline T-cell leukemia cell line and the unique structure of its long terminal repeat. Virology 1989; 169:458–61.
51. Mullins JI, Casey JW, Nicolson MO, Burck KB, Davidson N. Sequence arrangement and biological activity of cloned feline leukemia virus proviruses from a virus-productive human cell line. J Virol 1981; 38:688–703.

52. Post JE, Warren L. Reactivation of latent feline leukemia virus. In: Hardy WD Jr, Essex M, McClelland AJ, eds. Feline leukemia virus. New York: Elsevier-North Holland, 1980; 151–5.
53. Rojko JL, Hoover EA, Quackenbush SL, Olsen RG. Reactivation of latent feline leukaemia virus infection. Nature 1982; 298:385–8.
54. Madewell BR, Jarrett O. Recovery of feline leukaemia virus from non-viraemic cats. Vet Rec 1983; 112:339–42.
55. Pedersen NC, Meric SM, Ho E, Johnson L, Plucker S, Theilen GH. The clinical significance of latent feline leukemia virus infection in cats. Feline Pract 1984; 14:32–48.
56. Elder JH, Mullins JI. Nucleotide sequence of the envelope gene of Gardner-Arnstein feline leukemia virus B reveals unique sequence homologies with a murine mink cell focus-forming virus. J Virol 1983; 46:871–80.
57. Stewart MA, Warnock M, Wheeler A, et al. Nucleotide sequences of a feline leukemia virus subgroup A envelope gene and long terminal repeat and evidence for the recombinational origin of subgroup B viruses. J Virol 1986; 58:825–34.
58. Riedel N, Hoover EA, Gasper PW, Nicolson MO, Mullins JI. Molecular analysis and pathogenesis of the feline aplastic anemia retrovirus, feline leukemia virus C-Sarma. J Virol 1986; 60:242–50.
59. Donahue PR, Hoover EA, Beltz GA, et al. Strong sequence conservation among horizontally transmissible, minimally pathogenic feline leukemia viruses. J Virol 1988; 62:722–31.
60. Sarma PS, Log T, Jain D, Hill PR, Huebner RJ. Differential host range of viruses of feline leukemia-sarcoma complex. Virology 1975; 64:438–46.
61. Jarrett O. Feline leukaemia virus subgroups. In: Hardy WD Jr, Essex M, McClelland AJ, eds. Feline leukemia virus. New York: Elsevier-North Holland, 1980; 473–9.
62. Jarrett O, Russell PH. Differential growth and transmission in cats of feline leukaemia viruses of subgroups A and B. Int J Cancer 1978; 21:466 72.
63. Jarrett O, Golder MC, Toth S, Onions DE, Stewart MF. Interaction between feline leukaemia virus subgroups in the pathogenesis of erythroid hypoplasia. Int J Cancer 1984; 34:283–8.
64. Levy LS, Gardner MB, Casey JW. Isolation of a feline leukaemia provirus containing the oncogene *myc* from a feline lymphosarcoma. Nature 1984; 308: 853–6.
65. Mullins JI, Brody DS, Binari RC Jr, Cottere SM. Viral transduction of c-*myc* gene in naturally occurring feline leukaemias. Nature 1984; 308:856–8.
66. Fulton R, Forrest D, McFarlane R, Onions D, Neil JC. Retroviral transduction of T-cell antigen receptor $\beta$-chain and *myc* genes. Nature 1987; 326:190–4.
67. Besmer P. Acute transforming feline retroviruses. Curr Top Microbiol Immunol 1983; 107:1–27.
68. Onions DE, Jarrett O. Viral oncogenesis: lessons from naturally occurring animal viruses. Cancer Surv 1987; 6:161–80.
69. Neil JC, Forrest D, Doggett DL, Mullins JI. The role of feline leukaemia virus in naturally occurring leukaemias. Cancer Surv 1987; 6:117–37.

70. Overbaugh J, Donahue PR, Quackenbush SL, Hoover EA, Mullins JI. Molecular cloning of a feline leukemia virus that induces fatal immunodeficiency disease in cats. Science 1988; 239:906–10.
71. Tzavaras T, Stewart M, McDougall A, et al. Molecular cloning and characterization of a defective recombinant feline leukaemia virus associated with myeloid leukaemia. J Gen Virol 1990; 71:343–54.
72. Matsumoto Y, Tsujimoto H, Fukasawa M, et al. Molecular cloning of feline leukemia provirus genomes integrated in the feline large granular lymphoma cells. Arch Virol 1990; 111:177–85.
73. Francis DP, Essex M, Hardy WD Jr. Excretion of feline leukaemia virus by naturally infected pet cats. Nature 1977; 269:252–4.
74. Hardy WD Jr, Hess PW, MacEwen EG, et al. Biology of feline leukemia virus in the natural environment. Cancer Res 1976; 36:582–8.
75. Pederson NC, Theilen G, Keane MA, et al. Studies of naturally transmitted feline leukemia virus infection. Am J Vet Res 1977; 38:1523–31.
76. Hoover EA, Rojko JL, Olsen RG. Factors influencing host resistance to feline leukemia virus. In: Olsen RG, ed. Feline leukemia. Boca Raton, FL: CRC Press, 1981; 69–76.
77. Hoover EA, Olsen RG, Hardy WD Jr, Schaller JP, Mathes LE. Feline leukemia virus infection: age-related variation in response to cats to experimental infection. J Natl Cancer Inst 1976; 57:365–9.
78. Dornsife RE, Gasper PW, Mullins JI, Hoover EA. Induction of aplastic anemia by intra-bone marrow inoculation of a molecularly cloned feline retrovirus. Leuk Res 1989; 13:745–55.
79. Rojko JL, Hoover EA, Mathes LE, Krakowka S, Olsen RG. Influence of adrenal corticosteroids on the susceptibility of cats to feline leukemia virus infection. Cancer Res 1979; 39:3789–91.
80. Hoover EA, Rojko JL, Wilson PL, Olsen RG. Determinants of susceptibility and resistance to feline leukemia virus infection. I. Role of macrophages. J Natl Cancer Inst 1981; 67:889–98.
81. Hardy WD Jr. The feline leukemia virus. J Am Anim Hosp Assoc 1981; 17: 951–80.
82. Sarma PS, Log T. Viral interference in feline leukemia-sarcoma complex. Virology 1971; 44:352–8.
83. Jarrett O, Hardy WD Jr, Golder MC, Hay D. The frequency of occurrence of feline leukaemia virus subgroups in cats. Int J Cancer 1978; 21:334–7.
84. Lutz H, Pedersen NC, Higgins J, Troy FA, Theilen GH. Long-term immune response to feline leukemia virus components in cats after natural infection. In: Essex M, Todaro G, Hausen HZ, eds. Viruses of naturally occurring cancers. Cold Spring Harbor, NY: Cold Spring Harbor Laboratories, 1980; 653–64.
85. Snyder HW Jr, Singhal MC, Zucherman EE, Jones FR, Hardy WD Jr. The feline oncornavirus-associated cell membrane antigen (FOCMA) is related to, but distinguishable from, FeLV-C gp70. Virology 1983; 131:315–27.
86. Mathes LE, Olsen RG. Immunobiology of feline leukemia virus disease. In: Olsen RG, ed. Immunobiology of feline leukemia virus disease. Boca Raton, FL: CRC Press, 1981; 77–88.

87. McClelland AJ, Hardy WD Jr, Zuckerman EE. Prognosis of healthy feline leukemia virus infected cats. In: Hardy WD Jr, Essex M, McClelland AJ, eds. Feline leukemia virus. New York: Elsevier-North Holland, 1980; 121–6.
88. Trainin Z, Wernicke D, Ungar-Waron H, Essex M. Suppression of the humoral antibody response in natural retrovirus infections. Science 1983; 220:858–9.
89. Hoover EA, Mullins JI, Quackenbush SL, Gasper PW. Experimental transmission and pathogenesis of immunodeficiency syndrome in cats. Blood 1987; 70:1880–92.
90. Cockerell GL, Hoover EA, Krakowska S, Olsen RG, Yohn DS. Lymphocyte mitogen reactivity and enumeration of circulating B- and T-cells during feline leukemia virus infection in the cat. J Natl Cancer Inst 1976; 57:1095–9.
91. Thompkins MB, Ogilivie GK, Gast AM, Franklin R, Weigel R, Tompkins WAF. Interleukin-2 suppression in cats naturally infected with feline leukemia virus. J Biol Response Mod 1989; 8:86–96.
92. Kiehl AR, Fettman MJ, Quackenbush SL, Hoover EA. Effects of feline leukemia virus infection on neutrophil chemotaxis in vitro. Am J Vet Res 1987; 48: 76–80.
93. Mathes LE, Olsen RG, Hebebrand LC, et al. Immunosuppressive properties of virion polypeptide, a 15,000-dalton protein, from feline leukemia virus. Cancer Res 1979; 39:950–5.
94. Mathes LE, Olsen RG, Hebebrand LC, Hoover EA, Schaller JP. Abrogation of lymphocyte blastogenesis by a feline leukaemia virus protein. Nature 1978; 274:687–9.
95. Lafrado LJ, Lewis MG, Mathes LE, Olsen RG. Suppression of in vitro neutrophil function by feline leukaemia virus (FeLV) and purified FeLV-p15E. J Gen Virol 1987; 68:507–13.
96. Mitani M, Cianciolo GJ, Snyderman R, Yasuda M, Good RA, Day NK. Suppressive effect on polyclonal B-cell activation of a synthetic peptide homologous to a transmembrane component of oncogenic retroviruses. Proc Natl Acad Sci U S A 1987; 84:237–40.
97. Lafrado LJ, Olsen RG. Demonstration of depressed polymorphonuclear leukocyte function in nonviremic FeLV-infected cats. Cancer Invest 1986; 4:297–300.
98. Lafrado LJ, Dezzutti CS, Lewis MG, Olsen RG. Immunodeficiency in latent feline leukemia virus infections. Vet Immunol Immunopathol 1989; 21:39–46.
99. Swenson CL, Kociba GJ, Mathes LE, et al. Prevalence of disease in nonviremic cats previously exposed to feline leukemia virus. Am Vet Med Assoc 1990; 196:1049–52.
100. Toth SR, Onions DE, Jarrett O. Histopathological and hematological findings in myeloid leukemia induced by a new feline leukemia virus isolate. Vet Pathol 1986; 23:462–70.
101. Hause WR, Olsen RG. Clinical aspects of feline leukemia diseases. In: Olsen RG, ed. Feline leukemia. Boca Raton, FL: CRC Press, 1981; 89–114.
102. Schalm OW. Interpretations in feline bone marrow cytology. J Am Vet Med Assoc 1972; 161:1418–25.

103. Schalm OW, Jain NC, Carroll EJ. Veterinary hematology, 3rd ed. Philadelphia: Lea & Febiger, 1975; 565-91.
104. Hillman RS, Finch CA. Red cell manual, 5th ed. Philadelphia: F. A. Davis Co., 1985; 56-98.
105. Bennett JM, Catovsky D, Daniel MT, et al. Proposals for the classification of the myelodysplastic syndromes. Br J Haematol 1982; 51:189-99.
106. Bennett JM, Catovsky D, Daniel MT, et al. Proposed revised criteria for the classification of acute myeloid leukemia. Ann Intern Med 1985; 103:626-9.
107. Cotter SM, Hardy WD Jr, Essex M. Association of feline leukemia virus with lymphosarcoma and other disorders in the cat. J Am Vet Med Assoc 1975; 166:449-54.
108. Cotter SM. Anemia associated with feline leukemia virus infection. J Am Vet Med Assoc 1979; 175:1191-4.
109. Hardy WD Jr. Feline leukemia virus non-neoplastic diseases. J Am Anim Hosp Assoc 1981; 17:941-9.
110. Mackey L, Jarrett W, Jarrett O, Laird H. Anemia associated with feline leukemia virus infection in cats. J Natl Cancer Inst 1975; 54:209-17.
111. Maggio L, Hoffman R, Cotter SM, Dainiak N, Mooney S, Maffei LA. Feline preleukemia: an animal model of human disease. Yale J Biol Med 1978; 51:469-76.
112. Madewell BR, Jain NC, Weller RE. Hematologic abnormalities preceding myeloid leukemia in three cats. Vet Pathol 1979; 16:510-9.
113. Blue JT, French TW, Kranz JS. Non-lymphoid hematopoietic neoplasia in cats: a retrospective study of 60 cases. Cornell Vet 1988; 78:21-42.
114. Hoover EA, Kociba GJ, Hardy WD Jr, Yohn DS. Erythroid hypoplasia in cats inoculated with feline leukemia virus. J Natl Cancer Inst 1974; 53:1271-6.
115. Hoover EA, Kociba GJ. Bone lesions in cats with anemia induced by feline leukemia virus. J Natl Cancer Inst 1974; 53:1277-84.
116. Jarrett O. Natural occurrence of subgroups of feline leukemia virus. In: Essex M, Todaro G, Hausen HZ, eds. Viruses of naturally occurring cancers. Cold Spring Harbor, NY: Cold Spring Harbor Laboratory, 1980; 603-11.
117. Scott DW, Schultz RD, Post JE, Bolton GR, Baldwin CA. Autoimmune hemolytic anemia in the cat. J Am Anim Hosp Assoc 1973; 9:530-9.
118. Hardy WD Jr, McClelland AJ. Feline leukemia virus: its related diseases and control. Vet Clin North Am 1977; 7:93-103.
119. Swenson CL, Kociba GJ, O'Keefe DA, Crisp MS, Jacobs RM, Rojko JL. Cyclic hematopoiesis associated with feline leukemia virus infection in two cats. J Am Vet Med Assoc 1987; 191:93-6.
120. Lester SJ, Searcy GP. Hematologic abnormalities preceding apparent recovery from feline leukemia virus infection. J Am Vet Med Assoc 1981; 178:471-4.
121. Gabbert NH. Cyclic neutropenia in a feline leukemia-positive cat: a case report. J Am Anim Hosp Assoc 1984; 20:343-7.
122. Willard MD. Corticosteroid-responsive leukopenia and neutropenia associated with FeLV infection in 2 cats. Mod Vet Pract 1985; October:719-22.
123. Ward JM, Sodikoff CH, Schalm OW. Myeloproliferative disease and abnormal erythrogenesis in the cat. J Am Vet Med Assoc 1969; 155:879-88.

124. Schalm OW, Theilen GH. Myeloproliferative disease in the cat, associated with C-type leukovirus particles in bone marrow. J Am Vet Med Assoc 1970; 157:1686–96.
125. Herz A, Theilen GH, Schalm OW, Munn RJ. C-type virus in bone marrow cells of cats with myeloproliferative disorders. J Natl Cancer Inst 1970; 44:339–48.
126. Facklam NR, Kociba GJ. Cytochemical characterization of feline leukemic cells. Vet Pathol 1986; 23:155–61.
127. Jain NC, Kono CS, Madewell BR. Cytochemical studies of normal feline blood and bone marrow cells. Blut 1989; 58:195–9.
128. Fraser CJ, Joiner GN, Jardine JH, Gleiser CA. Acute granulocytic leukemia in cats. J Am Vet Med Assoc 1974; 165:355–9.
129. Henness AM, Crow SE. Treatment of feline myelogenous leukemia: four case reports. J Am Vet Med Assoc 1977; 171:263–6.
130. Stann SE. Myelomonocytic leukemia in a cat. J Am Vet Med Assoc 1979; 174: 722–5.
131. Jarrett WFH, Anderson LJ, Jarrett O, Laird HM, Stewart MF. Myeloid leukaemia in a cat produced experimentally by feline leukaemia virus. Res Vet Sci 1971; 12:385–7.
132. Cotter SM, Essex M. Animal model: feline acute lymphoblastic leukemia and aplastic anemia. Am J Pathol 1977; 87:265–8.
133. Francis DP, Cotter SM, Hardy WD Jr, Essex M. Comparison of virus-positive and virus-negative cases of feline leukemia and lymphoma. Cancer Res 1979; 39:3866–70.
134. Mackey L. Feline leukaemia virus and its clinical effects in cats. Vet Rec 1975; 96:5–11.
135. Onions D, Jarrett O, Testa N, Frassoni F, Toth S. Selective effect of feline leukaemia virus on early erythroid precursors. Nature 1982; 296:156–8.
136. Blue JT. Myelofibrosis in cats with myelodysplastic syndrome and acute myelogenous leukemia. Vet Pathol 1988; 25:154–;60.
137. Boyce JT, Hoover EA, Kociba GJ, Olsen RG. Feline leukemia virus-induced erythroid aplasia: in vitro hemopoietic culture studies. Exp Hematol 1981; 9:990–1001.
138. Abkowitz JL, Ott RL, Nakamura JM, Steinmann L, Fialkow PJ, Adamson JW. Feline glucose-6-phosphate dehydrogenase cellular mosiacism: application to the study of retrovirus-induced pure red cell aplasia. J Clin Invest 1985; 75:133–40.
139. Riedel N, Hoover EA, Dornsife RE, Mullins JI. Pathogenic and host range determinants of the feline aplastic anemia retrovirus. Proc Natl Acad Sci U S A 1988; 85:2758–62.
140. Abkowitz JL, Holly RD, Grant CK. Retrovirus-induced feline pure red cell aplasia: hematopoietic progenitors are infected with feline leukemia virus and erythroid burst forming cells are uniquely sensitive to heterologous complement. J Clin Invest 1987; 80:1056–63.
141. Kociba GJ, Halper JM. Demonstration of retroviral proteins associated with erythroid progenitors of cats with feline leukemia virus-induced erythroid aplasia. Leuk Res 1987; 11:1135–40.

142. Abkowitz JL. Retrovirus-induced feline pure red cell aplasia: pathogenesis and response to suramin. Blood 1991; 7:1442–51.
143. Abkowitz JL, Ott RL, Holly RD, Adamson JW. Lymphocytes and antibody in retrovirus-induced feline pure red cell aplasia. J Natl Cancer Inst 1987; 78:135–9.
144. Abkowitz JL, Holly RD, Adamson JW. Retrovirus-induced feline pure red cell aplasia: the kinetics of erythroid marrow failure. J Cell Physiol 1987; 132:571–7.
145. Testa NG, Onions D, Jarrett O, Frassoni F, Eliason JF. Haemopoietic colony formation (BFU-E, GM-CFC) during the development of pure red cell hypoplasia induced in the cat by feline leukaemia virus. Leuk Res 1983; 7:103–16.
146. Rojko JL, Cheney CM, Gasper PW, et al. Infectious feline leukemia virus is erythrosuppressive in vitro. Leuk Res 1986; 10:1193–9.
147. Wellman ML, Kociba GJ, Lewis MG, Mathes LE, Olsen RG. Inhibition of erythroid colony-forming cells by a $M_r$ 15,000 protein of feline leukemia virus. Cancer Res 1984; 44:1527–9.
148. Dornsife RE, Gasper PW, Mullins JI, Hoover EA. In vitro erythrocytopathic activity of an aplastic anemia-inducing feline retrovirus. Exp Hematol 1989; 17:138–44.
149. Abkowitz JL, Holly RD, Segal GM, Adamson JW. Multilineage, non-species specific hematopoietic growth factor(s) elaborated by a feline fibroblast cell line: enhancement by virus infection. J Cell Physiol 1986; 127:189–96.
150. Heard JM, Fichelson S, Sola B, Martial MA, Varet B, Levy JP. Multistep virus-induced leukemogenesis in vitro: description of a model specifying three steps within the myeloblastic malignant process. Mol Cell Biol 1984; 4:216–20.
151. Lewis MG, Duska GO, Stiff MI, Lafrado LJ, Olsen RG. Polymorphonuclear leukocyte dysfunction associated with feline leukaemia virus infection. J Gen Virol 1986; 67:2113–8.
152. Olsen RG, Lewis MG, Lafrado LJ, Mathes LE, Haffer K, Sharpee R. Feline leukemia virus: current status of the feline induced immune depression and immunoprevention. Cancer Metastasis Rev 1987; 6:243–60.
153. Wellman ML, Kociba GJ, Mathes LE, Olsen RG. Suppression of feline bone marrow fibroblast colony-forming units by feline leukemia virus. Am J Vet Res 1988; 49:227–30.
154. Dezzutti CS, Wright KA, Lewis MG, Lafrado LJ, Olsen RG. FeLV-induced immunosuppression through alterations in signal transduction: down regulation of protein kinase C. Vet Immunol Immunopathol 1989; 21:55–67.
155. Wright KA, Dezzutti CS, Lewis MG, Olsen RG. FeLV-induced immunosuppression through alterations in signal transduction: changes in intracellular free calcium levels. Vet Immunol Immunopathol 1989; 21:47–53.
156. Quackenbush SL, Mullins JI, Hoover EA. Colony forming T lymphocyte deficit in the development of feline retrovirus induced immunodeficiency syndrome. Blood 1989; 73:509–16.
157. Mullins JI, Chen CS, Hoover EA. Disease-specific and tissue-specific production of unintegrated feline leukaemia virus variant DNA in feline AIDS. Nature 1986; 319:333–6.
158. Weller SK, Temin HM. Cell killing by avian leukosis viruses. J Virol 1981; 39:713–21.

159. Keshet E, Temin HM. Cell killing by spleen necrosis virus is correlated with a transient accumulation of spleen necrosis virus DNA. J Virol 1979; 31:376–88.
160. Poss ML, Mullins JI, Hoover EA. Posttranslational modifications distinguish the envelope glycoprotein of the immunodeficiency disease-inducing feline leukemia virus retrovirus. J Virol 1989; 63:189–95.
161. Poss ML, Quackenbush SL, Mullins JI, Hoover EA. Characterization and significance of delayed processing of the feline leukemia virus FeLV-FAIDS envelope glycoprotein. J Virol 1990; 64:4338–45.
162. Keating A, Gordon MY. Hierarchical organization of hematopoietic microenvironments: role of proteoglycans. Leukemia 1988; 2:766–9.
163. Dexter TM. Regulation of hemopoietic cell growth and development: experimental and clinical studies. Leukemia 1989; 3:469–74.
164. Chapelle A, Vuopio P, Borgstrom GH. The origin of bone marrow fibroblasts. Blood 1978; 41:783–7.
165. Jacobson RJ, Salo A, Fialkow PJ. Agnogenic myeloid metaplasia: a clonal proliferation of hematopoietic stem cells with secondary myelofibrosis. Blood 1978; 51:189–94.
166. Linenberger ML. Infection of nonhematopoietic marrow stromal cells in vivo with feline leukemia virus (FeLV) (abstract). Blood 1990; 76(Suppl. 1):489a.
167. Meincke JE, Hobbie WV, Hardy WD Jr. Lymphoreticular malignancies in the cat: clinical findings. J Am Vet Med Assoc 1972; 160:1093–9.
168. Levy LS, Fish RE, Baskin GB. Tumorigenic potential of a *myc*-containing strain of feline leukemia virus in vivo in domestic cats. J Virol 1988; 62:4770–3.
169. Onions D, Lees G, Forrest D, Neil J. Recombinant feline viruses containing the *myc* gene rapidly produce clonal tumors expressing T-cell antigen receptor gene transcripts. Int J Cancer 1987; 40:40–5.
170. Doggett DL, Drake AL, Hirsch V, Rowe ME, Stallard V, Mullins JI. Structure, origin, and transforming activity of feline leukemia virus-*myc* recombinant provirus FTT. J Virol 1989; 63:2108–17.
171. Braun MJ, Deininger PL, Casey JW. Nucleotide sequence of a transduced *myc* gene from a defective feline leukemia provirus. J Virol 1985; 55:177–83.
172. Stewart MA, Forrest D, McFarlane R, Onions D, Wilkie N, Neil JC. Conservation of the c-*myc* coding sequence in transduced feline v-*myc* genes. Virology 1986; 154:121–34.
173. Bonham L, Lobelle-Rich PA, Henderson LA, Levy LS. Transforming potential of a *myc*-containing variant of feline leukemia virus in vitro in early-passage feline cells. J Virol 1987; 61:3072–81.
174. Neil JC, Fulton R, McFarlane R, et al. Receptor-mediated leukaemogenesis: hypothesis revisited. Br J Cancer 1988; 58:76–9.

# VI

# VIRUSES AS VECTORS FOR GENE THERAPY

# 12

# Viruses as Therapeutic Gene Transfer Vectors

**Arthur W. Nienhuis, Christopher Edward Walsh, and Johnson Liu**

*National Heart, Lung and Blood Institute*
*Bethesda, Maryland*

## INTRODUCTION

Viruses are maintained in nature by virtue of their ability to transfer and express genetic information in target cells. Whether integrated in the host cell chromosome or freely replicating as an episomal structure, the viral genome directs the synthesis of its encoded proteins, often with diminution or cessation of host protein synthesis and resulting cytopathogenicity and usually with production of new virus particles. Alternatively, virus entry into the cell may be followed by latent infection, with incorporation of a quiescent genome that may be activated later. As the capacity to manipulate DNA by recombinant techniques has increased along with knowledge of the molecular basis of inherited and acquired human diseases, experimental and potentially therapeutic applications of virally mediated gene transfer have been developed. Much effort has been made to capitalize on the inherent efficiency of viruses to transfer and express exogenous genes in target cells.

Murine retroviruses, adenovirus, and parvovirus/adeno-associated virus, various herpesviruses, and vaccinia virus are being developed for gene transfer purposes in humans. These viruses vary greatly in their ability to infect specific types of differentiated cells, in the size of the DNA fragment that can be accommodated into a recombinant genome, and in the fate of the genome once incorporated into the target cell. At present, no single vector

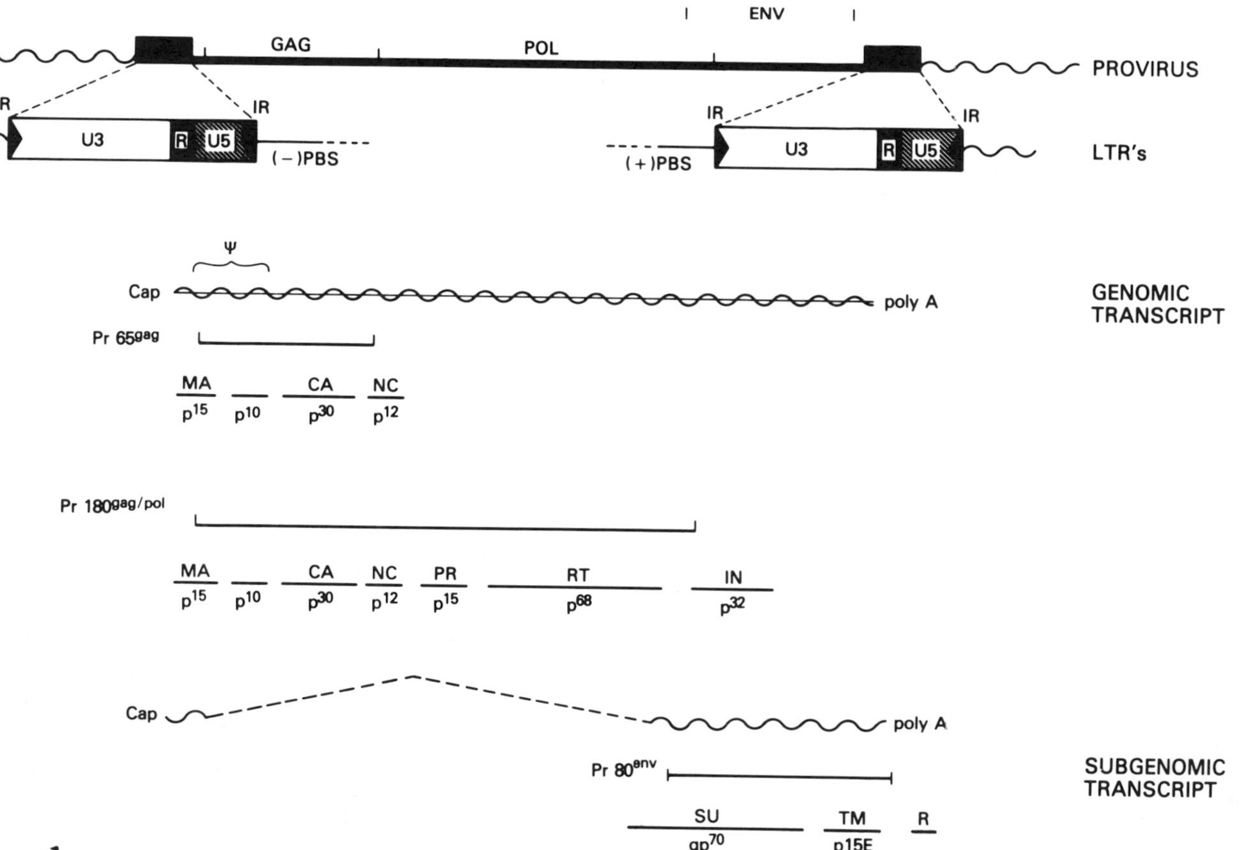
ENV
GAG
POL
PROVIRUS
IR
IR
U3
R
U5
(−)PBS
IR
IR
(+)PBS
U3
R
U5
LTR's
Ψ
Cap
poly A
GENOMIC TRANSCRIPT
Pr 65gag
MA
p15
p10
CA
p30
NC
p12
Pr 180gag/pol
MA
p15
p10
CA
p30
NC
p12
PR
p15
RT
p68
IN
p32
Cap
poly A
Pr 80env
SUBGENOMIC TRANSCRIPT
SU
gp70
TM
p15E
R

**Figure 1**

system is likely to be useful for all applications. Instead, specific vectors are being developed for particular experimental and therapeutic objectives. In all cases, recombinant viral vectors must be devoid of replication-competent helper virus and have minimal (if any) potential for damaging the target cell. The most progress in achieving these objectives has been made with retroviral and adenoviral vectors, although adeno-associated virus vectors also appear very promising.

The host range of viruses is often defined using rapidly dividing cell lines in vitro. Much more relevant for experimental and therapeutic applications is the capacity of specific viruses to infect primary cells under conditions that maintain the ability of the target cells to continue to function in vivo. For some applications, target cells are removed, maintained in culture during exposure to the viral vector, and then returned to the host. The hematopoietic stem cell is the prototype for this experimental approach, but similar strategies have been used for liver cells, fibroblasts, keratinocytes, and lymphocytes. Other desired targets for experimental or therapeutic applications, such as respiratory epithelium or brain cells, cannot be explanted, genetically modified, and returned to the host in a functional state. Attempts to achieve gene transfer into such cells necessarily has focused on the use of viruses whose natural tropism can be exploited to achieve gene transfer in vivo.

This chapter describes the basic biology and life cycle of viruses now in use as gene transfer vectors, with emphasis on the features of each virus that are relevant to specific in vivo uses. The current status of vector design and packaging systems for each is reviewed, along with the proposed experimental and therapeutic applications.

## RETROVIRUSES

Retroviruses have an RNA genome that, on viral entry into the cell, is converted into double-stranded DNA by reverse transcriptase before integration into a host cell chromosome (1,23). Once integrated, the provirus serves as a template for RNA polymerase II in generating RNA molecules that encode the structural proteins and enzymes required for new particle formation and that provide the genome for assembly into these viral particles (Fig. 1).

---

**Figure 1** Structure and expression of the murine leukemia virus genome virus (1,14,15). Transcriptional regulatory elements and the polyadenylation signal within the long terminal repeats (LTR) direct the synthesis of a genomic transcript that encodes GAG and POL proteins as shown. A spliced subgenomic transcript directs synthesis of the envelope protein components. See text for details and for definition of the abbreviations.

Packaged genome molecules are unspliced transcripts, whereas the mRNAs encoding proteins may be spliced or unspliced species. These properties—an RNA genome, reverse transcription, integration of a DNA provirus, and subsequent expression of this provirus in the host cells—are essential features of the diverse group of virus that make up the Retroviridae family (3, 4). This family includes the Oncovirinae, which may cause malignancies, particularly in rodents; the Lentivirinae, which cause various diseases, including acquired immunodeficiency syndrome (AIDS); and the nonpathogenic Spumavirinae. Oncovirinae have a "simple" genome that encodes only for structural proteins and enzymes, in contrast to the "complex" Lentivirinae genome, which also encodes for various regulatory proteins that control RNA transcription and processing.

The retroviral vectors currently in use for gene transfer into human cells are derived from members of the Oncovirinae subfamily, the murine leukemia viruses (MuLV) (5,6). Exogenous MuLV are transmitted horizontally in mice, either experimentally or by natural infection, whereas endogenous proviruses are transmitted vertically within the genome (3). Exogenous MuLV cause malignancy by two general mechanisms. Acutely transforming viruses have acquired coding sequences from a host cell protooncogene; these sequences have been modified by recombination and/or subsequent point mutation and can act as an oncogene in target cells (2). Replication-competent MuLV lack such transforming genes, and they cause tumors after long latency by establishing chronic productive infection (7). For these viruses, multiple integration events in target cells ultimately lead to protooncogene activation and/or inactivation of tumor suppressor genes by insertional mutagenesis. Tissue-specific enhancer and promoter elements determine the level of activity of the integrated proviral genome and the capacity for gene activation by insertional mutagenesis. The envelope protein may contribute to disease pathogenesis by abrogating growth factor dependence through interaction with a tissue-specific growth factor receptor (8). Thus the nature of the tumor produced by a specific replication-competent retrovirus depends on the properties of its envelope and transcriptional control elements and relies on viral propagation within a proliferating cell population.

The genome of many inbred mouse strains may contain as many as 50 different endogenous MuLV proviral genomes (9–13). Most are defective and cannot give rise to infectious viral particles. However, individual proviruses may be expressed, some in a developmentally specific pattern, and the encoded proteins may have important biologic effects. Retroviruses are mobile genetic elements; both exogenous and endogenous retroviruses may infect germ line cells and cause heritable mutations with specific phenotypes.

The oncovirinae have been the focus of intense study over the past two to three decades because of their ability to cause neoplasms in experimental animals (2). Although most human tumors do not reflect virus infection, the general principles regarding oncogenes and insertional mutagenesis deduced by study of RNA tumor viruses have greatly facilitated the understanding of human oncogenesis. Genetic engineering now permits conversion of these animal pathogens into agents potentially useful for human therapy (5,6).

## Organization and Function of the MuLV Genome

The use of MuLV for therapeutic gene transfer could only be attempted when sufficient information regarding genome structure and function was available to allow the design of vectors for gene transfer without transmission of replication-competent virus. Molecular cloning and sequencing of MuLV proviral genomes (14,15) became feasible about 10 years ago and provided the information necessary for the development of systems for retrovirally mediated gene transfer. Outlined in Figure 1 is the integrated proviral genome of the Moloney murine leukemia virus (MoMuLV), its genomic and subgenomic transcripts, and the encoded proteins. Most packaging systems and vectors in current use have employed components of MoMuLV (5,6). The general organization and function of other MuLV are similar, but the details provided here pertain specifically to MoMuLV.

The coding sequences of the genome are flanked by long terminal repeats (LTR) that contain the transcriptional control elements, polyadenylation signals, and sequences involved in replication and integration (1,14,15). There are three classes of virally encoded proteins, structural proteins (group-specific antigens, gag), various enzymatic activities, including reverse transcriptase (pol) integrase (In) and a protease and the major envelope proteins (env) (1,2,16). Each of these components is synthesized as a polyprotein that is subsequently cleaved by virally encoded or cellular proteases. The genomic transcript encodes gag and pol, whereas env is encoded by a subgenomic transcript that arises by RNA splicing.

Retroviral particles are diploid: each individual virion contains two full-length RNA molecules (3). Both molecules participate in the synthesis of a single DNA duplex, the precursor for the integrated provirus. Analysis of naturally occurring viral deletion mutants characterized by formation of empty capsids suggested the existence of a packaging signal (psi) that facilitates incorporation of retroviral RNA into capsids to the virtual exclusion of other cellular mRNAs (17). Deletional mutagenesis of the MoMuLV genome identified a 350 nucleotide region in the 5′-untranslated segment of the genomic transcript necessary for packaging (18). Subsequent work has shown that signals required for highly efficient packaging of a vector genome extend into the gag coding region (19,20). Indeed, incorporation of an 823 nucleotide segment of the MoMuLV genome into heterologous mRNAs leads to their incorporation into retroviral capsids (21). The packaging region is also thought to include the sites that interact specifically with gag-encoded proteins in the assembly of retroviral particles (17). The two molecules of RNA in each virion are intimately associated by chemical interaction within the packaging region of the genome, although the physical nature of the relationship has not been defined.

The gag proteins are synthesized on cytoplasmic ribosomes as a 65 kD precursor ($Pr65^{gag}$), subsequently cleaved after virion assembly into the p15 matrix (MA), p30 capsid (CA), and p12 nucleocapsid (NC) components (9, 16). The function of a fourth peptide, p12, derived from $Pr65^{gag}$ remains uncertain. Only NC has been shown to bind to the unspliced genomic transcript, presumably in the packaging region (9,17,22). Synthesis of the pol-region proteins from the MoMuLV genome transcript reflects infrequent suppression of the $Pr65^{gag}$ termination codon, with read-through translation to give a 180 kD precursor designated $Pr180^{gag/pol}$. Ultimately proteolytic cleavage of $Pr180^{gag/pol}$ yields, in addition to the gag-region proteins, p15 (protease), p68 (reverse transcriptase), and p32 (integrase). Each virion contains 3000–4000 molecules of the gag-region proteins and about 200–300 molecules of those encoded in the pol region (22).

The envelope region proteins are derived from a precursor, $Pr80^{env}$, that is translated from a spliced, subgenomic transcript (9). This precursor protein has a signal peptide leading to its synthesis on membrane-bound polysomes and establishment of $Pr80^{env}$ as a transmembrane protein. The intraluminal portion of the protein is glycosylated and cleaved by a cellular protease to yield gp70 (SU) and p15e (TM), which remain associated by non-covalent bonding. A complex involving several molecules of each forms, ostensibly to sequester the hydrophobic, membrane-fusionogenic N-terminal domain of p15e (9,17).

Assembly of virions may begin on intracellular membranes of the Golgi or occur only on cell surface membranes. The N-terminal portion of the gag precursor protein is required for particle assembly through interactions that must also involve the C-terminal cytoplasmic portion of p15e molecules (9,22). The details of this assesmbly process are poorly understood, but the outcome is a complex virion with a highly ordered capsid structure, enveloped in a cell membrane segment largely devoid of normal cellular proteins into which have been concentrated the virally encoded envelope proteins. Dimerization of the protease segments in $Pr180^{gag/pol}$ is required for this enzyme's activation (9,22,23). Proteolytic cleavages release the individual gag- and pol-encoded proteins after virion assembly is initiated. Conversion of the virion to an infectious particle coincides with the proteolytic release of the individual gag and pol proteins.

The U3 region of the LTR, so designated because its transcribed sequences are unique to the 3′ end of the proviral RNA, contain the MoMuLV enhancer and promoter elements (1,2). The U5 region, transcribed sequences of which are unique to the 5′ end of the viral RNAs, contains the polyadenylation signals for 3′ end formation. The U3 and U5 regions in the proviral LTR are separated by an 82 bp R region, transcribed sequences of which are found on both the 5′ and 3′ ends of the viral RNAs. These R regions, the tRNA binding site and a purine-rich track, are critical to reverse transcription and proviral integration, as described in a subsequent section.

MuLV exhibit a variable host range based on the structure of the envelope protein (gp70). Five types of viruses have been defined (9). Ecotropic viruses infect mouse cells and a few rodent cell lines, amphotropic viruses have a broad host range that includes human cells, and xenotropic viruses have a similarly broad host range but do not infect mouse cells. The two other types of viruses arise by recombination involving the genome of an exogenous virus and an endogenous provirus expressed during chronic productive viral infection in mice (7,9); these recombinant viruses are recognized by their expanded host range. For example, mink cell focus (MCF) viruses arise by recombination involving an exogenous ecotropic virus and an endogenous MCF or xenotropic expressed sequence (9–13). Recombination between an exogenous amphotropic virus and an endogenous MCF proviral transcript is represented by only a single example (24).

As discussed in more detail later, each type of MuLV is thought to rely on interaction with a specific cell surface molecule that acts as a receptor for initiating viral entry into cells (9). Specificity for receptor interaction resides in the N-terminal portion of gp70; the C-terminal portion of gp70 and the entire coding region of p15e are highly conserved among the MuLV.

Structural analysis, hybridization specificity, and sequence homology have allowed molecular classification of mouse endogenous proviruses (10–13). Most are of the xenotropic or MCF types. Some mouse strains have a few endogenous ecotropic proviruses, but endogenous amphotropic proviruses have not been described (9).

## Vector Production and Design

The utility of retroviruses as vectors for gene transfer relies entirely on the ability to engineer cell lines to produce retroviral particles to serve as vehicles for a vector genome without production of replication-competent virus (Fig. 2) (5,6,25). Cell lines are engineered to express a helper genome (or genomes) encoding viral proteins (18,26). A separate vector genome contains the gene to be transferred and also retains the cis-active elements necessary for RNA encapsidation, replication, and integration. The viral structural genes are

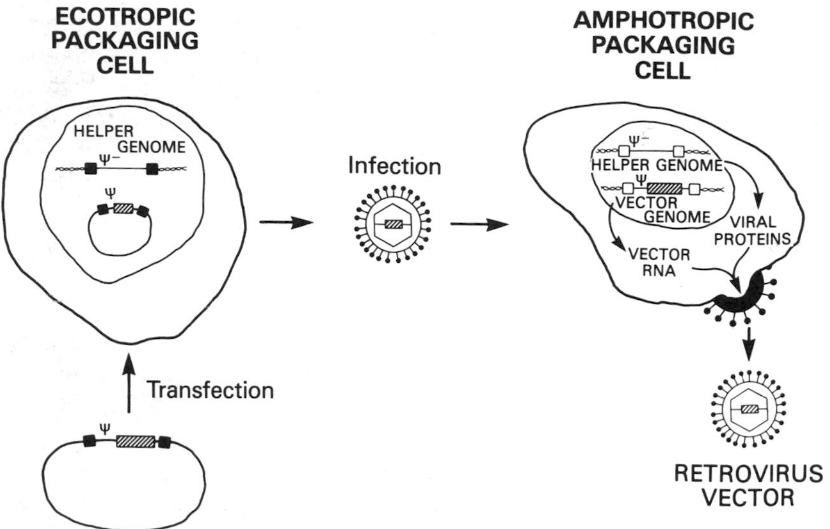


**Figure 2** Generation of vectors with amphotropic specificity by transfection (5,6,25). Plasmid DNA containing the recombinant proviral genome of interest is introduced into an ecotropic packaging cell by conventional methods of DNA transfer. The proviral genome is expressed before chromosomal integration, generating transcripts that are packaged to form ecotropic viral particles. After 48 h, the culture medium from these cells is removed and used to infect an amphotropic packaging cell line. Integration of the vector provirus allows stable production of retroviral particles. Many clones are screened to identify one that produces a high concentration of vector particles capable of transferring the recombinant genome into human cells without rearrangement.

expressed in RNA transcripts that lack the packaging signals required for incorporation into virions. Elimination of additional cis-required elements, including the LTR sequences and replication signals from helper transcripts, further reduces the probability of recombination to produce replication-competent virus or transfer of viral structural genes into target cells.

### Packaging Cell Lines and Producer Clones

The first widely used packaging cell lines were engineered by removal of the minimal packaging sequences from the proviral genome using recombinant DNA techniques (Fig. 2). This modified genome was transferred into mouse fibroblasts by conventional cotransfection with a selectable marker gene (10). Such engineered fibroblasts produce empty viral capsids; assembly of infectious virions begins only after introduction of the vector genome. The first packaging lines generated virus with ecotropic specificity, but substitution of amphotropic for ecotropic envelope coding sequences in the helper genome yielded packaging lines that produced vectors capable of infecting human cells (27,28). These first-generation packaging cells showed that retroviral vectors could be used for gene transfer. Unfortunately, recombination between helper and vector genomic RNAs led to the rapid emergence of replication-competent virus (29).

Several strategies have been employed to eliminate this potential for generation of replication-competent virus within vector producer clones (5, 6,25,30). Elimination of regions of homology between the helper and vector genome has been one general approach. Figure 3A is a diagram of a currently used vector backbone and helper genome combination. The vector genome has been mutated to convert the gag-region start codon to a termination codon. Two recombinant events and a point mutation would be required to generate a replication-competent virus from this combination (5,6). Vector producer clones based on these components have remained free of replication-competent virus during prolonged passage in vitro (31).

A second strategy to eliminate the production of replication-competent virus is by separating the coding sequences of the helper genome into two discrete transcriptional units (32–36). One of the first packaging lines to be developed was based on this approach (26), but because components of an avian virus were utilized, the line was not useful for gene transfer into mammalian cells. An example of newer packaging lines is shown in Figure 3B. At least three recombination events are required to generate replication-competent virus within producer clones derived from these packaging lines. Producer clones remain free of replication-competent viruses even when vector backbones are used that retain significant portions of the wild-type retroviral genome.

The efficiency of retroviral vector production is a critical quality of each producer clone (5,6,25). Generally, the ability to infect a desired target population is directly proportional to the concentration of infectious vector particles in the culture medium. Since no practical strategies have been developed to concentrate biologically active retroviruses, the rate of production of particles during expansion of the producer clone from subconfluency to confluency is of critical importance. Usually $10^6$–$10^7$ vector particles per ml culture medium are required for successful gene transfer. In practice, it is necessary to screen many retroviral clones producing each vector to identify one capable of sufficient virus production. Prolonged passage of a producer clone or the exact culture conditions under which it is maintained may also influence the rate of virus production, so that a high degree of standardization is needed to consistantly obtain useful vector preparations.

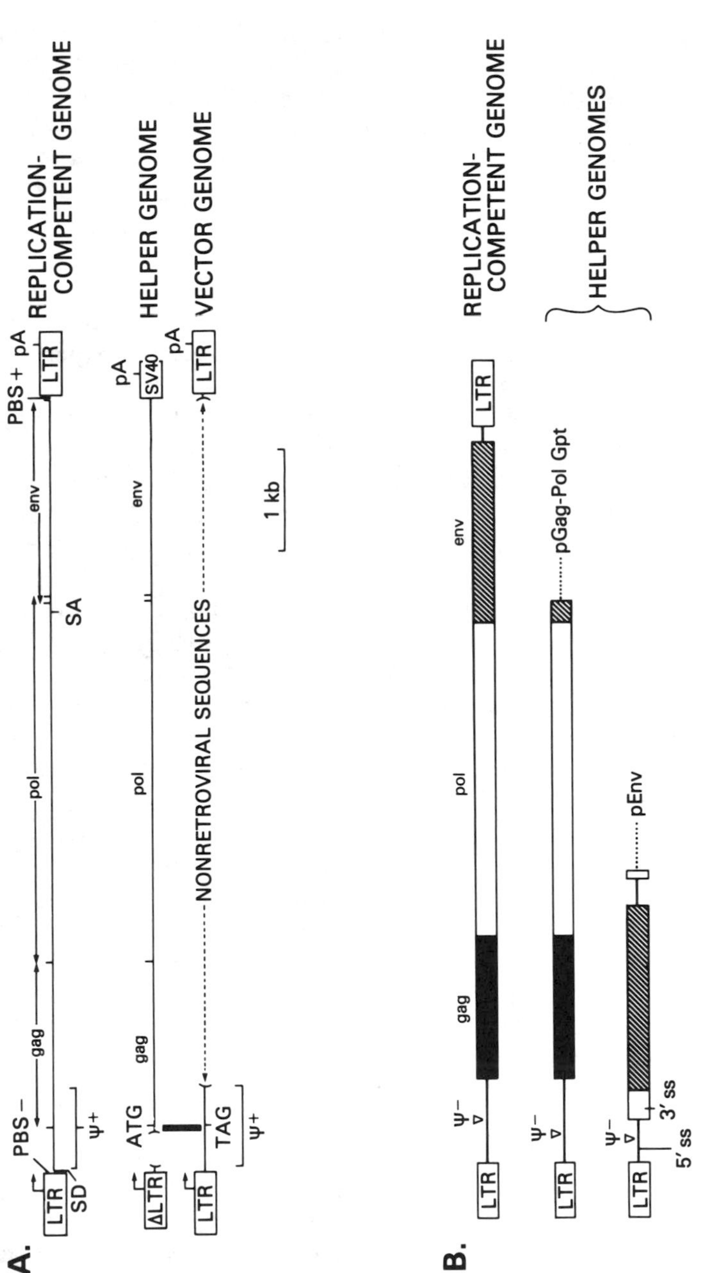
A.
LTR
SD
PBS−
ψ+
gag
pol
SA
env
PBS+
pA
LTR
REPLICATION-
COMPETENT GENOME
ΔLTR
ATG
gag
pol
env
SV40
pA
HELPER GENOME
LTR
TAG
ψ+
NONRETROVIRAL SEQUENCES
LTR
pA
VECTOR GENOME
1 kb
B.
LTR
ψ−
gag
pol
env
LTR
REPLICATION-
COMPETENT GENOME
LTR
ψ−
pGag-Pol Gpt
LTR
ψ−
5′ ss
3′ ss
pEnv
HELPER GENOMES

Figure 3

Introduction of the vector genome into packaging cells is best accomplished by retroviral infection (Fig. 2). Expression of envelope proteins specifically downmodulates the receptor for that type of virus, so that an ecotropic virus is used to introduce the vector genome into an amphotropic packaging cell line and an amphotropic virus is used to introduce the vector genome into an ecotropic packaging line (5,6,25,30). After construction of the vector genome in a bacterial plasmid, the plasmid DNA is introduced into a packaging line by calcium phosphate coprecipitation or some other standard method of DNA transfer. Within 48 h, infectious vector particles accumulate in the culture medium, which can then be used to infect the second packaging line. Individual clones containing the vector genome as a stable integratant is obtained. Clones are screened to identify those with one or a few unrearranged proviral vector genomes and a high capacity for virus production (Fig. 2).

One major advantage of this general strategy of trans infection is that the vector genomes are homogeneous and thus each diploid vector particle is homozygous for the vector genome. In contrast, other conventional strategies for DNA transfer result in integration of multiple copies of the genome, some of which may be rearranged. Heterogeneity in the vector RNA within producer clones results in the formation of heterozygous vector particles. Because both copies of the RNA genome participate in generation of the double-stranded proviral DNA genome (see later), further heterogeneity arises before integration in the target cell population. Often the integrated form of the vector genome in the target cell population is rearranged, resulting in inefficient gene transfer. The trans-infection technique allows derivation of producer clones that generate homozygous viral particles, sub-

---

**Figure 3** Modifications of the helper and vector genomes to eliminate production of replication-competent virus. (A) The vector genome in PA317 cells (30) was modified to eliminate a portion of the 5′ long terminal repeat (LTR) and to replace the 3′ LTR with a polyadenylation signal derived from the SV40 genome. The initiation codon of the GAG region in the LN vector was mutated to a terminator codon, leaving only 50 base pairs of homology in which a recombination event would generate a proviral genome having a functional 5′ end. Viral sequences at the 3′ end of the vector genome, present in earlier versions, were eliminated, thereby reducing the probability that replication-competent virus could be generated in a producer clone by recombination of the helper and vector genomes. (Adapted from Ref. 5.) (B) An example of a "split" packaging line (adapted from Ref. 33). Two separate genomes, one encoding the GAG and POL proteins and the other the envelope proteins, were introduced separately to create a packaging cell line. Such split packaging line have a very low probability of generating replication-competent virus by recombination of the expressed helper sequences with a vector genome.

stantially improving the possibility that the integrated provirus in the target cell population will be unrearranged and capable of expressing the gene product of interest.

### Vector Design

The primary consideration in vector design is to transfer the coding sequences of a particular protein into a target cell and then to obtain an adequate level of production of protein to achieve a specific experimental or therapeutic goal (5,6,25). Simple "single-gene" vectors utilize coding sequences in the form of a cDNA and rely on the retroviral LTR for transcriptional elements and RNA processing signals (Fig. 4). Vectors of more complex design may incorporate genes for more than one protein and utilize one or more independent promoters, rely on splicing to achieve expression of both genes, or utilize viral elements to create a polycistronic mRNA (37,38). MuLV can accommodate only about 8–9 kb of DNA in addition to the cis-active elements required for vector function; in practice, a minimal amount of DNA should be used to achieve expression of the desired gene product. Vector design ultimately relies on trial and error because the effect of any DNA sequence or configuration of control elements on vector production, replication, and integration is unpredictable. Recent reviews provide catalogs of the types of vectors already in use. Our summary focuses on a few general principles of vector design.

The choice of a vector "backbone" and packaging line should be guided by the objective of achieving stable production of vector particles free of replication-competent virus (Fig. 3). The goal of all applications of retrovirally mediated gene transfer is to achieve stable integration of the vector genome into the target population. Simultaneous infection with replication-competent virus has the potential of establishing a chronic productive infection with the possibility of subsequent secondary spread of the vector genome. For in vivo applications, replication-competent virus has the added risk of inducing neoplasms. As just summarized, available vector and packaging lines can be utilized to generate vector particles free of replication-competent virus, even with prolonged passage in vitro (5,6,25,31).

Another general consideration in vector design is whether to include a dominant selectable marker, such as the coding sequences for the phosphotransferase that confers resistance to G418 ($neo^R$). The $neo^R$ gene (or other dominant selectable marker genes) allows convenient identification of producer clones containing the vector genome during the trans-infection procedure. However, the need to express the $neo^R$ gene in producer cells and a second gene in the ultimate target population greatly complicates vector design. Indeed, the $neo^R$ gene may not be an innocent passenger, since expres-

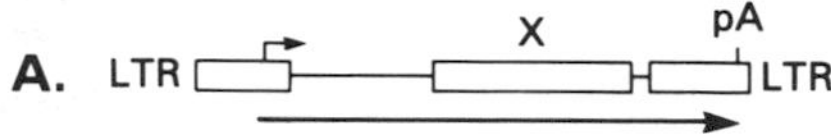


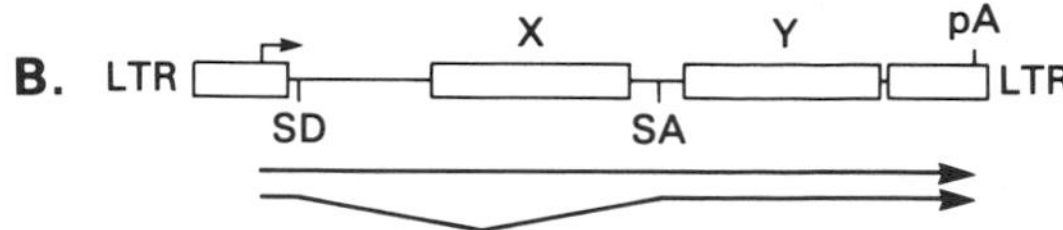


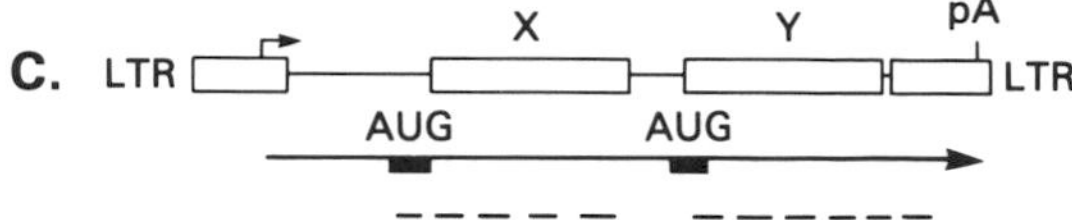


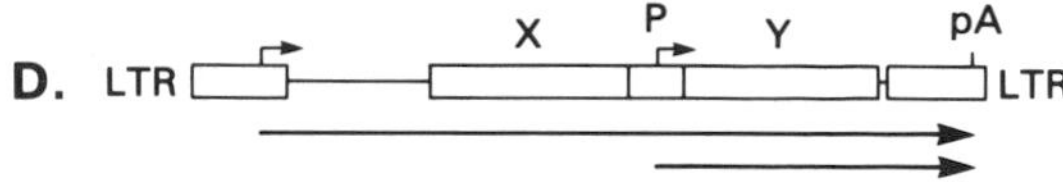


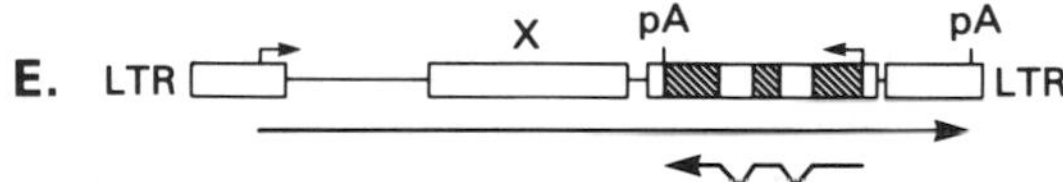


**Figure 4** Design of retroviral vectors (adapted from Ref. 6). (A) A simple vector with a single gene (X) under the control of the LTR promoter. (B) A vector having two genes (X and Y) under the control of the LTR promoter in which slicing is required for expression of the second genes (Y). (C) A vector design in which expression of two genes (X and Y) occurs from a polycistronic mRNA having the picornavirus translation initiation region (37,38). (D) A "double-promoter" vector in which one gene (X) is under the control of the LTR promoter and a second gene (Y) is transcribed from a second internal promoter. (E) A vector design in which a gene having its normal genomic structure with introns is expressed from its own promoter. This vector design has been used for the human $\beta$-globin gene (6) because regulatory elements required for high expression are contained within the introns.

sion of the neo$^R$ phosphotransferase may adversely affect some target cells (39). The neo$^R$ gene or other dominant selectable marker gene can readily be eliminated from vector design if the gene to be transferred itself encodes a protein that confers a selective advantage in vitro or one that can readily be detected in individual producer clones by enzymatic or immunologic assay. The trans-infection procedure can be performed with reasonable efficiency so that individual clones, obtained by limiting dilution, can be screened for the presence of the vector genome or for production of the gene product.

## Virus-Cell Interaction

### Receptors

As noted earlier, the tropism of specific types of murine retroviruses—ecotropic, amphotropic, or xenotropic—depends on the interaction of the virally encoded envelope protein, gp70, with a specific cell surface protein that acts as a viral receptor (9). The receptor for ecotropic viruses has been molecularly cloned and shown to be an integral membrane protein with multiple membrane spanning regions (40); this protein's normal function is a cationic amino acid transporter (41,42). The human counterpart of this protein, although highly homologous (87.6% at the amino acid level) (43), apparently has sufficient divergence to eliminate binding to the N-terminal sequences of ecotropic gp70 involved in receptor-virus interactions. The murine ecotropic virus receptor is widely expressed in many tissues, although the level of expression may be modulated. Activation of lymphocytes through a protein kinase C-dependent pathway increases receptor expression, whereas terminal differentiation of the human promyelocytic cell line, HL60, decreases expression of the human homolog (44). Receptor expression is generally higher in neoplastic than in normal cells. The infectivity of various target populations is thought to vary with the level of receptor expression. However, a recent test of this hypothesis yielded data suggesting that an accessory cellular factor(s) may also influence the frequency of viral infection, independently of the level of receptor-mediated virus binding (45,46).

A variety of different proteins can act as receptors in facilitating retroviral uptake by cells. The receptor for human immunodeficiency virus (HIV), CD4, is an accessory component of the T cell antigen receptor (47). A recently characterized human receptor for gibbon ape leukemia virus is homologous to a yeast phosphate permease (48); its function in human cells remains to be defined. The human receptor for murine amphotropic viruses has not been identified, although its gene has been localized to the pericentromeric region of human chromosome 8 (49).

### Retroviral Entry

Two distinct pathways have been defined for transfer of the contents of the retroviral particle into the cell following virus-receptor interaction (9). MoMuLV enters mouse cells by receptor-mediated endocytosis using a pathway that depends on endosome acidification (50). The encapsidated virus is thought to fuse with the endosome membrane to allow release of the nucleocapsid into the cell cytoplasm. Acidification facilitates disruption of the gp70-p15e complex and exposure of the N-terminal hydrophobic region of p15e, initiating fusion of virus envelope with the endosome membrane. A second pathway of retroviral entry is exhibited by HIV (51). HIV enters cells after interaction of its major envelope protein (gp120) with the external domain of CD4 induces exposure of a second env-encoded component, gp41. This hydrophobic protein induces fusion of the viral and cellular membranes, leading to transfer of the contents of the retroviral particle directly into the cytoplasm. The major role of CD4 appears to be in facilitating exposure of gp41. Indeed, the glycophospholipid-anchored external domain of CD4 appears to work nearly as well as the normal transmembrane form in facilitating entry of HIV into cells (52). Viruses that enter cells by membrane fusion may have the capacity to induce cellular syncytia (50).

There is evidence that certain viruses may enter cells using either pathway, depending on the properties of the target cell, such as a surface protease able to cleave the major envelope protein (50). The key element in facilitating transfer of the viral core into the target cell cytoplasm is the exposure of the transmembrane env component to induce fusion. Acidification may be required for these events for virus that enter through the endosome pathway.

### Reverse Transcription

The loss of the envelope coat after viral fusion with the cell or an endosomal membrane exposes the nucleocapsid to the ionic environment and nucleotide substrates within the cytoplasm, initiating reverse transcription (1–3, 53,54) (Fig. 5). A cellular tRNA is required as a primer for reverse transcriptase (RT) in initiating negative (−) strand synthesis. DNA synthesis begins at the 3′ boundary of the U5 region and extends to the 5′ end of the template RNA molecule, at which point the first of two required strand transfers occurs to allow continued DNA synthesis. Reverse transcriptase possesses an RNAse H function, resulting in degradation of the RNA template as DNA synthesis progresses. DNA sequences complementary to the R region are thus exposed, allowing the nascent DNA strand to anneal to the R region at the 3′ end of an RNA template molecule (Fig. 5). The first strand transfer event can be either an intra- or intermolecular event. Progression of DNA

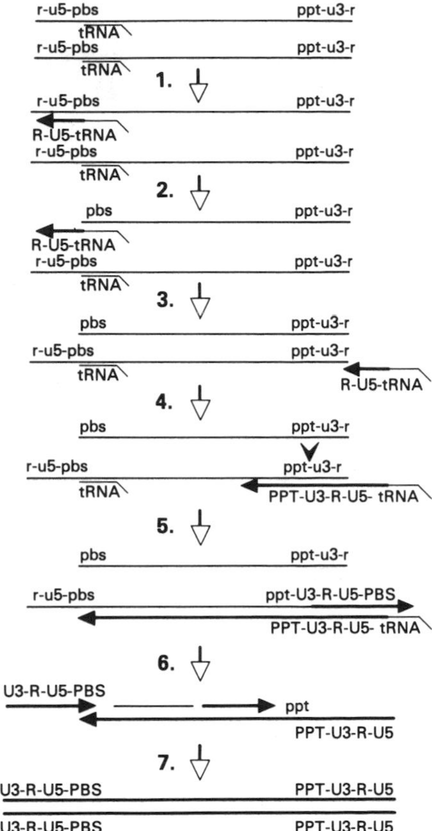


**Figure 5** Reverse transcription of the retroviral genome (adapted from Ref. 53). Negative-strand DNA synthesis begins on one or both of viral RNa templates (1) using a tRNA as a primer. After extension of DNA (heavy line) to the 5′ end of the genome step, the RNase H activity of reverse transcriptase degrades the RNA template, exposing the R region of the DNA (step 2), allowing base pairing with the corresponding region at the 3′ end of the RNA genome (step 3). This strand transfer may be either intramolecular, as shown, or intermolecular to the other RNA molecule. Extension of the DNA molecule beyond the polypurine track (ppt; step 4) and its degradation release a primer to initiate synthesis of the (+) strand (step 5). An intramolecular strand transfer (step 6) allows continued synthesis of the (+) strand on the DNA template. As shown (step 7), the final product is a double-stranded DNA molecule with duplicated long terminal repeats that serves as the substrate for integration. See text for further details.

synthesis beyond the 5′ end of the U5 region exposes the primer binding site for positive (+) strand synthesis. Purine-rich RNA oligonucleotides released by the RNAse H action of reverse transcriptase act as primers to initiate (+) strand DNA synthesis. The second strand transfer event occurs as (+) strand synthesis reaches the end of the (−) strand DNA molecule. The RNA sequences of the tRNA molecule that acted as a primer are degraded, and sequences complementary to the (−) strand are exposed. This second strand transfer event appears to be intramolecular. The (+) strand synthesis is initiated at multiple sites on a (−) strand DNA template(s), with subsequent joining of the fragments together by DNA ligation. Template switches may occur during (−) or (+) strand synthesis, accounting for the frequency of homologous recombination during retrovirus replication.

The product of reverse transcriptase is most often a linear DNA molecule with duplicated long terminal repeats (1–3,53,54). Current evidence suggests that this molecule is the substrate for integration. In addition, circular molecules having either a single or tandemly repeated LTR are also formed, but their relevance to the retroviral life cycle is unknown.

Genetic therapy requires efficient gene transfer with high fidelity. In nature, retroviruses exhibit genetic instability with an evolutionary premium on their ability to acquire diversity during replication (3). There is ample opportunity for homologous recombination because both RNA molecules of the diploid virion participate in formation of the DNA genome. The RNA to DNA to RNA life cycle of a retrovirus requires two enzymes, reverse transcriptase and RNA polymerase II, that are error prone and lack an editing function. Estimates suggest that each replication cycle introduces one point mutation per retroviral genome (3).

The use of retroviruses as vectors for genetic therapy requires efforts to control this propensity to generate genetic diversity. As noted earlier, the use of producer clones with only one or a few unrearranged integrated vector genomes allows formation of homogeneous vector particles with two identical genomes, minimizing the consequences of recombination during reverse transcription. The ability of producer clones to generate vector particles capable of transferring and expressing the gene of interest in target cells can serve to verify that deleterious point mutations have not occurred during its derivation.

### Integration

Integrase, a virally encoded enzyme, binds to either end of the linear DNA product of reverse transcription (55,56). Inverted repeats at the ends of the LTR provide a 9 base pair recognition sequence for enzyme binding (57). Two nucleotides are removed to create a recessed 3′ terminus. Integrase also mediates a staggered endonuclease cleavage of the target cell DNA and is thought to ligate the 5′ extended end of genomic DNA to the recessed 3′ hydroxyl end of the proviral genome. Integration is completed by gap repair and ligation. The integration mechanism eliminates two nucleotides from each end of the linear proviral genome and creates a four nucleotide direct repeat in genomic DNA at its boundaries with the provirus (55–57).

The integrated form of the provirus is consistent and highly precitable; a linear genome is flanked by LTRs from which two nucleotides have been excised. Replication through an RNA intermediate ensures that the missing terminal nucleotides are regenerated in creating the next proviral integration template. In contrast, the integration site within the host cell DNA appears to lack sequence specificity. Local features of chromatin structure, nucleosome organization, and replication or transcriptional activity may influence the exact site of proviral insertion so that integration is not completely random (58). The integration site of each provirus in host cell DNA provides a unique marker that can be used to identify the progeny, both in vitro and in vivo, of the cell in which the integration event occurred.

## Applications

Retrovirally mediated gene transfer requires an active state of cell division; quiescent cells are refractory to transduction (59,60). Virus binding and internalization probably occur independently of cell cycle status, but the reverse transcription and/or integration steps apparently require activities, present only in dividing cells, that complement the viral enzymatic activities. This requirement for cell division has limited the applicability of retroviral vectors for therapeutic gene transfer, and current efforts have focused on inducing an active state of cell proliferation in vitro to make usually quiescent target cells susceptible to retrovirally mediated gene transfer.

### Hematopoietic Stem Cells

These cells have the capacity to reconstitute the entire lymphohematopoietic system after bone marrow transplantation (61,62). Many genetic diseases, such as the thalassemias, sickle cell anemia, chronic granulomatous disease, and severe combined immunodeficiency, are caused by defects in cells derived from the hematopoietic stem cell and can be cured by bone marrow transplantation (63). Even tissue macrophages are replaced after bone marrow transplantation with cells derived from the graft. These considerations made the hematopoietic stem cell one of the first and a highly desired target for therapeutic gene transfer.

Early experiments demonstrated that retroviruses could transfer genes into the self-renewing stem cells that gave rise to spleen colonies when injected into irradiated mice (64), and later gene insertion into long-term repopulating stem cells was also achieved (65,66). The efficiency of gene transfer remained low until recombinant cytokines became available, which could be used to stimulate division of the usually quiescent stem cell in vitro (67,68). With current protocols, approximately 20% of murine stem cells are successfully transduced, and most mice that are recipients of a vector-infected marrow graft have circulating genetically modified cells for months or even years following transplantation (64,69). Redesigned vectors that rely on strong viral or cellular promoters have resulted in persistent, long-term gene expression.

Retrovirally mediated gene transfer into stem cells of larger animal species, necessary before genetic therapy in humans, has been difficult to achieve (64,69–73). Recently, purification of marrow cells by positive immunoselection and the use of recombinant cytokines during 3–6 days in culture in vitro with or without autologous stroma has resulted in a higher transduction efficiency. Of all circulating myeloid and lymphoid cells, 1–10% contained the proviral genome after autologous reconstruction with infected marrow cells (Ref. 74 and K. Mcdonagh and A. W. Nienhuis, unpublished observations). Expression of the gene for adenosine deaminase (ADA), an enzyme that is deficient in some patients with severe combined immunodeficiency, has been demonstrated months after autologous transplantation of nonhuman primates with retrovirally transduced cells (75). These preclinical data support the development of protocols for retrovirally mediated gene transfer into human stem cells. Clinical studies are scheduled to begin during 1993.

### Lymphocytes

The first cells to be transduced with a retroviral vector and returned to the patients from whom they were obtained were tumor-infiltrating lymphocytes (TIL) (76,77). Treatment protocols for patients with malignant melanoma or kidney cancer had been developed that involved recovery of lymphocytes from excised neoplastic lesions, expansion of these cells in vitro, and reinfusion in an effort to exploit the putative tumor immune response for therapeutic benefit. The life span and migration characteristics of the reinfused TIL could be determined because the integrated retroviral genome provided a permanent marker of the transduced cells and their progeny. Retrovirally marked TIL were shown to persist in circulation for several weeks and could be found infiltrating recurrent tumor deposits (77).

These studies paved the way for subsequent therapeutic gene transfer protocols. Peripheral blood lymphocytes from two patients with ADA deficiency were harvested by apheresis, expanded by stimulation with interleukin-2 and an antibody to the T cell receptor, transduced with a retroviral vector containing the coding sequences for human ADA, and reinfused after 7–9 days in vitro (78). This procedure was repeated at 4–6 week intervals. An increase in circulating T cells, the appearance of isohemagglutinins, and the establishment of normal reactivity on immune testing provided evidence for the therapeutic benefit of this procedure (79). The transduced proviral genome and human ADA activity were demonstrated in circulating lymphocytes, establishing that gene transfer was the mechanism for the observed therapeutic effect. Other protocols have been developed that involve insertion of genetic elements into lymphocytes to render cells resistant to human immunodeficiency virus as a treatment for acquired immunodeficiency syndrome (80,81) and by insertion of cytokine genes, like the gene for tumor necrosis factor, into TIL for cancer therapy (82,83).

### Liver Cells

In animal models, ablation of a portion of the liver surgically or by injection of an hepatotoxin, such as carbon tetrachloride, results in liver regeneration (84). During the regenerative phase, hepatocytes are susceptible to infection by retroviral vectors injected into the portal vein. A practical clinical protocol has been developed based on the observation that hepatocytes, when explanted into tissue culture, divide two to three times and can be transduced with a retroviral vector (85,86). The cultured hepatocytes engraft within the liver parenchyma with reasonable efficiency after injection into the spleen or portal vein.

One candidate disease for treatment by hepatocyte-targeted gene therapy is familial hypercholesterolemia (FHC) (87). Individuals homozygous for this disorder have very high serum cholesterol and suffer from premature coronary disease. The receptor for low-density lipoprotein (LDL), the major transport form for cholesterol in the plasma, is missing in individuals with homozygous familial FHC. In an animal model for this disorder, the Watanabe rabbit, excision and culture of 20% of the liver as a single-cell suspension, transduction of the hepatocytes, and reinjection resulted in a 30–40% lowering of the serum cholesterol level (88). One patient with homozygous LDL receptor deficiency has also undergone somatic cell gene therapy using this protocol. The outcome of this clinical experiment is not yet known.

### Cancer Cells

The pathogenesis of human neoplasms reflects somatic mutations in protooncogenes and tumor suppressor genes (89,90). Normal growth regulatory mechanisms are compromised, and the cancer grows in an uncontrolled fashion. Several strategies have been proposed to use retrovirally mediated gene transfer to inhibit tumor cell growth (76,77). In animal models, expression of cytokine genes may invoke an inflammatory response that results in tumor regression (91–94). Alternatively, expression of HLA antigens or, preferably, tumor-specific antigens following introduction of the appropriate gene into a tumor cell population may also allow the retrovirally transduced stem cells to invoke an inflammatory or immune response on reimplantation into the patient.

One approved gene therapy protocol involves implantation of retroviral producer cells within the lesions of patients with brain tumors (95). These producer cells generate a vector containing the coding sequences for the herpes simplex thymidine kinase gene. Cells expressing this gene become sensitive to the antiviral agent, gancyclovir. If a significant fraction of the rapidly dividing tumor cells become infected during the 1–2 weeks following implantation of the retroviral producer cells, treatment with gancyclovir could destroy both the retroviral producer cells and the retrovirally transduced brain tumor cells. A "bystander" effect, whereby nontransduced tumor cells are also killed by the invoked inflammatory response, has made this strategy quite successful in controlling tumor growth in animal models.

### Other Targets for Retrovirally Mediated Gene Transfer

Myoblasts (96), fibroblasts (97), endothelial cells (98,99), and keratinocytes (100) are among the cell populations that can be explanted and induced to divide in vitro while retaining the capacity to reestablish themselves in an animal after reimplantation. Each has been a target for retrovirally mediated gene transfer in animal models, and some success has been achieved with myoblasts. When injected into skeletal muscle, these cells find their way through the basal lamina and fuse with existing myocytes. Human growth hormone has been produced for several weeks in mice that have received genetically modified myoblasts (96). This approach has been proposed as a strategy for correcting a deficiency in serum protein, for example, patients with hemophilia who lack a coagulation factor.

## Safety Issues

The primary concern regarding the use of retroviral vectors in humans is the possibility that these agents may induce neoplasms. As discussed earlier, murine retroviruses cause various types of neoplasms in rodent species (7). Acutely transforming retroviruses have acquired a cellular protooncogene during passage in vivo. Mutation of this gene, either in the course of recombination with retroviral sequences or later, converts it to an oncogene. Retroviruses can also cause neoplasms by insertional mutagenesis. The integrated proviral genome may disrupt a cellular gene required for growth control, or the transcriptional control elements present within the LTR may activate a protooncogene either by an enhancer effect or by transcription from the LTR promoter (7). Generally, retroviruses that induce neoplasms by this mechanism do so only after long latency. Chronic productive infection in vivo is necessary to allow integration of multiple proviral genomes into the target population. Ultimately, a clonal population emerges that has accumulated two or more critical insertional mutations, which result in neoplastic transformation.

Vectors in current use are replication defective (5,6,25). Ideally, the proviral genome integrates only once in each target cell. In practice, two or three integration events may occur. The probability that a single provirus will damage or activate a gene involved in growth regulation has been estimated at 1 in $10^6$. Since two or more mutations are required for transformation, the probability that any single cell transduced with a retroviral vector will be transformed has been estimated as less than 1 in $10^{12}$.

Early generation vector and packaging cell combinations regularly gave rise to replication-competent virus through recombination between the vector and helper genome (29,30). The potential for such replication-competent virus to cause disease was established in a nonhuman primate model (74). Rhesus monkeys received an autologous transplant of retrovirally transduced bone marrow cells, enriched in repopulating stem cells by immunoselection. Before bone marrow transplantation, the animals received a dose of radiation capable of ablating the myeloid and lymphoid systems. Of eight animals transplanted according to this protocol, three developed rapidly progressive lymphoma. These animals had failed to develop a humoral antibody response and were chronically viremic. The genome of the tumor cells was riddled with 50–100 proviral insertions (74).

The presumed pathogenic mechanism for these lymphomas is insertional mutagenesis. The majority of viral genomes cloned from the serum of one animal had the structure of the predicted vector-helper recombinant arising from the components present in the producer cell. Based on these observations, screening procedures have been intensified to verify that clinically certified vector preparations are free of replication-competent virus.

## ADENOASSOCIATED VIRUSES

Initially identified in the 1960s as a contaminant of adenovirus tissue culture preparations, adenoassociated virus (AAV) was determined to be a distinct virus that required a helper virus (adenovirus or herpesvirus) for replication (101–103). Although a member of the Parvoviridae family and structurally similar to animal parvoviruses, AAV is unique in many respects. AAV is dependent upon coinfection with a second autonomous virus for productive infection. Thus, AAV, a so-called dependovirus, lacks regulatory and structural gene functions provided by the helper virus. AAV has developed mechanisms to promote its biologic continuity by integration into the host cell genome and establishment of a latent state. AAV infects a broad range of host cell types and has been isolated from both primate and nonprimate species. AAV has never been associated with human disease. This viral commensalism represents a key feature required for a safe and useful gene transduction vector.

AAV is among the smallest and structurally simplest of the DNA viruses. Five serotypes of AAV have been identified, of which AAV-2 has been best characterized. AAV-2 is not enveloped, and its linear single-stranded DNA genome is encapsidated within an icosahedral protein coat. Infectious particles (20–26 nm diameter) are resistant to heat (56°C at 1 h), broad pH range, protease activity, and detergents. Particles have been purified on cesium chloride isopyknic density gradients (at a density of 1.41 g/cm$^3$) and are easily separated from accompanying adenovirus (104).

AAV is a defective virus that requires coinfection with an unrelated helper virus for viral replication and subsequent viral production. Infection of permissive cells with AAV in the presence of helper virus allows productive AAV generation and host cell lysis (105). Adenovirus and herpesvirus provide the necessary helper functions (106,107). Without an appropriate helper virus, productive infection does not occur and the AAV chromosome integrates into the host cell genome to produce a latent state (108). The AAV proviral state is stable, as documented by multiple (>150) passages of latent cell lines (109). If a latent cell is subsequently infected with helper virus, however, the AAV genome is rescued from the host cell genome and virus production occurs, thus completing the AAV life cycle.

Viral integration appears to have no apparent effect on cell growth or morphology (110). The establishment of a latent genome that can be later rescued ensures the survival of AAV in the absence of helper virus. The natural history of AAV infection is not well understood because of the lack of an associated disease. Epidemiologic surveys have shown that 85% of adults are positive for serum antibodies to AAV capsid proteins, presumably indicating previous AAV infection (111,112). AAV isolates have only been obtained from patients with symnptoms of adenoviral infection (113). The range of permissive host cells has largely been derived from tissue culture cells. Human AAV replicates in nonhuman cells if the appropriate helper virus is added: human AAV infects and replicates in murine cells if murine adenovirus is used as helper virus, suggesting that the specificity of the helper virus determines host cell range during a productive infection. Latency or integration of the AAV provirus has been studied in only a limited number of transformed cell lines (114).

## Genomic Organization

The AAV genome is a linear single-stranded DNA molecule that contains 4680 base pairs and is organized similarly to other parvoviruses. The left half of the genome contains coding sequences for regulatory proteins; the right side of the genome codes for three AAV structural proteins forming the capsid coat (Fig. 6). The virion is composed of three capsid polypeptides, VP1, VP2, and VP3, with molecular weights of 87, 73, and 62 kD, respectively

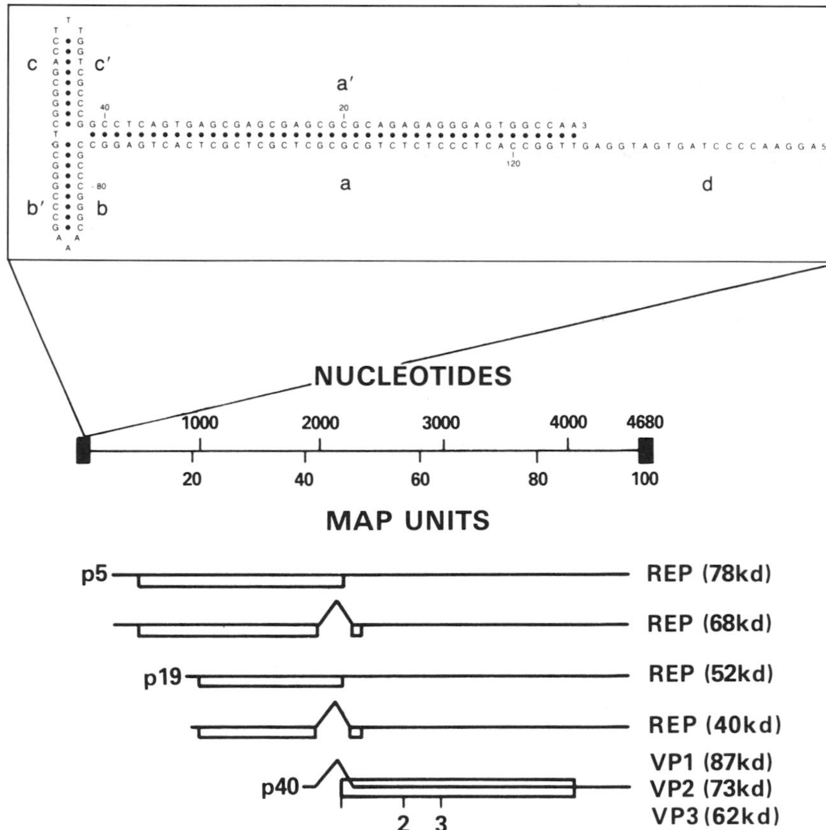


**Figure 6** The wild-type AAV genome. (Top) Sequence of the AAV inverted terminal repeat in the hairpin configuration. (Bottom) The AAV genome flanked by inverted terminal repeat sequences with viral promoters defined as p5, p19, and p40. The mRNA transcripts and corresponding translated REP and CAP (VP) proteins are indicated. Genome map units and nucleotide number are indicated. (Modified from K. Berns, Ref. 163.)

(115,116). VP3 represents 90% of the total virion protein; VP1 and VP2 constitute approximately 5% each. The three proteins have extensive overlapping sequences but differ primarily at the amino-terminal regions (117, 118). The relative amounts of each protein present in the intracellular pool reflect their distribution in AAV particles. AAV particles assemble and accumulate in the nucleus of the infected cell and form aggregates when viewed by electron microscopy. The architecture of AAV particles has not been characterized, but the crystalline structure of canine parvovirus has been reported and may be similar (119).

Because of the small size of the AAV genome, overlapping reading frames are utilized to produce multiple protein products. Left-sided gene products have been termed *rep* because mutations in this region block DNA replication (120), and the right-sided gene products are termed *cap*, for capsid proteins. The genome is separated by a central intron and flanked by inverted terminal repeat sequencies (ITR) that have evolved as the primar strand for DNA polymerase and as the origin of replication. A highly conserved feature of the parvoviruses are the termini containing palindromic sequences. AAV terminal repeat sequences are identical at both the 3′ and 5′ ends and consist of 145 base pairs. The palindromic sequences within the terminal repeat include 125 base pairs of DNA (Fig. 6). Both parental and daughter DNA strands (plus and minus) are equally packaged or encapsidated. The AAV genome contains two promoters at the left end (map positions 5 and 19) from which the four *rep* transcripts are derived. The p40 promoter, at map unit 40 (0–100 map units), initiates coat protein gene transcripts (121). Polyadenylation signals are located near the right end at map position 94 (122).

The current model for AAV genome replication utilizes the palindromic terminal sequencies as 3′-OH primers for DNA replication and allows for replication of the terminus (for review see Ref. 123). The palindromic sequences permit self priming or "hairpin transfer," which does not require RNA priming for the synthesis of a duplex linear molecule (Fig. 7). One end is covalently joined and subsequently opened by the enzymatic action of the *Rep* (68 kD) protein, which functions as a nickase at a site opposite the original 3′ terminus (at base 125). This creates a new 3′-OH primer, which allows the end to be repaired. The terminal repeat is denatured with the return of the original hairpin configuration, which generates new replicative intermediates and displaces single-stranded progeny molecules. DNA progeny strands supplied by strand displacement replication are subsequently packaged in the host cell nucleus with the three capsid proteins (VP1, VP2, and VP3) to form mature infectious particles. These proteins do not appear to have a direct role in AAV replication (replication occurs in the absence of capsid proteins); however, in the absence of capsid proteins or intact capsids,

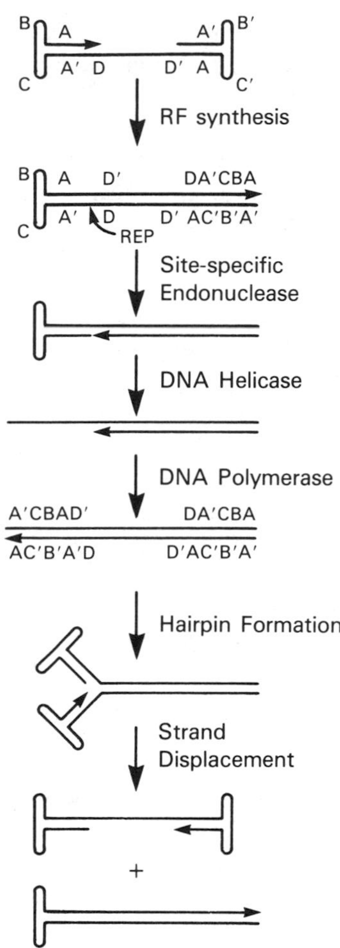


**Figure 7** Replication mechanism of AAV. The hairpin configuration at the 3′ end of the AAV genome acts as the primer for replication. A double-stranded replicative form (RF) is generated and cleaved specifically by a nickase (endonuclease, such as Rep68). The duplex molecule is subsequently denatured, generating a new progency single-stranded molecule and a RF intermediate used for further replication. (Modified from N. Muzyczka, Ref. 123; see text for details.)

single-stranded AAV progeny do not accumulate. Pulse-chase experiments indicate that empty capsids are rapidly formed in infected cells, and empty capsids serve as precursors to DNA-containing particles (124).

Tissue culture cells infected only with AAV contain low levels of AAV transcripts and protein and no detectable AAV replication (125); coinfection with helper virus induces AAV mRNA and protein synthesis and assembly into AAV virions. A number of early adenoviral genes are involved in the AAV helper function. The AdE1A product induces transcription from the p5 and p19 promoters and *rep* protein synthesis (126,127). *rep* acts to induce transcription at all three promoters, producing a 1–2 log increase in mRNA synthesis. The human kidney cell line 293, transformed by adenovirus, constitutively expresses E1A and is permissive for AAV viral production. Coinfection with adenovirus in these cells augments AAV production, indicating that other adenoviral genes are required for AAV efficient gene expression. AdE1B and E4 gene products work in a cooperative fashion to allow accumulation of AAV mRNA, whereas AdE2A and Ad VA RNAs are involved with transport of mRNA to the cytoplasm and efficient translation (128–133). The requirement for helper virus is not absolute and can be abrogated under certain conditions. Evidence that cellular factors are involved in replication is shown in experiments in which the exposure of nonpermissive cell lines to heat, ultraviolet irradiation, cycloheximide, hydroxyurea, or carcinogens enables cells to become permissive for AAV replication in the absence of helper virus infection (134,135).

## Vector Design

The use of AAV as a viral transduction vector was initially demonstrated by using an infectious molecular clone of the wild-type (wt) AAV (136). When transfected into human cells in the presence of adenovirus, the AAV sequence was rescued from the plasmid, and a lytic cycle occurred. A deletion mutant of AAV replaced a portion of the *cap* region with a bacterial antibiotic resistance gene controlled by the simian virus 40 (SV40) early promoter. Recombinant AAV stocks were produced by transfecting the recombinant plasmid into cells infected with adenovirus. The necessary *rep* and *cap* gene proteins required for recombinant AAV replication and encapsidation were supplied in trans by co-transfection with a second "helper" plasmid containing these genes. Both wild-type and recombinant AAV (rAAV) virions were produced. Contaminating adenovirus was inactivated by heating at 56°C, and the recombinant AAV particles were used to infect human cell lines. Recombinant viral stocks contained $10^6$ infectious particles per ml, comparable with retroviral vector titers. Geneticin-resistant cells were isolated with a transduction frequency of 0.5–5.0%. Tratschin and coworkers, using a similar strategy, engineered a bacterial chloramphenicol acetyltransferase or neomycin resistance gene downstream from the endogenous AAV p40 or p19 promoters (137). The recombinant genome integrated stably into the host genome and was maintained with serial passages. When these latently infected cells were superinfected with adenovirus, the recombinant provirus could be rescued and replicated in the cell. Similar vectors and similar transduction frequencies were obtained in a variety of human myeloid leukemia and lymphoblastoid cell lines (114).

These experiments showed that AAV was feasible as a transduction vehicle, but it suffered several disadvantages: (1) a size limitation of foreign DNA that could be inserted, (2) poor transduction efficiency compared to other viral vectors, (3) the generation of wild-type AAV virions, and (4) potential rescue of the provirus if superinfection with adenovirus occurred.

## Packaging Systems

In an attempt to improve rAAV packaging, Samulski et al. (138) developed an infectious plasmid (p*sub*201$^+$) that incorporated restriction enzyme sites flanking the viral coding domain, allowing for insertion of nonviral sequences between the two ITR. A similar approach utilized an infectious plasmid (d13-94) that retained only the terminal repeat sequences, a SV40-neomycin gene cassette could be inserted between the terminal repeats and used as selectable marker for both vectors (139). Recombinant AAV stocks were generated using a complementary plasmid containing the AAV coding sequences to supply the missing AAV gene products in trans. rAAV infection of human cell lines yielded transduction frequencies of 80%f (139,140). The increased transduction efficiency was thought to be due to *rep* deletion, previously shown to suppress heterologous promoters (141,142). These studies also demonstrated that only the AAV ITR were required for replication, packaging, and integration.

To supply the necessary replication and packaging proteins, a complementary plasmid (pAAV/Ad) is cotransfected that contains no sequence homology with the recombinant plasmid (p*sub*201$^+$) (Fig. 8) (140). The complementing plasmid includes the wild-type AAV genome flanked by adenoviral terminal repeat sequences, preventing mobilization of this helper genome and eliminating wild-type AAV contamination. Recombinant titers of $10^4$–$10^5$ per ml were generated. The recombinant virus stably integrated into host cell genome and could not be rescued from cells with adenovirus superinfection. Lacking *rep* for excision and replication, *both* wild-type AAV and adenovirus are required for rescue. This new packaging system eliminated wild-type AAV production, increased packaging size capability to ~5 kb, improved transduction efficiency, and reduced the possibility of proviral rescue.

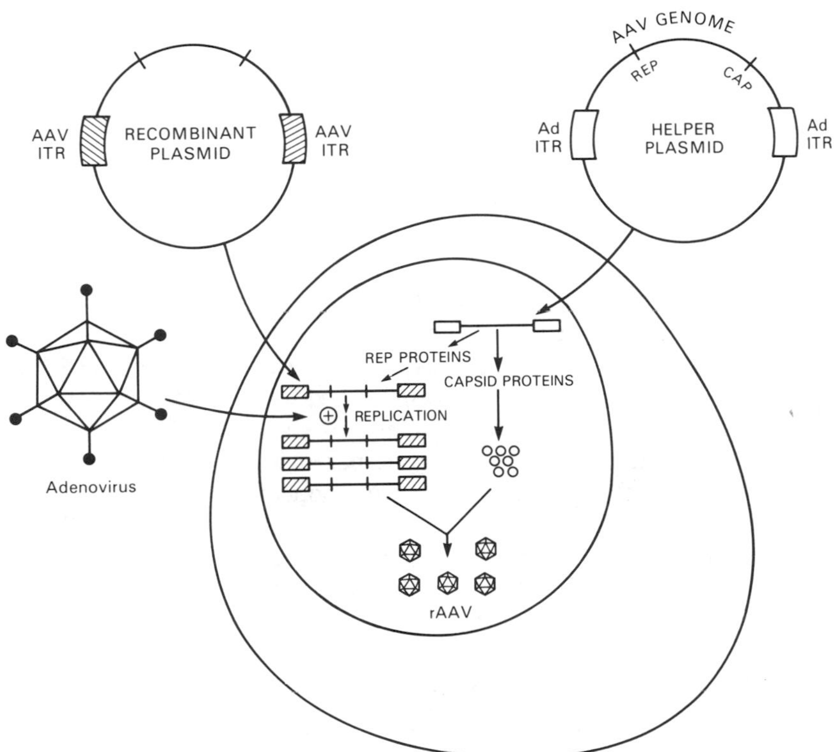


**Figure 8** Generation of helper-free recombinant adenoassociated virions. A producer cell line is cotransfected with "helper" and recombinant AAV (rAAV) plasmids. The helper plasmid generates REP and CAP protein synthesis. REP protein maintains rAAV plasmid replications, which are subsequently encapsidated, forming infectious rAAV particles. Adenoviral infection provides the necessary replication and packaging functions (see text for details).

This packaging system still produced contaminating infectious adenovirus and yielded low-titer recombinant preparations.

Recombinant virion production, although improved, is still hampered by the necessity for both cotransfection of recombinant and helper plasmids and infection with helper virus in a permissive cell line (such as 293 or HeLa). Cell lysis and death due to viral replication of both AAV and adenovirus limits recombinant virion generation. In an attempt to develop a packaging cell line analogous to the retroviral system, a HeLa cell line was developed that contained the integrated AAV genome lacking the terminal repeat sequences (143). Transfection with the recombinant plasmid-containing gp120 gene and adenovirus infection yielded recombinant titers of only $10^3$–$10^4$ per ml. The low titer may reflect low wt AAV genome copy per cell (usually one to two copies) compared to multiple copies after plasmid transfection. Other approaches for AAV packaging cell lines using the insertion of adenoviral early genes or *rep* genes into permissive cells are currently being evaluated (R. J. Samulski, personal communication).

## Virus-Cell Interaction

Limited information exists concerning the infectious entry of AAV into host cells. After binding to a specific cell surface receptor, AAV uncoats and delivers its genome to the nucleus. Ultrastructural studies have revealed that virions are taken up in endocytotic vesicles and an acidified environment promotes uncoating (144). Indirect evidence of specific host cell receptors was described by the inhibition of porcine parvovirus infection in permissive cells after incubation of the host cells with monoclonal antibody to membrane proteins (145). A polypeptide of 40 kD was characterized by immunoblot. A putative receptor binding site of canine parvovirus was described after analysis of its crystalline three-dimensional structure using high-resolution electron microscopy (119).

## Fate of Recombinant Genome

Latent infections were produced in vitro by infecting continuous lines of human cells with high multiplicities of wild-type AAV-2 in the absence of helper virus. Cultures remained latently infected for >150 passages, and several clones were isolated and characterized (146). The proviral DNA was found to be covalently linked to cellular DNA in tandem concatamers. Genomic blotting of several clones revealed that the viral-cellular junction fragments were of a different size, suggesting that wild-type AAV integration occurred randomly (or at several different sites) into the human genome (147). Two AAV-cellular junctions were isolated from a bacteriophage library and sequenced. The flanking cellular sequences were present one or two times in the human genome (148). In each case, the inverted terminal repeat was at or near the junction with cellular DNA, and sequence analysis showed evidence of deletion and/or rearrangements in the terminal repeat sequences. Evidence for extensive DNA rearrangements found in latent cell lines led to a reevaluation of random wild-type AAV integration. Using the flanking sequences as probes, normal cell sequences were consistently disrupted: 15 of 21 independently derived clones of latently infected human cells showed evidence that at least one copy of the original sequence had been altered in size as a result of viral DNA integration. The cellular target sequence for integration was mapped to a 7 kbp region of chromosome 19. Biotinylated probes visualized the unoccupied target site at 19q13.3-qter. This represents the first example of site-specific integration by a mammalian DNA virus (149).

These results have been confirmed and extended by employing a protein-DNA binding enrichment technique to isolate AAV proviral DNA from latent human cell lines (150). Nucleotide comparison of clonal cellular sequences demonstrate viral-cellular junction rearrangements involving deletion of portions of the terminal repeats. An unrearranged preintegration junction cellular sequence used as a probe confirmed the sequence location at chromosome 19. Amplification by polymerase chain reaction (PCR) using AAV and junction-specific primers generated viral-junction breakpoints that lay within a 100 bp sequence on chromosome 19. In situ analysis of latently infected cell chromosomes using AAV-specific probes further demonstrated that viral DNA integrated into only one locus. Both single- and multiple-copy number insertion patterns were located within this integration region.

The minimal elements required for AAV integration are currently being delineated. AAV vectors containing only the ITR integrate at high frequency, indicating that AAV integration relies on host cellular enzymes. However, work in our laboratory demonstrated a lack of site-specific integration with recombinant vectors containing only AAV termini (151) when clones were selected for $neo^R$ resistence, perhaps as a result of selection pressure or the absence of additional viral trans-acting sequences required for targeted integration.

## Application of AAV Gene Transfer

### Cultured Cells

Interest in AAV as a general gene transduction vector has led to its use in a variety of cell types. The expression of the cystic fibrosis transmembrane conductance regulator (CFTR) gene using an AAV vector in bronchial epithelial cells corrected defective $Cl^-$ secretion (152). The correction of ornithine transcarbamylase enzymatic activity in cultured hepatocytes has been reported using an AAV vector (153). In addition, human and nonhuman vascular smooth muscle cells have been used as targets for AAV gene transfer (154). rAAV virions carrying a SV40 promoter driving a glucocerebrosidase gene (the defective gene in Gaucher's disease) transduced NIH 3T3 cells. Gene expression was detected by cell-specific staining for the enzymatic activity and western blotting of the appropriate molecular weight protein (R. J. Samulski, unpublished results). An AAV vector carrying an adenovirus polIII promoter linked to the TAR element of HIV was constructed and used to infect human T lymphocytes. PCR analysis of the TAR sequences showed high-level mRNA expression in several of the transduced T cell clones

(T. Shimada, unpublished results). AAV may be useful as a vehicle for gene therapy directed at limiting or entirely abrogating HIV viral transcription in HIV-infected lymphocytes.

Our laboratory has utilized the AAV system to introduce a human $\gamma$-globin gene into human erythroleukemia cells (K562) and achieved high-level globin gene expression (151). K562 cells provide a model for the study of globin gene regulation. Recently described important cis-acting regulatory elements, collectively termed the locus control region (LCR), control globin gene expression (155). These sites are located several kilobases both 5′ and 3′ to the $\beta$-gene cluster on chromosome 11. When linked to globin genes, LCR sites enhance globin gene expression to a level equivalent to that of endogenous globin genes in transfected cells and transgenic animals (156, 157). Retroviral vectors incorporating LCR elements are unstable, thus limiting their utility as genetic transfer vectors for globin.

A human $^{A}\gamma$-globin gene linked to the HS 2 portion of the LCR and the neo$^{R}$ gene was subcloned into p*sub*201. This construct was used to generate recombinant AAV and infect K562 cells. Neo$^{R}$ clones were obtained and characterized by genomic blotting. One or two unrearranged copies of the viral genome were transferred, but integration analysis revealed random insertion into the host cell genome. RNA expression using both a RNase protection and PCR method showed nearly endogenous levels of expression from the transferred globin gene. This result indicates that rAAV can transfer regulatory elements required for the control of gene expression.

### Primary Cells

Transduction of murine hematopoietic progenitor cells using a recombinant AAV vector carrying a dominant selectable neo$^{R}$ gene has been reported (158). Adult B10.BR/cd murine bone marrow cells were incubated with rAAV for 2 h, and cells were grown in vitro in methylcellulose in either the absence or presence of G418. Transduction efficiency was calculated at ~0.5–1.5% based on the number of drug-resistant colonies per total colonies. Despite the poor transduction, this experiment suggested that primary cells could be infected with rAAV. rAAV constructs carrying the parvovirus B19 viral sequences were also infectious for erythroid progenitor cells from human bone marrow (159). Unselected human bone marrow was used for viral infection. Results were expressed only as a decrease in the number of erythroid colonies grown in vitro, presumarly because of the specific inhibitory effect of B19 genome expression on erythroid cell growth.

We recently demonstrated transduction of $\beta$-galactosidase gene by an rAAV and its expression in human hematopoietic cells (160). CD34$^{+}$-selected human and rhesus pluripotential cells were incubated with rAAV and grown in methylcellulose culture. Using DNA extracted from single colonies and

PCR amplification, the β-galactosidase coding sequences were detected in 35–90% of individual colonies. No significant toxicity to colony formation was observed. Gene transfer and stable expression have been described using murine hematopoietic cells (161). These results are consistent with the documented tropism of parvoviruses for hematopoietic cells (162).

### Safety Issues

One of the salient features of the AAV system is the lack of any demonstrable pathology when appropriate cells are infected with either wild-type or recombinant AAV. No epidemiologic data currently exist suggesting AAV as an etiologic agent of any disease. However, wild-type adenovirus required for the generation of rAAV is quite capable of causing serious disease, particularly in immunocompromised hosts. rAAV packaging systems will need to be modified to eliminate adenoviral contamination.

### Summary

Recombinant AAV is among the newest of possible genetic transfer vectors. This once obscure virus possesses unique properties that distinguish it from all other vectors. Its major advantage is the lack of pathogenicity in humans. Wild-type AAV has the unique ability to selectively integrate into the mammalian genome at a specific region, thus reducing concerns of insertional mutagenesis and oncogenic potential. Its ability to carry regulatory elements without interference from the viral genome allows greater control of transferred gene expression. In vitro experiments demonstrate that rAAV vectors can transduce primary hematopoietic cells and support the development of this vector system for gene transfer. Disadvantages include the inferior packaging systems, which yield low numbers of recombinant virions, and contamination with wild-type adenovirus. The small genome limits packaging to ~5 kb, ruling out transfer of larger genomes. Recombinant AAV particles do not appear to demonstrate the same site-specific genome integration as wild-type virions.

## ADENOVIRUS

In 1953, Rowe and colleagues isolated a cytopathogenic agent from human adenoidal tissue undergoing degeneration in tissue culture (164). Named adenovirus, this agent has been studied for 40 years. Among the more than 40 serotypes, some cause infections of the conjunctivae, upper and lower respiratory tract, gastrointestinal system, and urinary tract; others have not been linked to any human disease. Molecular analysis of adenoviruses has been spurred by the discovery that some serotypes can cause tumors in animals and transform tissue culture cells (165). Adenoviruses are among the best studied viruses of eukaryotes, and adenovirus vectors were among the first to be engineered for gene transfer. Recently, there has been renewed interest in using these vectors for genetic therapy in humans.

## Structure and Genomic Organization

Adenovirus virions are 60–90 nm in diameter. The icosahedral particles have a dense core surrounded by the capsid. The core contains the DNA molecule. The major capsid proteins are the hexon, penton base, and fiber. The penton complex at each of the 12 icosahedral vertices is composed of a wide penton base and a protruding fiber (166). The adenovirus serotypes 2 (Ad2) and 5 (Ad5) have been studied most extensively as vectors. These viruses contain a linear DNA genome of 36 kb with inverted terminal repeats. DNA sequences near the termini contain the replication origins and packaging signals.

Adenoviruses exhibit two phases of gene expression during the lytic life cycle, early and late, which are separated by the onset of viral DNA replication 6–7 h postinfection (Fig. 9). Over 30 early-phase transcripts have been identified from five noncontiguous regions (E1, E2a, E2b, E3, and E4) (167). Late-phase transcripts initiate at the single major late promoter (MLP) situated at map unit 17, generating polycistronic transcripts that are alternatively

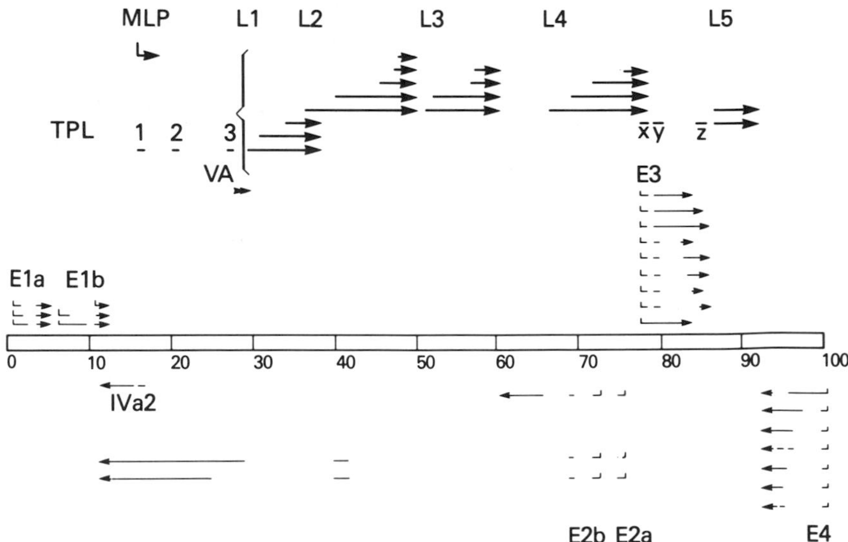


**Figure 9** Transcription map of adenovirus (see text).

processed to result in mRNA species with an identical 5′-untranslated leader sequence, the tripartite leader (TPL) (168,169). In addition to the viral mRNA, two short 160 nucleotide (nt) RNAs are transcribed by RNA polymerase III (170). These virus-associated (VA) RNAs, VA-RNA I and II, accumulate to high levels (approximately $10^5$–$10^6$ copies per cell) late in infection. Late in infection, between 20 and 40% of pulse-labeled total RNA is viral. Viral infection eventually results in shutoff of host protein synthesis, and only viral proteins are synthesized (171,172). By 48–72 h after infection, the cell is lysed with a burst of virus production.

## Vector Design

Adenovirus recombinants can be divided into helper-independent and helper-dependent vectors (173). Since the inclusion of wild-type helper virus would lead to cell lysis, we focus on strategies for the generation of helper-independent vectors. The DNA packaging limit for adenoviruses is a maximum of 2 kb of foreign DNA into the wild-type virus genome. To permit packaging of larger DNA inserts, Ad mutants with deletions in the early region (such as E1) have been used to create space for exogenous DNA insertion. The human 293 cell line contains the left 14% of the Ad5 viral genome, including the E1 region, and can complement viruses that lack E1 (174). Recombinant viruses with deletions in the E1 region, which can be propagated in complementing cell lines, are termed conditional (defective), that is, conditional for propagation only in 293 cells (173). Alternatively, because the E3 region is not essential for virus replication, recombinant viruses with deletions in the E3 region are termed nonconditional; that is, they can propagate without complementing E3 protein (175).

A typical adenovirus vector is depicted in Figure 10. This conditional (defective) version has a 2.6 kb deletion in the E1 region to render the virus unable to replicate. The E3 region has been deleted to create space for the exogenous DNA. A cassette is inserted into the left end of the construct and contains the 5′-inverted terminal repeat, the Ad origin of replication, the encapsidation signal, the E1A enhancer, the MLP, and the tripartite leader sequences, followed by the foreign cDNA and a polyadenylation signal from the SV40 virus. The TPL sequences are included to increase the efficiency of translation (176).

## Packaging Systems

Typically, a part of the dispensible E3 region and/or E1 region is substituted with foreign genes. This recombinant clone contains the entire upstream region of the genome. The clone is linearized at a site downstream from the inserted gene, followed by separation into upstream and downstream frag-

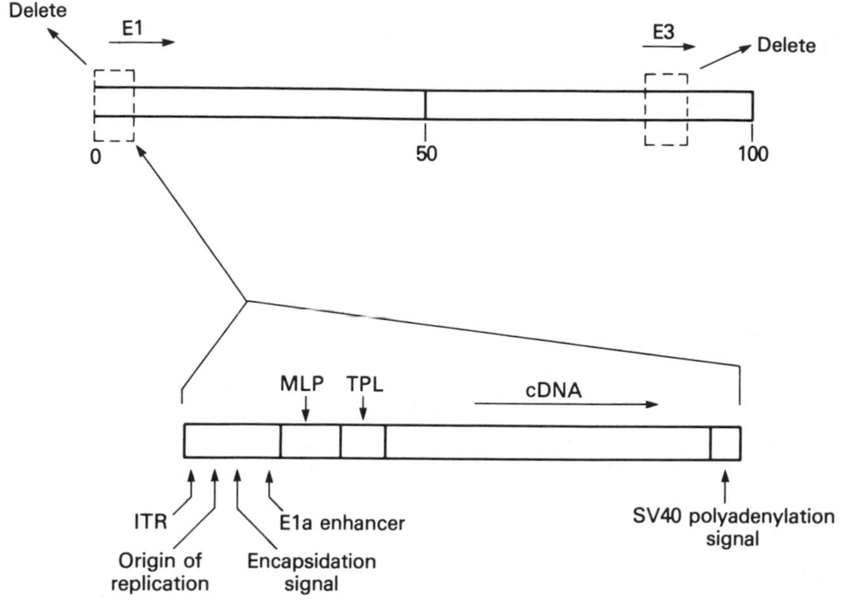


**Figure 10** Typical cassette for defective adenovirus vector. The cassette shows the ITR, the adenovirus origin of replication, the encapsidation signal, and the E1a enhancer upstream from the major late promoter (MLP), which drives the inserted gene.

ments. Ligated DNA is then transfected into 293 cells; DNA molecules with corresponding upstream and downstream fragments yield virus. Alternatively, a plasmid containing the recombinant sequence and an adenoviral subgenomic fragment (or deletion mutant) can be introduced into 293 cells without ligation (177). Infectious recombinant virions are created by recombination in vivo at the overlapping site (178). With either method, plasmid DNA sequences upstream from the viral DNA are deleted in the process of viral replication. This method of generating adenovirus stock should yield a helper-free recombinant virus that is defective and replicates only in 293 cells.

## Virus-Cell Interaction and Pathway of Viral Entry

Adenovirus enters the cell through an unidentified receptor and is transported through the cytoplasm within an endosome. Once in the endosome, acidification alters the hydrophobicity of the adenoviral capsid proteins and allows the capsid proteins (particularly the penton base protein) to disrupt the vesicle membrane and escape lysosomal degradation (179). Subsequently, the virus extrudes from the endosome, uncoats, and enters the nucleus.

A novel strategy that capitalizes on the efficient cellular entry mechanism of the adenovirus is the coupling of adenovirus capsid to a polylysine-transferrin (180) or to a polylysine-antibody (181) mixture that contains the DNA to be transferred. Theoretically, the polylysine-transferrin conjugate would be delivered in conjunction with adenovirus to achieve co-internalization in the same endosome in which adenoviral disruption of the vesicle would free the conjugate (182). Using a complex carrying the firefly luciferase reporter gene, Curiel et al. demonstrated markedly increased gene expression with adenovirus-mediated endosomal lysis (180). In related experiments, a monoclonal antibody was made competent to carry DNA by the attachment of a polylysine residue (181). The antibody was specific for an adenovirus epitope, thus complexing the DNA to the exterior of the virion. These molecular conjugate vectors were used to deliver the firefly luciferase gene to human airway epithelial cells via a receptor-mediated endocytosis pathway. Direct association of the adenovirus with the complex also permitted polylysine-transferrin gene transfer to chicken bone marrow cells. Presumably, these molecular conjugate vectors have no packaging size constraint and may be designed without codelivery of the viral genome (183).

## Fate of the Recombinant Genome

The replicative cycle of wild-type adenovirus infection has been well studied. Wild-type adenovirus has a profound effect on host cell macromolecular synthesis and eventually leads to cell lysis and death. There is no evidence that adenoviral DNA integrates into the host genome during this stage of infection (184). However, adenovirus can transform cells of rodent, human, and simian origin (185). In contrast to lytic infection, transformation is characterized by stable integration into the host genome (186). Recombinant adenoviral vectors can also stably transduce cells via selection with drugs or enzymes (187) and have been found to be integrated in a structure colinear with that of the input viral genome. In contrast, the fate of the recombinant genome of defective viruses that do not carry selectable markers, such as neomycin resistance, is unclear. These recombinant genomes may exist in an extrachromosomal state. Surprisingly, the status of the viral DNA has been studied in only one instance, after gene transfer to mouse muscle tissue (188). Southern blot analysis of DNA detected a fragment corresponding to the left end of the recombinant genome, indicating persistence of the viral DNA in a linear form following infection. The episomal state of the recombinant genome implies that expression of the foreign gene will be transient and dependent upon replicative turnover of the infected cell.

## Applications

### Respiratory Epithelial Cells

Although adenoviruses are not restricted to respiratory epithelial cells, they clearly productively infect such cells in vivo (189). The lining of the respiratory tract contains a heterogeneous mixture of epithelial cells that are potential targets for the introduction of genes (190). Only a small portion of airway cells are actively proliferating, however, and most are terminally differentiated, a potential limitation for the use of conventional retroviral vectors.

Two disorders that lead to pathology of the lung epithelial cells are $\alpha_1$-antitrypsin ($\alpha_1$-AT) deficiency and cystic fibrosis. $\alpha_1$-AT deficiency is a genetic disorder characterized by decreased amounts of the protease inhibitor, $\alpha_1$-AT (191). $\alpha_1$-AT is a 52 kD glycoprotein that serves as the major inhibitor of neutrophil elastase, a serine protease capable of destroying the connective tissue of the alveolar wall. Consequently, a deficiency of $\alpha_1$-AT predisposes affected individuals to emphysema, as well as hepatitis and cirrhosis. CF is a common genetic disorder characterized by abnormal ion transport by epithelial cells of the pancreas, gastrointestinal tract, liver, and lung (192). The clinical manifestations of CF predominantly reflect desiccation of respiratory secretions and subsequent lung pathology. The gene responsible for CF was recently identified and cloned; the encoded protein, called the cystic fibrosis transmembrane conductance regulator, functions as a $Cl^-$ channel responsible for secreting $Cl^-$ from the cell (193).

Rosenfeld et al. developed an adenovirus vector to deliver the human $\alpha_1$-AT gene (194) and the CFTR gene (195) to epithelial cells of the cotton rat respiratory tract. Replication-defective vectors carrying a human $\alpha_1$-AT gene were introduced into the tracheae of cotton rats. $\alpha_1$-AT protein was detected in lung lavage fluid for up to 7 days following the treatment at concentrations of 10–1000 ng/ml of $\alpha_1$-AT. Unfortunately, it remains unclear whether this concentration of $\alpha_1$-AT is sufficient to correct the clinical manifestations of $\alpha_1$-AT deficiency, and the bioactivity of the $\alpha_1$-AT protein was not reported. Based on this preliminary study, the same investigators prepared replication-defective vectors carrying the CFTR cDNA driven by the adenovirus MLP (195). The recombinant vector was introduced into the lungs of cotton rats, and expression of human CFTR mRNA transcripts and protein was detected in the airway epithelium. Assays using polymerase chain amplification suggested that CFTR mRNA was expressed in rats for several months.

### Liver Cells

As previously mentioned, adenovirus exhibit a broad host range specificity and efficiently penetrate many cell types (173). Adenoviruses are capable of infecting and expressing genes in hepatoma cell lines and primary mouse hepatocytes (196). A defective adenovirus recombinant was constructed to carry the rat ornithine transcarbamylase (OTC) cDNA under the control of the adenovirus MLP (197) and injected intravenously into newborn Spf-ash mutant mice defective in OTC protein synthesis, with resultant hyperammonemia, orotic aciduria, growth retardation, and sparse fur. An increase in OTC activity was detected and accompanied by a diminution of orotic acid in the urine. OTC mRNA transcripts were detectable for over 1 year following the injection, suggesting the long-term presence of the transferred gene. More recently, *Escherichia coli* $\beta$-galactosidase and human $\alpha_1$-AT protein have been produced after intraportal injection of rats with replication-deficient recombinant adenoviruses containing these genes (198). These data are promising because, like respiratory epithelial cells, hepatocytes proliferate slowly and may be less susceptible to retroviral transduction.

### Muscle Cells

Transfer of the $\beta$-galactosidase gene into mouse skeletal and cardiac muscles after intravenous administration has been demonstrated using recombinant adenovirus (188). Expression of $\beta$-galactosidase was observed for at least 12 months despite the extrachromosomal state of the virus.

## Safety Issues

The safety of adenovirus vectors is related to the fate of the recombinant genome. Since the defective viruses not expressing selectable genes probably do not integrate into host DNA, the potential for insertional mutagenesis is theoretically low. By rendering the recombinant virus replication deficient, lysis of the infected cell should be impossible. However, rescue of the recombinant replication function, either by host cell provision of E1A function in trans or by concurrent wild-type adenoviral infection, could conceivably lead to uncontrolled transmission of recombinant adenovirus. The potential hazards of viral dissemination in an immunologically competent host are unknown.

## Summary

Many questions remain about the ability of adenoviruses to serve as vectors for gene therapy, primarily involving the fate of the virus. Available data suggest that replication-deficient recombinant adenoviruses do not integrate into the cellular genome. Thus, therapy for cystic fibrosis, for example, may require repeated instillation of the recombinant virus, possibly by aerosolized preparation. The host immune system may either prevent viral infection or, alternatively, initiate an inflammatory reaction in the lung tissue that may be harmful to the host. In addition to these concerns, the ability to deliver sufficient levels of functional protein to the genetically deficient host has not been determined in any of the studies cited to date.

## HERPESVIRUSES

The members of the family Herpesviridae have been classified into alphaherpesvirinae, betaherpesvirinae, and gammaherpesvirinae (199). Because this nomenclature divides herpesviruses on the basis of host range and reproductive cycle, we retain this subclassification in our discussion of herpesvirus vectors.

The alphaherpesvirinae, including herpes simplex virus types 1 and 2 (HSV-1 and HSV-2), have a variable host range and can efficiently lyse cells and establish latent infections, primarily in neural ganglia. The betaherpesvirinae, including HCMV, characteristically have a long reproductive cycle, and infected cells become enlarged (cytomegalia); these viruses can establish latency in secretory glands, the lymphoreticular system, and kidneys. The gammaherpesvirinae, including Epstein-Barr virus and herpesvirus saimiri, replicate primarily in lymphoblastoid cells, as well as some epithelioid and fibroblastic cells; latent virus is frequently demonstrated in lymphoid tissue. Because the Herpesviridae can establish latent infection in neural or lymphoreticular tissues, several members have been used to transfer foreign genetic material.

A typical herpesvirion consists of a core of DNA that forms a torus surrounded by an icosadeltahedral capsid of 100–110 nm, an amorphous tegument, and a membrane envelope from which viral glycoprotein spikes project (199). The majority of herpesvirus DNAs are linear double-stranded molecules. The DNAs differ with respect to their size and base compositions, as well as their sequence arrangement. For this reason, we consider the herpesviruses individually.

### Herpes Simplex Virus

We first consider the neurotropic genera of the herpes simplex viruses (HSV-1 and HSV-2). Postmitotic neurons can be latently infected by the neurotropic herpesviruses. HSV latency is thought to occur in the following stages (200): primary infection at a peripheral site with viral replication; retrograde ascent of virus through sensory nerve axons to neuronal cell bodies in sensory or autonomic ganglia; and establishment of latency within the nuclei of neurons. Reactivation from latency can occur, with descent of virus back to the peripheral site and replication and shedding of infectious virus. Serologic studies have indicated that, although more than 90% of adults have been infected with HSV, only a small proportion suffer from symptomatic reactivation of virus (201). In the immunocompromised host, reactivation of HSV can lead to esophagitis, pneumonia, or, rarely, widespread dissemination.

### Genomic Organization and Life Cycle

The HSV genome consists of a single molecule of linear, double-stranded DNA (dsDNA) of approximately 150 kb (Fig. 11) (200). The dsDNA can be divided into two covalently joined strands, the long (L) and the short (S). Each strand contains a unique (U) sequence bounded by inverted repeat elements. The genome contains about 70 genes that are coordinately regulated in a cascade fashion in productively infected cells (202). Three major classes of mRNA and their respective polypeptides are synthesized: immediate early ($\alpha$ or IE), early ($\beta$ or E), and late ($\gamma$ or L). The five IE genes are transcribed in the absence of de novo viral protein synthesis; efficient IE transcription is stimulated by a viral structural protein Vmw65 (also known as VP16) in a process that requires recognition of the so-called TAATGARAT motif (203–205). The IE proteins, notably the product of IE 1 gene, Vmw110 (or ICP0), in turn transactive E and L genes. The IE gene products are believed to determine whether an infected cell establishes either the productive or latent state.

During viral latency, the viral genome persists in a circular or concatameric extrachromosomal state (206). Initial studies incorrectly concluded that viral genes were not expressed in latently infected tissues. Subsequently, several groups demonstrated HSV-specific RNA transcripts within latently

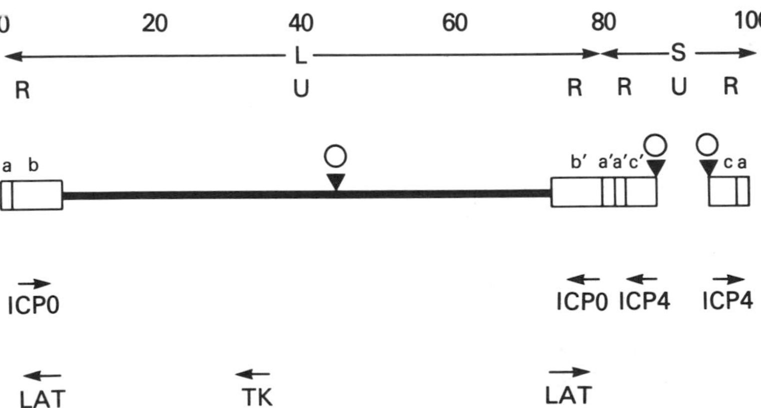


**Figure 11** Transcription map of herpesvirus (see text).

infected ganglia (207). These latency-associated transcripts (LAT) were found to map to only a single portion of the viral genome that partly overlaps one end of the IE 1 gene; the LAT transcripts are synthesized from the opposite DNA strand, being complementary to the 3′ end of IE 1 mRNA (208–211). The IE 1 gene product, Vmw110 (ICP0), as previously mentioned, is an important regulatory of gene expression. It has been suggested that the juxtaposition and interaction of antisense LAT and sense IE 1 transcripts is a means of regulating ICP0 mRNA and protein synthesis, thereby enhancing the latent state.

## Vector Design

Two types of HSV vectors have been developed: plasmid derived (usually helper dependent) and virus derived (212). Plasmid-derived vectors consist of plasmids bearing an HSV-1 origin of replication and an HSV-1 packaging signal (213). These defective amplicons retain only the cis-acting sequences required for replication and packaging and can be polymerized in an HSV-1-infected cell into DNA large enough to be packaged (Fig. 12). The major

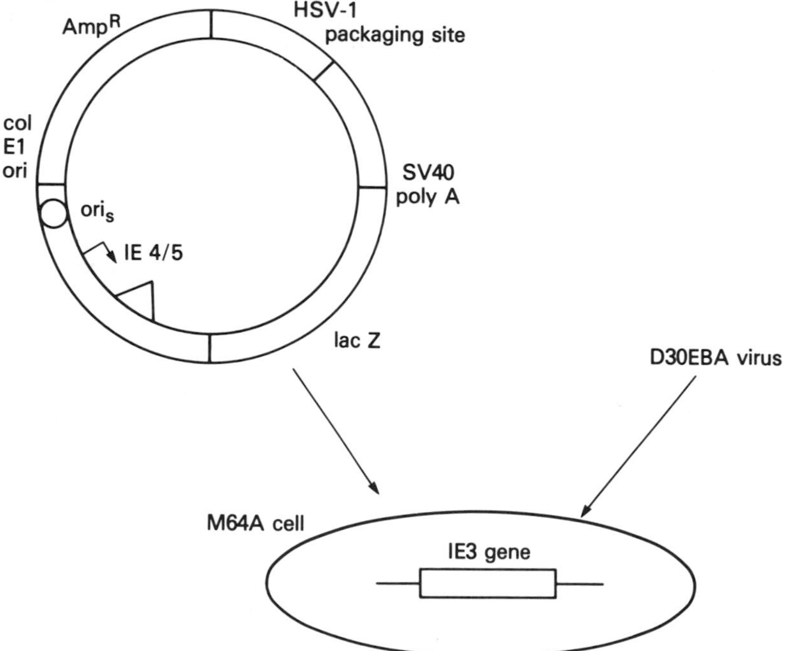


**Figure 12** Packaging system for plasmid-derived herpesvirus vector (see text).

problem with plasmid-derived vectors is that they are dependent upon wild-type helper virus for replication; the wild-type virus should result in shutdown of host cell protein synthesis and lysis of the infected cell (214). To overcome this problem, defective vectors were constructed that expressed the foreign DNA, under the control of an HSV-1 IE promoter, early in infection (215). By superinfecting with a helper virus containing a temperature-sensitive mutation in the major IE protein, Vmw175, the IE promoter driving the foreign gene will be more active at the nonpermissive temperature (37°C), thus allowing expression of the foreign gene without causing lysis of the cell at body temperature (see later).

An alternative approach to plasmid-derived vectors directly introduced the foreign gene into a conditionally dispensible region of the genome and purified the recombinant virus by plaque purification (216). These virus-derived recombinants are engineered by direct alterations, and three general schemes have been used: growth selection, marker insertion, and direct detection (212). The most commonly used type of growth selection is for loss or gain of HSV-1 thymidine kinase (TK) activity. This selectable marker enzyme phosphorylates thymidine and other nucleoside analogs. Both $TK^-$ and $TK^+$ viruses can be selected for by a variety of strategies. The exogenous DNA can then be inserted into the domain of the viral tk gene to engineer the recombinent virus. For the purposes of this discussion we have divided virus-derived HSV vectors into three categories: replication compromised, replication defective, and replication competent but highly attenuated.

**Packaging Systems**

The packaging systems for plasmid-derived vectors can be illustrated by methods used to produce pHSVlac (215). LacZ is a convenient marker gene because the encoded bacterial enzyme, β-galactosidase, can be detected histochemically; pHSVlac contains the lacZ gene under the control of the HSV-1 IE 4/5 promoter. Typically, pHSVlac has been packaged into HSV-1 virions by using a temperature-sensitive (ts) mutant, HSV-1 strain 17 ts K, as helper virus. ts K contains a mutation in the IE3 gene that encodes the major regulatory protein; the mutant is thus incapable of DNA replication and unable to produce progeny virus at 37°C. Typically, CV1 cells were transfected with pHSVlac DNA. Following a 24 h incubation period at 37°C, HSV-1 ts K was added to supply helper function. The cells were then incubated at 31°C, the permissive temperature for the mutant, thus generating viral stock of both the recombinant and temperature-sensitive mutant.

An efficient packaging system for HSV-1 vectors was documented using a deletion mutant, D30EBA, as helper virus; virus was grown on the complementing cell line M64A (217). D30EBA is a HSV-1 strain 17 deletion mutant that lacks the IE3 gene. M64A cells were genetically engineered to carry the IE3 gene. pHSVlac virus was prepared in the following manner: M64A cells were transfected with pHSVlac DNA and then infected 1 day later with D30EBA virus. Since pHSVlac contains the packaging signal and capsid sequences, progeny virus included D30EBA and pHSVlac virus.

### Virus-Cell Interaction and Pathway of Viral Entry

The virus initiates infection by binding to a specific receptor on the cell surface followed by fusion of the virion envelope with the cell membrane (218, 219). The viral nucleocapsid then migrates into the nucleus, where the viral DNA is released and transcribed as described. Following this acute replicative phase of infection, HSV-1 becomes latent in neurons.

In addition to neurons, other cell types may support HSV entry and/or replication. A fibroblastic cell line with a high level of receptors for basic fibroblast growth factor (bFGF) has been reported to be more susceptible to HSV-1 infection, suggesting that bFGF receptor serves as a portal of entry (220). These data have been disputed; however, it may be possible to improve viral entry through the use of agents that change the ionic charge potential of target cell membranes.

### Fate of the Recombinant Genome

During latency, the viral genome remains in the nucleus as a nonintegrated episome coated with nucleosomes (206,221). As alluded to previously, transcription occurs from only one region of the viral genome, known as the LAT sequence (208,221). LAT transcript production can therefore serve as a marker of latent infection.

### Applications

*Central Nervous System.* One of the earliest models of HSV gene transfer developed in a specific attempt to transfer a therapeutically important human gene to the central nervous system (CNS) used a nondefective virus-derived vector expressing the hypoxanthine phosphoriboxyltransferase (HPRT) cDNA (222). Complete deficiency of the purine salvage enzyme HPRT leads to a devastating human neurologic disease, Lesch-Nyhan syndrome, in which uric acid is overproduced (223,224). Notably, restoration of HPRT activity in the circulation via bone marrow transplantation does not cure the neurologic syndrome (225–227); thus, Lesch-Nyhan syndrome represents a paradigm for vectors that can target the CNS. The human HPRT gene was delivered to $HPRT^-$ rat neuroma cells in vitro by inserting the HPRT cDNA into the viral tk gene. Herpesvirus vectors, which replace the tk gene with a foreign gene, have been described; these can support productive infection in neuroma cells, which have endogenous tk enzyme activity. Having documented transient HPRT expression in the rat neuroma cells, the same vector was found to express HPRT mRNA in mouse brains in vivo after intracranial inoculation (228). In the latter case, however, high doses of this vector induced encephalitis and death of animals. Consequently, subsequent efforts have focused on the development of attenuated HSV vectors.

Four models of HSV-1-mediated gene transfer have been described that permit the introduction of genes into postmitotic neurons. The first model utilized plasmid-derived amplicons (213). Defective HSV-1 amplicons have been used to express lacZ in cultured cortical and hippocampal neurons (215, 229,230), as well as striatal neurons (231). Dysfunction of neurons from the corpus striatum is thought to lead to Huntington's disease and Parkinson's disease, and vectors targeting the striatum could be very useful. For example, vectors based on this design may permit localized delivery of tyrosine hydroxylase to striatal neurons of patients with Parkinson's disease (232).

In the second model, a replication-compromised virus, typically $ICP0^-$, contains a foreign gene, such as the *E. coli* lacZ, under the control of an IE viral promoter (212). Infection of neurons would proceed with retrograde ascent and expression of the foreign gene in the primary and then secondary neurons after lysis and release of virus from primary neurons. Vectors expressing foreign genes driven by the IE promoter would be useful only for short-term expression because the promoters are active only during the acute phase of viral infection (less than 10 days postinfection). The ability of these vectors to express foreign genes in vivo has not been demonstrated.

In the third model, replication-defective virus, lacking an immediate early gene required for viral replication ($ICP4^-$), carries lacZ under the control of the LAT promoter (212). The objective of these experiments was to establish a nonlytic gene delivery system: following transport to the neuronal nucleus, the vector would stably express the foreign gene in only the latently infected primary neuron. This type of vector has been used successfully in dorsal root ganglia after sciatic nerve inoculation (233), trigeminal ganglia after corneal scarification, and neurons in the hypoglossal nucleus after injection into the tongue (233). A recombinant HSV-1 vector construct containing the rat $\beta$-glucuronidase (GUSB) cDNA under the control of the LAT promoter was employed to investigate GUSB expression in the CNS of MPS VII mice infected by corneal inoculation (234). MPS VII mice lack the GUSB enzyme and serve as models for the human genetic disease mucopolysaccharidosis (Sly disease), a lysosomal storage disorder that leads to accumulation of glycosaminoglycans in numerous body tissues. The metabolic defect results in a severe degenerative syndrome in the CNS of affected individuals. Analogous to the situation in Lesch-Nyhan syndrome, the delivery of the defective enzyme (GUSB) in Sly disease via bone marrow transplantation does not correct the CNS pathology, thus spurring the development of neuron-specific vectors (235). Cells expressing GUSB enzymatic activity were detected in the trigeminal ganglia and brainstems of latently infected MPS VII mice for up to 4 months post-inoculation. Unfortunately, too few cells were corrected to alter the disease phenotype of the animals, pointing to the need for further improvement in the vector system.

In the fourth model, replication-competent but highly attenuated strains of HSV are employed. These may be capable of establishing latency in a greater number of neurons than replication-defective vectors. Stereotactic inoculation of an attenuated HSV vector into the hippocampus and caudate lobe of rat brain has been described (236). Virus attenuation was accomplished by inactivation of the viral gene Us3 via insertion of a lacZ reporter gene. The lacZ gene was driven by the glycoprotein C late promoter. The attenuated virus caused little detectable damage to hippocampal neurons, and transient lacZ expression was detected in a proportion of dentate gyrus neurons following hippocampal injection. That these vectors established latent infection was suggested by the appearance of LAT transcripts in the brain 10 months after infection.

*Nonrecombinant Mutants and CNS Neoplasms.* Finally, HSV mutants can be genetically engineered to be deficient in the virus-encoded enzyme thymidine kinase. The mutants can replicate in dividing cells but are severely impaired for replication in nondividing cells in the mammalian nervous system. Such a mutant (dlsptk) demonstrated killing in two long-term human glioma lines and three short-term glioma cell populations (237). Subcutaneous and subrenal human gliomas implanted in nude mice were growth inhibited after intraneoplastic injection of dlsptk, and nude mice with intracranial gliomas had prolonged survival following intraneoplastic inoculation of dlsptk.

### Safety Issues

The current focus of HSV vector development is generating a vector capable of infecting a larger number of neurons but without causing neuropathologic damage via replication function. The most promising vectors in this regard make use of replication-defective or replication-competent but highly attenuated strains. Until these can be engineered and tested in animal models, the relative risks of recombinant HSV vectors will remain unclear.

## Human Cytomegalovirus

Human cytomegalovirus (HCMV) is a widely distributed pathogen that latently infects humans. Between 59 and 79% of the adult population have antibodies to HCMV, and approximately 95% of blood donors carry viral DNA as detected by the polymerase chain reaction. Infection in the immunologically normal host is most often asymptomatic. Those with symptomatic disease may suffer from a mononucleosis syndrome (see Chap. 6). Infected individuals may shed virus from a variety of body fluids, including saliva, semen, tears, urine, cervical secretions, and breast milk. In the immunocompromised host, HCMV can produce life-threatening disease, including retinitis, pneumonitis, and gastrointestinal ulceration. Those at risk include bone marrow and solid organ transplant recipients, patients with AIDS, and developing fetuses.

How HCMV establishes latency is still not entirely clear (Chap. 6). The initiation of HCMV infection following transmission by blood or granulocyte transfusion suggests that bone marrow-derived hematopoietic cells may serve as a reservoir for latent virus. These reports indicated that HCMV can infect myeloid cells of peripheral blood and bone marrow, suggesting a natural tropism that might be exploited for delivering foreign genetic material to hematopoietic cells.

### Genome Organization

The genome of HCMV is linear and double stranded, with some 240 kb of DNA and a coding capacity for at least 100 proteins. Reminiscent of other herpesviruses, the viral genome includes immediate early ($\alpha$), early ($\beta$), and late ($\gamma$) genes that are regulated by complex transcriptional and posttranscriptional signals. The early $\beta_{2.7}$ gene promoter has been widely studied in recombinant viral constructs.

### Vector Design

Manipulation of the HCMV genome has proven to be challenging. In particular, a modified *E. coli* lacZ gene was inserted into one of the two copies of the $\beta_{2.7}$ gene to create the recombinant human CMV-RC256 isolate (238). This Towne strain-based recombinant virus expresses copious amounts of $\beta$-galactosidase and has served as a model for HCMV expression vectors.

### Packaging System

At the present time, packaging systems for CMV vectors are limited. RC256 was engineered by insertion of the lacZ gene into the viral genome via homologous recombination with CMV (Towne strain) DNA. The progeny virus was plated onto fresh human fibroblast cells and plaque purified on the basis of the blue staining of the lacZ gene.

### Fate of the Recombinant Genome

Like HSV, CMV is thought to function in an extrachromosomal state, although this has not been documented for the recombinant vectors. One difference between CMV and the large DNA viruses, such as adenovirus and HSV, is that CMV does not result in shutdown of host cell machinery. Thus, although CMV does lyse infected fibroblasts, the target cell of CMV in vivo is not known and may not be lysed by permissive infection.

### Safety Issues

Although the HCMV genome contains several putative transforming regions, tumors have not been observed following HCMV infection. Furthermore, the HCMV Towne strain has been safely used as a vaccine for immunization of bone marrow transplant candidates (239). At the present time, CMV-based vectors are not sufficiently refined to assess their safety.

### Applications

Maciejewski et al. used the recombinant RC256 isolate to study the ability of HCMV to infect primitive human bone marrow progenitors (240). After RC256 infection of progenitor cells, lacZ activity was demonstrated in infected $CD34^+$ target cells and in the progeny generated in culture from $CD34^+$ cells. HCMV late antigen was detected in infected precursor cells, and virus was released from colonies derived from $CD34^+$ cells. $\beta$-Galactosidase activity appeared to correlate with myelomonocytic differentiation. Presumably, these replication-competent viruses may induce a cytopathic effect to varying degrees in cells of different types.

### Summary

One motivation for developing herpesvirus vectors stemmed from a need to transfer foreign DNAs more than 5 kb in size. Plasmid-derived, helper-dependent herpesvirus vectors theoretically could accomodate 150 kb of DNA. As indicated, these DNA molecules are arranged in multiple repeat units. Inclusion of foreign sequences into a unit repeat could lead to amplification of the foreign sequence in the recombinant virion following co-transfection of cells with helper virus DNA.

Second, since herpesviruses can establish latent infections of neural tissue, they should prove useful in gene therapy targeting the CNS. At the present time, herpesvirus-based systems are still being refined; thus, the utility of these viruses in treating neurologic disorders is difficult to assess.

Finally, as with the adenoviruses, the herpesviruses can establish persistent infection without integrating into the cellular genome and do not seem to require an actively replicating host cell to initiate infection. The large DNA viruses thus have some distinct advantages over retroviral vectors, which may be exploited in future experiments.

## REFERENCES

1. Varmus HE. Form and function of retroviral proviruses. Science 1982; 216:812–20.
2. Varmus H. Retroviruses. Science 1988; 240:1427–35.

3. Katz RA, Skalka AM. Generation of diversity in retroviruses. Annu Rev Genet 1990; 24:409–45.
4. Teich N. Taxonomy of retroviruses. In: Weiss R, Teich N, Barums H, Coffin J, eds. RNA tumor viruses. Cold Spring Harbor, NY: Cold Spring Harbor Laboratory Press, 1985; 1–16.
5. Miller AD, Rosman GJ. Improved retroviral vectors for gene transfer and expression. Biotechniques 1989; 7:980–2, 984–6, 989–90.
6. Miller AD. Retroviral vectors. Curr Top Microbiol Immunol 1992; 158:1–24.
7. Tsichlis PN, Lazo PA. Virus-host interactions and the pathogenesis of murine and human oncogenic retroviruses. Curr Top Microbiol Immunol 1991; 171: 95–171.
8. Tsichlis PN, Bear SE. Infection by mink cell focus-forming viruses confers interleukin 2 (IL-2) independence to and IL-2-dependent rat T-cell lymphoma line. Proc Natl Acad Sci U S A 1991; 88:4611–5.
9. Hunter E, Swanstrom R. Retrovirus envelope glycoproteins. Curr Top Microbiol Immunol 1990; 157:187–253.
10. Stoye JP, Coffin JM. The four classes of endogenous murine leukemia virus: structural relationships and potential for recombination. J Virol 1987; 61:2659–69.
11. Stoye JP, Coffin JM. Polymorphism of murine endogenous proviruses revealed by using virus class-specific oligonucleotide probes. J Virol 1988; 62:168–75.
12. Laigret F, Repaske R, Boulukos K, Rabson AB, Khan AS. Potential progenitor sequences of mink cell focus-forming (MCF) murine leukemia viruses: ecotropic, xenotropic, and MCF-related viral RNAs are detected concurrently in thymus tissues of AKR mice. J Virol 1988; 62:376–86.
13. Amanuma H, Laigret F, Nishi M, Ikawa Y, Khan AS. Identification of putative endogenous proviral templates for progenitor mink cell focus-forming (MCF) MuLV-related RNAs. Virology 1988; 164:556–61.
14. Shinnick TM, Lerner RA, Sutcliffe JG. Nucleotide sequence of Moloney murine leukaemia virus. Nature 1981; 293:543–8.
15. Shoemaker C, Goff S, Gilboa E, Paskind M, Mitra SW, Baltimore D. Structure of a cloned circular Moloney murine leukemia virus DNA molecule containing an inverted segment: implications for retrovirus integration. Proc Natl Acad Sci U S A 1980; 77:3932–6.
16. Leis J, Baltimore D, Bishop JM, et al. Standardized and simplified nomenclature for proteins common to all retroviruses. J Virol 1988; 62:1808–9.
17. Linial ML, Miller AD. Retroviral RNA packaging: sequence requirements and implications. Curr Top Microbiol Immunol 1990; 157:125–52.
18. Mann R, Mulligen RC, Baltimore D. Construction of a retrovirus packaging mutant and its use to produce helper-free defective retrovirus. Cell 1983; 33: 153–9.
19. Armentano D, Yu SF, Kantoff PW, von Ruden T, Anderson WF, Gilboa E. Effect of internal viral sequences on the utility of retroviral vectors. J Virol 1987; 61:1647–50.
20. Bender MA, Palmer TD, Gelinas RE, Miller AD. Evidence that the packaging signal of Moloney murine leukemia virus extends into the gag region. J Virol 1987; 61:1639–46.

21. Adam MA, Miller AD. Identification of a signal in a murine retrovirus that is sufficient for packaging of non retroviral RNA into virions. J Virol 1988; 62: 3802–6.
22. Lever AM, Richardson JH, Harrison GP. Retroviral RNA packaging. Biochem Soc Trans 1991; 19:963–6.
23. Skalka AM. Retroviral proteases: first glimpses at the anatomy of a processing machine. Cell 1989; 56:911–3.
24. Ott D, Friedrich R, Rein A. Sequence analysis of amphotropic and 10A1 murine leukemia viruses: close relationship to mink cell focus-inducing viruses. J Virol 1990; 64:757–66.
25. McLachlin JR, Cornetta K, Eglitis MA, Anderson WF. Retroviral-mediated gene transfer. Prog Nucleic Acid Res Mol Biol 1990; 38:91–135.
26. Watanabe S, Temin HM. Construction of a helper cell line for avian reticuloendotheliosis virus cloning vectors. Mol Cell Biol 1983; 3:2241–9.
27. Cone RD, Mulligan RC. High-efficiency gene transfer into mammalian cells: generation of helper-free recombinant retrovirus with broad mammalian host range. Proc Natl Acad Sci U S A 1984:6349–53.
28. Miller AD, Law MF, Verma IM. Generation of helper-free amphotropic retroviruses that transduce a dominant-acting, methotrexate-resistant dihydrofolate reductase gene. Mol Cell Biol 1985; 5:431–7.
29. Miller AD, Trauber DR, Buttimore C. Factors involved in production of helper virus-free retrovirus vectors. Somat Cell Mol Genet 1986; 12:175–83.
30. Miller AD, Buttimore C. Redesign of retrovirus packaging cell lines to avoid recombination leading to helper virus production. Mol Cell Biol 1986; 6:2895–902.
31. Muenchau DD, Freeman SM, Cornetta K, Zwiebel JA, Anderson WF. Analysis of retroviral packaging cell lines for generation of replication-competent virus. Virology 1990; 176:262–5.
32. Danos O, Mulligan RC. Safe and efficient generation of recombinant retroviruses with amphotropic and ecotropic host ranges. Proc Natl Acad Sci U S A 1988; 85:6460–4.
33. Markowitz D, Goff S, Bank A. A safe packaging line for gene transfer: separating viral genes on two different plasmids. J Virol 1988; 62:1120–4.
34. Markowitz D, Goff S, Bank A. Construction and use of a safe and efficient amphotropic packaging cell line. Virology 1988; 167:400–6.
35. Takahara Y, Hamada K, Housman DE. A new retrovirus packaging cell for gene transfer constructed from amplified long terminal repeat-free chimeric proviral genes. J Virol 1992; 66:3725–32.
36. Miller AD, Garcia JV, von Suhr N, Lynch CM, Wilson C, Eiden MV. Construction and properties of retrovirus packaging cells based on gibbon ape leukemia virus. J Virol 1991; 65:2220–4.
37. Adam MA, Ramesh N, Miller AD, Osborne WR. Internal initiation of translation in retroviral vectors carrying picornavirus 5′ nontranslated regions. J Virol 1991; 65:4985–90.
38. Morgan RA, Couture L, Elroy-Stein O, Ragheb J, Moss B, Anderson WF. Retroviral vectors containing putative internal ribosome entry sites: development of a

polycistronic gene transfer system and applications to human gene therapy. Nucleic Acids Res 1992; 20:1293–9.
39. Von Melchner H, Housman DE. The expression of neomycin phosphotransferase in human promyelocytic leukemia cells (HL60) delays their differentiation. Oncogene 1988; 2:137–40.
40. Albritton LM, Tseng L, Scadden D, Cunningham JM. A putative murine ecotropic retrovirus receptor gene encodes a multiple membrane-spanning protein and confers susceptibility to virus infection. Cell 1989; 57:659–66.
41. Kim JW, Closs EI, Albritton LM, Cunningham JM. Transport of cationic amino acids by the mouse ecotropic retrovirus receptor. Nature 1991; 352:725–8.
42. Wang H, Kavanaugh MP, North RA, Kabat D. Cell-surface receptor for ecotropic murine retroviruses is a basic amino-acid transporter. Nature 1991; 352: 729–31.
43. Yoshimoto T, Yoshimoto E, Meruelo D. Molecular cloning and characterization of a novel human gene homologous to the murine ecotropic retroviral receptor. Virology 1991; 185:10–7.
44. Yoshimoto R, Yoshimoto E, Meruelo D. Enhanced gene expression of the murine ecotropic retroviral receptor and its human homolog in proliferating cells. J Virol 1992; 66:4377–81.
45. Miller DG, Miller AD. Tunicamycin treatment of CHO cells abrogates multiple blocks to retrovirus infection, one of which is due to a secreted inhibitor. J Virol 1992; 66:78–84.
46. Wang H, Paul R, Burgeson RE, Keene DR, Kabat D. Plasma membrane receptors for ecotropic murine retroviruses require a limiting accessory factor. J Virol 1991; 6468–77.
47. Maddon PJ, Dalgleish AG, McDougal JS, Clapham PR, Weiss RA, Axel R. The T4 gene encodes the AIDS virus receptor and is expressed in the immune system and the brain. Cell 1986; 47:333–48.
48. Johann SV, Gibbons JJ, O'Hara B. GLVR1, a receptor for gibbon ape leukemia virus, is homologous to a phosphate permease of *Neurospora crassa* and is expressed at high levels in the brain and thymus. J Virol 1992; 66:1635–40.
49. Garcia JV, Jones C, Miller AD. Localization of the amphotropic murine leukemia virus receptor gene to the pericentromeric region of human chromosome 8. J Virol 1991; 65:6316–9.
50. McClure MO, Sommerfelt MA, Marsh M, Weiss RA. The pH independence of mammalian retrovirus infection. J Gen Virol 1990; 71:767–73.
51. Maddon PJ, McDougal JS, Clapham PR, et al. HIV infection does not require endocytosis of its receptor, CD4. Cell 1988; 54:865–74.
52. Diamond DC, Finberg R, Chaudhuri S, Sleckman BP, Burakoff SJ. Human immunodeficiency virus infection is efficiently mediated by a glycolipid-anchored form of CD4. Proc Natl Acad Sci U S A 1990; 87:5001–5.
53. Hu WS, Temin HM. Retroviral recombination and reverse transcription. Science 1990; 250:1227–33.
54. Panganiban AT, Fiore D. Ordered interstrand and intrastrand DNA transfer during reverse transcription. Science 1988; 241:1064–9.
55. Grandgenett DP, Mumm SR. Unraveling retrovirus integration. Cell 1990; 60:3–4.

56. Sandmeyer SB, Hansen LJ, Chalker DL. Integration specificity of retrotransposons and retroviruses. Annu Rev Genet 1990; 24:491–518.
57. Bushman FD, Craigie R. Sequence requirements for integration of Moloney murine leukemia virus DNA in vitro. J Virol 1990; 64:5645–8.
58. Pryciak PM, Varmus HE. Nucleosomes, DNA-binding proteins, and DNA sequence modulate retroviral integration target site selection. Cell 1992; 69:769–80.
59. Miller DG, Adam MA, Miller AD. Gene transfer by retrovirus vectors occurs only in cells that are actively replicating at the time of infection. Mol Cell Biol 1990; 10:4239–42.
60. Springett GM, Moen RC, Anderson S, Blaese RM, Anderson WF. Infection efficiency of T lymphocytes with amphotropic retroviral vectors in cell cycle dependent. J Virol 1989; 63:3865–9.
61. Spangrude GJ, Smith L, Uchida N, et al. Mouse hematopoietic stem cells. Blood 1991; 78:1395–402.
62. Ogawa M. Differentiation and proliferation of hematopoietic stem cells. Blood 1993; Submitted for publication.
63. Williams DA, Lemischka IR, Nathan DG, Mulligan RC. Introduction of new genetic material into pluripotent haematopoietic stem cells of the mouse. Nature 1984; 310:476–80.
64. Karlsson S. Treatment of genetic defects in hematopoietic cell function by gene therapy. Blood 1991; 78:2481.
65. Dick JE, Magli MC, Huszar D, Phillips RA, Bernstein A. Introduction of a selectable gene into primitive stem cells capable of long-term reconstitution of the hemopoietic system of W/Wv mice. Cell 1985; 42:71–9.
66. Lemischka IR, Raulet DH, Mulligen RC. Developmental potential and dynamic behavior of hematopoietic stem cells. Cell 1986; 45:917–27.
67. Bodine DM, Karlsson S, Nienhuis AW. Combination of interleukins 3 and 6 preserves stem cell function in culture and enhances retrovirus-mediated gene transfer into hematopoietic stem cells. Proc Natl Acad Sci U S A 1989; 86:8897–901.
68. Lim B, Apperley JF, Orkin SH, Williams DA. Long-term expression of human adenosine deaminase in mice transplanted with retrovirus-infected hematopoietic stem cells. Proc Natl Acad Sci U S A 1989; 86:8892–6.
69. Nienhuis AW, Bodine D, Donahue R, McDonagh K, Sorrentino B. Progress toward gene insertion into hematopoietic stem cells. In: Thomas ED, ed. Applications of basic science to hematopoiesis and treatment of disease. New York: Raven Press, 1992; In press.
70. Bodine DM, McDonagh KT, Brandt SJ, et al. Development of a high-titer retrovirus producer cell line capable of gene transfer into rhesus monkey hematopoietic stem cells. Proc Natl Acad Sci U S A 1990; 87:3738.
71. Schuening FG, Kawahara K, Miller AD, et al. Retrovirus-mediated gene transduction into long-term repopulating marrow cells of dog. Blood 1991; 78:2568.
72. Carter RF, Abrams-Ogg ACG, Dick JE, et al. Autologous transplantation of canine long-term marrow culture cells genetically marked by retroviral vectors. Blood 1992; 79:356.

73. Kantoff PW, Flake AW, Eglitis MA, et al. In utero gene transfer and expression: a sheep transplantation model. Blood 1980; 73:1066.
74. Donahue RE, Kessler SW, Bodine D, et al. Helper virus induced T cell lymphoma in nonhuman primates after retroviral mediated gene transfer. J Exp Med 1992; 176:1125–35.
75. Bodine D, Moritz T, Luskey B, et al. Expression of the adenosine deaminase (ADA) gene after transduction into rhesus monkey repopulating stem cells. Blood 1992; 80:72a.
76. Culver KW, Anderson WF, Blaese RM. Lymphocyte gene therapy. Hum Gene Ther 1991; 2:107–9.
77. Rosenberg SA, Aebersold P, Cornetta K, et al. Gene transfer into humans—immunotherapy of patients with advanced melanoma, using tumor-infiltrating lymphocytes modified by retroviral gene transduction. N Engl J Med 1990; 323: 570–8.
78. Anderson FW, Blaese RM, Culver K. The ADA human gene therapy clinical protocol. Hum Gene Ther 1990; 1:331–62.
79. Blaese M, Anderson WF. Personal communication, 1992.
80. Sullenger BA, Gallardo HF, Ungers GE, Gilboa E. Overexpression of TAR sequences renders cells resistant to human immunodeficiency virus replication. Cell 1990; 63:601–8.
81. Malim MH, Bohnlein S, Hauber J, Cullen BR. Functional dissection of the HIV-1 Rev trans-activator–derivation of a trans-dominant repressor of Rev function. Cell 1989; 58:205–14.
82. Rosenberg SA. Gene therapy of cancer. Important Adv Oncol 1992; 17–38.
83. Rosenberg SA. Karnofsky Memorial Lecture. The immunotherapy and gene therapy of cancer. J Clin Oncol 1992; 10:180–99.
84. Kaleko M, Garcia JV, Miller AD. Persistent gene expression after retroviral gene transfer into liver cells in vivo. Hum Gene Ther 1991; 2:27–32.
85. Kay MA, Baley P, Rothenberg S, et al. Expression of human alpha 1-antitrypsin in dogs after autologous transplantation of retroviral transduced hepatocytes. Proc Natl Acad Sci U S A 1992; 89:89–93.
86. Wilson JM, Chowdhury NR, Grossman M, et al. Temporary amelioration of hyperlipidemia in low density lipoprotein receptor-deficient rabbits transplanted with genetically modified hepatocytes. Proc Natl Acad Sci U S A 1990; 87:8437–41.
87. Grossman M, Wilson JM. Frontiers in gene therapy: LDL receptor replacement for hypercholesterolemia. J Lab Clin Med 1992; 119:457–60.
88. Chowdhury JR, Grossman M, Gupta S, Chowdhury NR, Baker JR Jr, Wilson JM. Long-term improvement of hypercholesterolemia after ex vivo gene therapy in LDLR-deficient rabbits. Science 1991; 254:1802–5.
89. Lowy D. Molecular aspects of oncogenesis. In: Stamatoyannopoulos G, Nienhuis AW, Majerus P, Varmus HR, eds. Molecular basis of blood diseases, 2nd ed. Philadelphia: W. B. Saunders, In Press, 1993.
90. Witte O. Oncogenic mechanisms of hemannumological neoplasm. In: Stamtoyannopoulos G, Nienhuis A, Majerus P, Varmus HE, eds. Molecular basis of blood diseases, 2nd ed. Philadelphia: W. B. Saunders, In Press, 1993.

91. Tepper RI, Pattengale PK, Leder P. Murine interleukin-4 displays potent antitumor activity in vivo. Cell 1989; 57:503–12.
92. Fearon ER, Pardoll DM, Itaya T, et al. Interleukin-2 production by tumor cells bypasses T helper function in the generation of an antitumor response. Cell 1990; 60:397–403.
93. Gansbacher B, Zier K, Daniels B, Cronin K, Bannerji R, Gilboa E. Interleukin 2 gene transfer into tumor cells abrogates tumorigenicity and induces protective immunity. J Exp Med 1990; 172:1217–24.
94. Blankenstein I, Wuin ZH, Uberla K, et al. Tumor suppression after tumor cell-targeted tumor necrosis factor alpha gene transfer. J Exp Med 1991; 173: 1047–52.
95. Culver KW, Ram Z, Wallbridge S, Ishii H, Oldfield EH, Blaese RM. In vivo gene transfer with retroviral vector-producer cells for treatment of experimental brain tumors. Science 1992; 256:1550–2.
96. Dhawan J, Pan LC, Pavlath GK, Travis MA, Lanctot AM, Blau HM. Systemic delivery of human growth hormone by injection of genetically engineered myoblasts. Science 1991; 254:1509–12.
97. Palmer TD, Rosman GJ, Osborne WR, Miller AD. Genetically modified skin fibroblasts persist long after transplantation but gradually inactivate introduced genes. Proc Natl Acad Sci U S A 1991; 88:1330–4.
98. Nabel EG, Plautz G, Boyce FM, Stanley JC, Nabel GJ. Recombinant gene expression in vivo within endothelial cells of the arterial wall. Science 1989; 244:1342–4.
99. Dichek DA, Nussbaum O, Degen SJ, Anderson WF. Enhancement of the fibrinolytic activity of sheep endothelial cells by retroviral vector-mediated gene transfer. Blood 1991; 77:533–41.
100. Jensen PK, Bolund L. Tissue culture of human epidermal keratinocytes: a differentiating model system for gene testing and somatic gene therapy. J Cell Sci 1991; 100(2):255–9.
101. Hoggan MD, Blacklow NR, Rowe WP. Studies of small DNA viruses found in various adenovirus preparations: physical, biological, and immunological characteristics. Proc Natl Acad Sci U S A 1966; 55:1467–74.
102. Melnick JL, Mayor HD, Smith KO, Rapp F. Association of 20 millimicron particles with adenoviruses. J Bacteriol 1965; 90:271–4.
103. Atchison RW, Casto BC, Hammond WM. Adenovirus-associated defective virus particles. Science 1965; 149:754–6.
104. Arella M, Garzon S, Bergeron J, Tijssen P. Physicochemical properties, production, and purification of parvoviruses. In: Tijssen P, ed. Handbook of parvoviruses. Boca Raton, FL: CRC Press, 1989; 11–30.
105. Berns KI, Bohenzky RA. Adeno-associated viruses: an update. Adv Virol Res 1987; 32:243–306.
106. Buller RH, Janik JE, Sebring ED, Rose JA. Herpes simplex virus types 1 and 2 completely help adenovirus-associated virus replication. J Virol 1981; 40:241–7.
107. Casto BC, Armstrong JA, Atchinson RW, Hammon WMcD. Studies on the relationship between adeno-associated virus type 1 (AAV-1) and adenoviruses.

II. Inhibition of adenovirus plaques by AAV; its nature and specificity. Virol 1967; 33:452–8.
108. Hoggan MD, Thomas GF, Johnson FB. Continuous carriage of adenovirus-associated virus genome in cell culture in the absence of helper adenovirus. In: Silvestri LG, ed. Proc 4th Lepetit Colloquim. Amsterdam: North-Holland, 1972; 243–9.
109. Berns KI, Pinkerton TC, Thomas GF, Hoggan MD. Detection of adeno-associated virus (AAV)-specific nucleotide sequences in DNA isolated from latently infected Detroit 6 cells. Virology 1975; 68:556–60.
110. Handa H, Shiroki K, Shimojo H. Complementation of adeno-associated virus with temperature-sensitive mutants of human adenovirus types 12 and 5. Virology 1977; 82:84–92.
111. Hoggan MD. Adeno-associated viruses. Prog Med Virol 1970; 12:211–39.
112. Blacklow NR, Hoggan MD, Serano MS, et al. A seroepidemiologic study of adenovirus-associated virus infections in infants and children. Am J Epidemiol 1971; 94:359–66.
113. Blacklow NR, Hoggan MD, Rowe WP. Serological evidence for human infection with adeno-associated viruses. J Natl Cancer Inst 1968; 40:319–27.
114. Lebkowski JS, McNally MM, Okarma TB, Lerch LB. Adeno-associated virus: a vector system for efficient introduction of DNA into a variety of mammalian cell types. Mol Cell Biol 1988; 8:3988–96.
115. Rose JA, Maizel JK, Shatkin AJ. Structural proteins of adenovirus-associated viruses. J Virol 1971; 8:766–70.
116. Salo RJ, Mayor HD. Structural polypeptides of parvoviruses. Virology 1977; 78:340–5.
117. Becerra SP, Rose JA, Hardy M, Baroudy BM, Anderson CW. Direct mapping of adeno-associated virus capsid proteins B and C: as possible ACG initiation codon. Proc Natl Acad Sci U S A 1985; 82:7919–23.
118. Becerra SP, Koczot F, Fabisch P, Rose JA. Synthesis of adeno-associated virus structural proteins requires both alternative mRNA splicing and alternative initiations from a single transcript. J Virol 1988; 62:2745–54.
119. Tsao J, Chapman MS, Agbandjo M, et al. The three-dimensional structure of canine parvovirus and its functional implications. Science 1991; 25:1456–64.
120. Hermonat PL, Labow MA, Wright R, Berns KI, Muzyczka N. Genetics of adeno-associated virus: isolation and preliminary characterization of adeno-associated virus type 2 mutants. J Virol 1984; 51:329–39.
121. Green MR, Roeder RG. Definition of a novel promoter for the major adenovirus-associated virus mRNA. Cell 1980; 22:231–43.
122. Srivastava A, Lusby EW, Berns KI. Nucleotide sequence and organization of the adeno-associated virus 2 genome. J Virol 1983; 45:555–64.
123. Muzyczka N. In vitro replication of adeno-associated virus DNA. Semin Virol 1991; 2:281–90.
124. Myers MW, Carter B. Adeno-associated virus replication. The effect of L-canavanine or a helper virus mutation on accumulation of viral capsids and progeny single-stranded DNA. J Biol Chem 1981; 265:567–70.

125. Redemann BE, Mendelson E, Carter BJ. Adeno-associated virus Rep protein synthesis during productive infection. J Virol 1989; 63:873–82.
126. Chang L-S, Shi Y, Shenk T. Adeno-associated virus p5 promoter contains an adenovirus E1A inducible element and a binding site for the major late transcription factor. J Virol 1989; 63:3479–88.
127. Tratschin JD, Tal J, Carter B. Negative and positive regulation in trans of gene expression from adeno-associated virus vectors in mammalian cells by a viral Rep gene product. Mol Cell Biol 1985; 5:3251–60.
128. Samulski RJ, Shenk T. Adenovirus E1B 55-$M_r$ polypeptide facilitates timely cytoplasmic accumulation of adeno-associated virus mRNAs. J Virol 1988; 62:206–10.
129. Laughlin CA, Jones N, Carter BJ. Effect of deletions in adenovirus region 1 genes upon replication of adeno-associated virus. J Virol 1982; 41:868–76.
130. McPherson RA, Ginsberg HS, Rose JA. Adeno-associated virus helper activity of adenovirus DNA binding protein. J Virol 1982; 44:666–73.
131. West MHP, Trempe JP, Tratschin JD, Carter BJ. Gene expression in adeno-associated virus vectors: the effects of chimeric mRNA structure, helper virus, and adenovirus VAI RNA. Virology 1987; 60:38–42.
132. Janik JE, Huston MM, Cho K, Rose JA. Efficient synthesis of adeno-associated virus structural proteins requires both adenovirus DNA binding protein and VAI RNA. Virology 1989; 168:320–9.
133. Janik JE, Huston MM, Rose JA. Locations of adenovirus genes required for the replication of adenovirus-associated virus. Proc Natl Acad Sci U S A 1981; 78:1925–9.
134. Yakinoghi AO, Heilbronn R, Burkle A, Schlehofer J, zan-Hausen H. DNA amplification of adeno-associated virus as a response to cellular genotoxic stress. Cancer Res 1988; 48:3123–9.
135. Yakobson B, Koch T, Winocour E. Replication of adeno-associated virus in synchronized cells without the addition of a helper virus. J Virol 1987; 61:972–81.
136. Hermonat PL, Muzyczka N. Use of adeno-associated virus as a mammalian DNA cloning vector: transduction of neomycin resistance into mammalian tissue culture cells. Proc Natl Acad Sci U S A 1984; 81:6466–70.
137. Tratschin JD, Miller IL, Smith MG, Carter BJ. Adeno-associated virus vector for high-frequency integration, expression, and rescue of genes in mammalian cells. Mol Cell Biol 1985; 5:3251–60.
138. Samulski RJ, Chang L-S, Shenk T. A recombinant plasmid from which an infectious adeno-associated virus genome can be excised in vitro and its use to study viral replication. J Virol 1987; 61:3096–101.
139. McLaughlin SK, Collis P, Hermonat PL, Muzyczka N. Adeno-associated virus general transduction vectors: analysis of proviral structures. J Virol 1988; 62:1963–73.
140. Samulski RJ, Chang L-S, Shenk T. Helper-free stocks of recombinant adeno-associated viruses: normal integration does not require viral gene expression. J Virol 1989; 63:3822–8.

141. Labow MA, Graf LH, Berns KI. Adeno-associated virus gene expression inhibits cellular transformation by heterologous genes. Mol Cell Biol 1987; 7: 1320–5.
142. Antoni BA, Rabson AB, Miller IL, Trempe JP, Chejanovsky N, Carter BJ. Adeno-associated virus Rep inhibits human immunodeficiency virus type 1 production in human cells. J Virol 1991; 65:396–404.
143. Vincent KA, Moore GK, Haigwood NL. Replication and packaging of HIV envelope genes in a novel adeno-associated virus vector system. In: Brown F, Channock RM, Ginsberg HS, Lerner RA, eds. Vaccines 90. Cold Spring Harbor, NY: Cold Spring Harbor Laboratory Press, 1990; 353–9.
144. Basak S, Turner H. Infectious entry pathway for canine parvovirus. Virol 1992; 186:368–76.
145. Harding MJ, Molitor TW. A monoclonal antibody which recognizes cell surface antigen and inhibits porcine parvovirus replication. Arch Virol 1992; 123: 323–33.
146. Berns KI, Pinkerton TC, Thomas GF, Hoggan MD. Detection of adeno-associated virus (AAV)-specific nucleotide sequences in DNA isolated from latently infected Detroit 6 cells. Virology 1975; 68:556–60.
147. Cheung AK-M, Hoggan MD, Hauswirth WW, Berns KI. Integration of the adeno-associated virus genome into cellular DNA in latently infected human Detroit 6 cells. J Virol 1980; 33:739–48.
148. Kotin RM, Siniscalco M, Samulski RJ, et al. Site-specific integration by adeno-associated virus. Proc Natl Acad Sci U S A 1990; 87:2211–5.
149. Kotin RM, Menninger JC, Ward DC, Berns KI. Mapping and direct visualization of a region-specific viral DNA integration site on chromosome 19q13-qter. Genomics 1991; 10:831–4.
150. Samulski RJ, Zhu X, Xiao X, et al. Targeted integration of adeno-associated virus (AAV) into chromosome 19. EMBO J 1991; 10:3941–50.
151. Walsh CE, Liu JM, Young N, Xiao X, Nienhuis AW, Samulski RJ. Regulated high level expression of a human $\gamma$-globin gene introduced into erythroid cells by a novel adeno-associated virus (AAV) vector. Proc Natl Acad Sci U S A 1992; 89:7257–61.
152. Egan M, Flotte T, Afione S, et al. Defective regulation of outwardly rectifying $Cl^-$ channels by protein kinase A corrected by insertion of CFTR. Nature 1992; 358:581–4.
153. Jones SN, Grompe M, Samulski RJ, Caskey CT. Adeno-associated virus-mediated transduction of ornithine transcarbamylase activity in murine hepatoma cells. Am J Hum Genet 1991; 49:436a.
154. March KI, Hirshmann J, Bauriedel G, Samulski RJ. The adeno-associated virus as a gene transfer vector for human and non-human vascular smooth muscle cells. Clin Res 1992; 40:358a.
155. Orkin SH. Globin gene regulation and switching: circa 1990. Cell 1990; 63: 665–72.
156. Collis P, Antoniou M, Grosveld F. Definition of the minimal requirements with the human $\beta$-globin gene and the dominant control region for high level expression. EMBO J 1990; 9:233–40.

157. Fraser P, Hurst J, Collis P, Grosveld F. DNase 1 hypersensitive sites 1, 2 and 3 of the human B-globin dominant control region direct position-independent expression. Nucleic Acids Res 1990; 8:3503–8.
158. Laface D, Hermonat P, Wakeland E, Peck A. Gene transfer into hematopoietic progenitor cells mediated by an adeno-associated virus vector. Virology 1989; 162:483–7.
159. Srivastava CH, Samulski RJ, Lu L, Larsen SH, Srivastava A. Construction of a recombinant human parvovirus B19: adeno-associated virus 2 (AAV) DNA inverted terminal repeats are functional in an AAV-B19 hybrid virus. Proc Natl Acad Sci U S A 1989; 86:8078–82.
160. Goodman, S., Nienhuis, A. W. Unpublished results, 1992.
161. He H, Wei JF, Ohasshi T, et al. Transduction and expression of the human glucocerebrosidase gene. Blood 1991; 78:191a.
162. Srivastava A, Lu L. Replication of B19 parvovirus in highly enriched hematopoietic progenitor cells from normal human marrow. J Virol 1988; 62:3059–63.
163. Berns K. Parvovirus replication. Microbiol Rev 1990; 54:316–29.
164. Rowe WP, Huebner RJ, Gillmore LK, Parrott RH, Ward TG. Isolation of a cytopathogenic agent from human adenoids undergoing spontaneous degeneration in tissue culture. Proc Soc Exp Biol Med 1953; 84:570–3.
165. Flint SJ. Transformation by adenoviruses. In: Tooze J, ed. DNA tumor viruses: molecular biology of tumor viruses. Cold Spring Harbor, NY: Cold Spring Harbor Laboratory Press, 1981; 547–76.
166. Stewart PL, Burnett RM, Cyrklaff M, Fuller SD. Image reconstruction reveals the complex molecular organization of adenovirus. Cell 1991; 67:145–54.
167. Berk AJ. Adenovirus promoters and E1A transactivation. Annu Rev Genet 1986; 20:45–79.
168. Berget SM, Moore C, Sharp P. Spliced RNA segments at the 5′ terminus of adenovirus 2 late mRNA. Proc Natl Acad Sci U S A 1977; 74:3171–5.
169. Chow LT, Roberts JM, Lewis JB, Broker TR. A map of cytoplasmic RNA transcripts from lytic adenovirus type 2, determined by electron microscopy of RNA-DNA hybrids. Cell 1977; 11:819–36.
170. Thimmappaya B, Weinberger C, Schneider RJ, Shenk T. Adenovirus VAI RNA is required for efficient translation of viral mRNAs at late times after infection. Cell 1982; 31:543–51.
171. Bello LJ, Ginsberg HS. Inhibition of host protein synthesis in type 5 adenovirus-infected cells. J Virol 1967; 1:843–50.
172. Flint SJ, Broker TR. Lytic infection by adenoviruses. In: Tooze J, ed. Molecular biology of tumor viruses. Cold Spring Harbor, NY: Cold Spring Harbor Laboratory Press, 1981; 443–546.
173. Berkner KL. Expression of heterologous sequences in adenoviral vectors. Curr Top Microbiol Immunol 1992; 158:39–66.
174. Graham FL, Smiley J, Russell WC, Nairn R. Characteristics of a human cell line transformed by DNA from human adenovirus type 5. J Gen Virol 1977; 36:59–72.

175. Graham FL, Prevec L. Manipulation of adenovirus vectors. In: Murray EJ, ed. Methods in molecular biology. Clifton, NJ: Humana Press, 1991; 109–28.
176. Berkner KL, Schaffhausen BS, Roberts TM, Sharp PA. Abundant expression of polyomavirus middle T antigen and dihydrofolate reductase in an adenovirus recombinant. J Virol 1987; 61(4):1213–20.
177. Berkner KL, Sharp PA. Generation of adenovirus by transfection of plasmids. Nucleic Acids Res 1983; 11:6003–20.
178. Hanahan D, Gluzman Y. Rescue of functional replication origins from embedded configurations in a plasmid carrying the adenovirus genome. Mol Cell Biol 1984; 4:302–9.
179. Seth P, Fitzgerald D, Willingham M, Pastan I. Pathway of adenovirus entry into cells. In: Crowell RL, Lonberg-Holm K, eds. Virus attachment and entry into cells. Washington, DC: American Society for Microbiology, 1986; 191–5.
180. Curiel DT, Agarwal S, Wagner E, Cotten M. Adenovirus enhancement of transferrin-polylysine-mediated gene delivery. Proc Natl Acad Sci U S A 1991; 88:8850–4.
181. Curiel DT, Wagner E, Cotten M, et al. High-efficiency gene transfer mediated by adenovirus coupled to DNA-polylysine complexes. Hum Gene Ther 1992; 3:147–54.
182. Wagner E, Zatloukal K, Cotten M, et al. Coupling of adenovirus to transferrin-polylysine/DNA complexes greatly enhances receptor-mediated gene delivery and expression of transfected genes. Proc Natl Acad Sci U S A 1992; 89:6099–103.
183. Cotton M, Wagner E, Zatloukal K, Phillips S, Curiel DT, Bernstiel ML. High-efficiency receptor-mediated delivery of small and large (48 kilobase) gene constructs using the endosome-disruption activity of defective or chemically inactivated adenovirus particles. Proc Natl Acad Sci U S A 1992; 89:6094–8.
184. Horwitz MS. Adenoviridae and their replication. In: Fields BN, Knipe DM, eds. Virology. New York: Raven Press, 1990; 1679–740.
185. Graham FL. Transformation by and oncogenicity of human adenoviruses. In: Ginsberg HS, ed. The adenoviruses. New York: Plenum Press, 1984; 339–98.
186. Van Doren K, Gluzman Y. Efficient transformation of human fibroblasts by adenovirus-simian virus 40 recombinants. Mol Cell Biol 1984; 4:1653–6.
187. Karlsson S, Van Doren K, Schweiger SG, Nienhuis AW, Gluzman Y. Stable gene transfer and tissue-specific expression of a human globin gene using adenoviral vectors. EMBO J 1986; 5:2377–85.
188. Stratford-Perricaudet LD, Makeh I, Perricaudet M, Briand P. Widespread long-term gene transfer to mouse skeletal muscles and heart. J Clin Invest 1992; 90:626–30.
189. Straus SE. Adenovirus infections in humans. In: Ginsberg HS, ed. The adenoviruses. New York: Plenum Press, 1984; 451–96.
190. Hazinski TA. Prospects for gene therapy in acute lung injury. Am J Med Sci 1992; 304:131–5.
191. Crystal RG. Gene therapy strategies for pulmonary disease. Am J Med 1992; 92(6A):44S–51S.

192. Boat TF, Welsh MG, Beaudet AL. Cystic fibrosis. In: Scriver CR, Beaudet AL, Sly WS, Valle D, eds. Metabolic basis of inherited disease. New York: McGraw-Hill, 1992; 2649–80.
193. Riordan JR, Rommens JM, Karem B-S, et al. Identification of the cystic fibrosis gene: cloning and characterization of complementary DNA. Science 1989; 245:1066–73.
194. Rosenfeld MA, Siegfried W, Yoshimura K, et al. Adenovirus-mediated transfer of a recombinant alpha 1-antitrypsin gene to the lung epithelium in vivo. Science 1991; 252:431–4.
195. Rosenfeld MA, Yoshimura K, Trapnell BC, et al. In vivo transfer of the human cystic fibrosis transmembrane conductance regulator gene to the airway epithelium. Cell 1992; 68:143–55.
196. Friedman JM, Babiss LE, Clayton DF, Darnell JE Jr. Cellular promoters incorporated into the adenovirus genome: cell specificity of albumin and immunoglobulin expression. Mol Cell Biol 1986; 6:3791–7.
197. Stratford-Perricaudet LD, Levrero M, Chasse JF, Perricaudet M, Briand P. Evaluation of the transfer and expression in mice of an enzyme-encoding gene using a human adenovirus vector. Hum Gene Ther 1990; 1:241–56.
198. Jaffe HA, Danel C, Longenecker G, et al. Adenovirus-mediated in vivo gene transfer and expression in normal rat liver. Nature Gen 1992; 1:372–8.
199. Kovler MB, Desrosiers RC, Fleckenstein B, et al. The family Herpesviridae: an update. Arch Virol 1992; 123:425–49.
200. Roizman B, Sears AE. Herpesviruses and their replication. In: Fields BN, Knipe DM, eds. Virology. New York: Raven Press, 1990; 1795–842.
201. Corey L, Spear PG. Infections with herpes simplex viruses. N Engl J Med 1986; 314:686–91, 749–57.
202. McGeoch DJ, Preston VG, Weller SK, Schaffer PA. Herpes simplex viruses. In: O'Brian SJ, ed. Genetic maps. Book 1. Viruses. Cold Spring Harbor, NY: Cold Spring Harbor Laboratory Press, 1990; 115–20.
203. Preston CM, Frame MC, Campbell MEM. A complex formed between cell components and an HSV structural polypeptide binds to a viral immediate early gene regulatory DNA sequence. Cell 1988; 52:425–34.
204. Campbell MEM, Palfreyman JW, Preston CM. Identification of herpes simplex virus DNA sequences which encode a trans-acting polypeptide responsible for stimulation of immediate-early transcription. J Mol Biol 1984; 180:1–19.
205. O'Hare P, Goding CR. Herpes simplex virus regulatory elements and the immunoglobulin octamer domain bind a common factor and are both targets for virion transactivation. Cell 1988; 52:435–45.
206. Mellerick DM, Fraser NW. Physical state of the latent herpes simplex virus genome in a mouse model system: evidence suggesting an episomal state. Virology 1987; 158:265–75.
207. Hill TJ. Herpes simplex virus latency. In: Roizman B, ed. The herpesviruses. New York: Plenum Press, 1985; 175–240.
208. Stevens JG, Wagner EK, Devi-Rao GB, Cook ML, Feldman LT. RNA complementary to a herpesvirus alpha gene mRNA is prominent in latently infected neurons. Science 1987; 235:1056–9.

209. Deatly AM, Spivack JG, Lavi E, O'Boyle DR, Fraser NW. Latent herpes simplex virus type 1 transcripts in peripheral and central nervous system tissues of mice map to similar regions of the viral genome. J Virol 1988; 62:749-56.
210. Croen KD, Ostrave JM, Dragovic LJ, Smialek JE, Strauss SE. Latent herpes simplex virus in human trigeminal ganglia: detection of an immediate early gene "antisense" transcript by in situ hybridization. N Engl J Med 1984; 317: 1427-32.
211. Stevens JG, Haarr L, Porter DD. Prominence of the herpes simplex virus latency associated transcript in trigeminal ganglia from seropositive humans. J Infect Dis 1988; 158:117-23.
212. Breakefield XO, DeLuca NA. Herpes simplex virus for gene delivery to neurons. New Biologist 1991; 3:203-18.
213. Spaete RR, Frenkel N. The herpes simplex virus amplicon: analyses of cis-acting replication functions. Proc Natl Acad Sci U S A 1985; 82:694-8.
214. Latchman DS. Herpes simplex virus life cycle and the design of viral vectors. In: Collins M, ed. Methods in molecular biology, Vol. 8. Practical molecular virology: viral vectors for gene expression. Clifton, NJ: Humana Press, 1991; 175-90.
215. Geller AI, Breakefield XO. A defective HSV-1 vector expresses *Escherichia coli* β-galactosidase in cultured peripheral neurons. Science 1988; 241:1667-9.
216. Shih M-F, Arsenakis P, Tiollais P, Roizman B. Expression of hepatitis B virus S gene by herpes simplex virus type 1 vectors carrying alpha- and beta-regulated gene chimeras. Proc Natl Acad Sci U S A 1984; 81:5867-70.
217. Geller AI, Keyomarsi K, Bryan J, Pardee AB. An efficient deletion mutant packaging system for defective herpes simplex virus vectors: potential applications to human gene therapy and neuronal physiology. Proc Natl Acad Sci U S A 1990; 87:8950-4.
218. Vahlne A, Svennerholm B, Lycke E. Evidence of herpes simplex virus type-selective receptors on cellular plasma membranes. J Gen Virol 1979; 44:217-25.
219. Morgan C, Rose WM, Mednis B. Electron microscopy of herpes simplex virus type 1 entry. J Virol 1968; 2:507-16.
220. Kaner RJ, Baird A, Mansukhani A, et al. Fibroblast growth factor receptor is a portal of cellular entry for herpes simplex virus type 1. Science 1990; 248: 1410-2.
221. Deshmane SL, Fraser NW. During latency, herpes simplex virus type 1 DNA is associated with nucleosomes in a chromatin structure. J Virol 1989; 63:943-7.
222. Deatly AM, Spivack JG, Lavi E, Fraser NW. RNA from an immediate early region of the type 1 herpes simplex virus genome is present in the trigeminal ganglia of latently infected mice. Proc Natl Acad Sci U S A 1987; 84:3204-8.
223. Palella TD, Silverman LJ, Schroll CT, Homa FL, Levine M, Kelley WN. Herpes simplex virus-mediated human hypoxanthine-guanine phosphoribosyltransferase gene transfer into neuronal cells. Mol Cell Biol 1988; 8(1):457-60.
224. Lesch M, Nyhan WL. A familial disorder of uric acid metabolism and central nervous system function. Am J Med 1964; 36:561-70.
225. Seegmiller JE, Rosenbloom FM, Kelley WN. Enzyme defect associated with a sex-linked human neurological disorder and excessive purine synthesis. Science 1967; 155:1682-4.

226. Edwards NL, Jeryc W, Fox IH. Enzyme replacement in the Lesch-Nyhan syndrome with long-term erythrocyte transfusions. Adv Exp Med Biol 1984; 165A: 23–6.
227. Nyhan WL, Parkman R, Page T, et al. Bone marrow transplantation in Lesch-Nyhan disease. Adv Exp Med Biol 1986; 195A:167–70.
228. Palella TD, Hidaka Y, Silverman LJ, Levine M, Glorioso J, Kelley WN. Expression of human HPRT mRNA in brains of mice infected with a recombinant herpes simplex virus-1 vector. Gene 1989; 80:137–44.
229. Freese A, Geller AI, Neve R. HSV-1 vector mediated neuronal gene delivery. Biochem Pharmacol 1990; 40:2189–99.
230. Geller AI, Freese A. Infection of cultured central nervous system neurons with a defective herpes simplex virus 1 vector results in stable expression of *Escherichia coli* beta-galactosidase. Proc Natl Acad Sci U S A 1990; 87:1149–53.
231. Freese A, Geller A. Infection of cultured striatal neurons with a defective HSV-1 vector: implications for gene therapy. Nucleic Acids Res 1991; 19: 7219–23.
232. O'Malley KL, Anhalt MJ, Martin BM, Kelsoe JR, Winfield SL, Ginns EI. Isolation and characterization of the human tyrosine hydroxylase gene: identification of 5′ alternative splice sites responsible for multiple mRNAs. Biochemistry 1987; 26:6910–4.
233. Dobson AT, Margolis TP, Sedarati F, Stevens JG, Feldman LT. A latent, nonpathogenic HSV-1-derived vector stably expresses beta-galactosidase in mouse neurons. Neuron 1990; 5:353–60.
234. Wolfe JH, Deshmane SL, Fraser NW. Herpesvirus vector gene transfer and expression of $\beta$-glucuronidase in the central nervous system of MPS VII mice. Nature Gen 1992; 1:379–84.
235. Birkenmeier EH, Barker JE, Vogler CA, et al. Increased life span and correction of metabolic defects in murine mucopolysaccharidosis type VII after syngeneic bone marrow transplantation. Blood 1991; 78:3081–92.
236. Fink DJ, Sternberg LR, Weber PC, Mata M, Goins WF, Glorioso JC. In vivo expression of $\beta$-galactosidase in hippocampal neurons by HSV-mediated gene transfer. Hum Gene Ther 1992; 3:11–9.
237. Martuza RL, Malick A, Markert JM, Ruffner KL, Coen DM. Experimental therapy of human glioma by means of a genetically engineered virus mutant. Science 1991; 252:854–6.
238. Spaete RR, Mocarski E. Insertion and deletion mutagenesis of the human cytomegalovirus genome. Proc Natl Acad Sci U S A 1987; 84:7213–7.
239. Plotkin SA, Mortimer EA. Cytomegalovirus vaccines. Vaccines 1988; 513–6.
240. Maciejewski JP, Bruening EE, Donahue RE, Mocarski ES, Young NS, St Jeor SC. Infection of hematopoietic progenitor cells by human cytomegalovirus. Blood 1992; 80:170–8.

# Index